Medicinal Substances in Jerusalem from Early Times to the Present Day

Efraim Lev

Translated by

Rebecca Toueg

BAR International Series 1112
2003

Published in 2016 by
BAR Publishing, Oxford

BAR International Series 1112

Medicinal Substances in Jerusalem from Early Times to the Present Day

ISBN 978 1 84171 490 5

BAR Publishing is the trading name of British Archaeological Reports (Oxford) Ltd. British Archaeological Reports was first incorporated in 1974 to publish the BAR Series, International and British. In 1992 Hadrian Books Ltd became part of the BAR group. This volume was originally published by Archaeopress in conjunction with British Archaeological Reports (Oxford) Ltd / Hadrian Books Ltd, the Series principal publisher, in 2003. This present volume is published by BAR Publishing, 2016.

Printed in England

BAR
PUBLISHING

BAR titles are available from:

BAR Publishing
122 Banbury Rd, Oxford, OX2 7BP, UK
EMAIL info@barpublishing.com
PHONE +44 (0)1865 310431
FAX +44 (0)1865 316916
www.barpublishing.com

CONTENTS

List of Illustrations

Sources for the Illustrations

Fi Hayuia al-Tibb (De Materia Medica) by Pedanios Dioscorides; The New-York Public Library, Spencer, Pres. Ms. 39, (no. 1).

The Israel Academy of Sciences and Humanities (no. 6, 7, 8, 9, 10, 11, 11, 12, 13, 14, 15, 16, 17, 18, 19, 20, 21, 22, 23, 24, 25, 26, 27, 28, 29, 30, 31, 32).

Prof. Alex Carmel private collection (35).

Other pictures are from the author's private collection (no. 2, 3, 4, 5, 40, 41).

List of Tables

Foreword

Jerusalem has always been a unique city. Hundreds of millions of people, believers of the three main monotheistic religions Christianity, Islam and Judaism, have always looked forward to visiting, living, dying or even being buried in the Holy City. Throughout its long history, this city was subject to different kings, sultans and leaders that ruled the city and its inhabitants. Simultaneously, the population of the city changed in origin, habitat, language, culture and in other aspects of life such as quality of the medical system, physicians and remedies that were used.

This book is a reflection of the growing academic interest in the history of this fascinating city in general and of medicine in Jerusalem in particular. The interest that the academic community has had in the subject of medicine in the holy city can be measured by the number of articles and books that have been published, academic courses and seminars that have been taught and conventions that have been held in various academic institutes in Israel.

The book deals with natural curative substances and healing materials used by the residents of Jerusalem throughout the ages. But it concerns the use of *materia medica* at the Land of Israel and throughout the Levant in this time span.

When I began working on this book I examined mainly the medieval and early Ottoman sources, but new researches were conducted by me and in collaboration with some other colleagues in order to get the whole picture of using natural substances for healing. Several new documents were revealed and studied, for example the Franciscan inventory lists, the Dr. Titus Tobler List, the list of medicinal substances in the British hospital for the Jews and the ethno-pharmacological survey of traditional folk medicine in Jerusalem.

It is an intensive and systematic historical study of the medicinal substances that were used by the inhabitants and the visitors of the City of Jerusalem. It deals with the description of the various substances and their uses. It also deals with comparisons of such uses in traditional and folk medicine of several ethnic groups of present day in the region and in other parts of the world.

Another interesting aspect of the study, the geographical origin of the substances, is dealt with as well. It was found that most of the medicinal substances that had been used during the Middle Ages and early Ottoman period were of local origin; others were brought from different countries, a fact that shed light on the well-developed trade relations in medicinal substances throughout the Muslim world, from India to the shore of Spain. Shortly after America was discovered and medicinal plants such as quinine were found, they were spread throughout the old world by the European traders and by European delegations and missionaries groups acting in the Levant, the Land of Israel and Jerusalem.

The study clearly shows that there was intensive medical activity in Jerusalem throughout the years thanks to its centrality among the different nations and religions and due to the political considerations of its rulers.

The book is composed of nine chapters divided into two parts. The introduction gives a short description of the history of medicine in Jerusalem, including basic chronological information about the medical systems, hospitals and physicians who operated in the city.

Part A includes six chapters dealing with information gathered from different historical sources of the medieval and early Ottoman periods (10th-18th century): Chapter One defines of the different historical periods dealt with here, the geographical area examined and detailed background of the sources that have been used, primary as well as secondary. Chapter Two begins with an introduction on healing with animal substances in the ancient world and concentrates on their uses in Jerusalem throughout history. Twenty-three substances of animal origin are presented in the table, out of which five are described in detail. Chapter Three focuses on the medicinal uses of non-organic materials in the holy city and it begins with an introduction on such uses in the old world. Evidence for the use of fourteen such substances have been traced, but only seven are presented in detail. Chapter Four, which is the longest chapter of the book, presents the use of plant origin substances in Jerusalem, since plants have always been the main part of any *materia medica* inventory in the world. After presenting the history of healing with plants, a table describing one hundred and seventy-four medicinal plants, for which there is clear evidence of their uses in Jerusalem is presented. Detailed information on fifty-seven plants follows the table. Chapter Five deals with three medicinal substances of unclear origin and Chapter Six summarises and concludes the first part of the book, which deals mainly with eclectic information concerning the time span of 10th-18th century.

Part B consists of three chapters which deal with specific subject matters including institutes and historical periods that deserve special attention concerning the uses of medicinal substances in the city of Jerusalem: Chapter Seven describes the unique episode of the Franciscan pharmacy in the holy city, a subject which is under intensive research at this time. Chapter Eight focuses on the nineteenth century and presents two lists of medicinal materials that were used in 19th century Jerusalem according to the Swiss physician Dr. Titus Tobler. For the first time it gives the complete list of medicinal substances used by the British medical missionaries delegation that operated in city. A short description of the medical conditions and medical system and institutions is also presented. The last chapter deals with the twentieth century. A list of traditional and folk medicine substances, which are still used in Jerusalem, is presented and this phenomenon is discussed.

Three appendices provide information concerning the historical periods dealt with in the book, the sources, which are mentioned and quoted in, Part One and the list of medicinal substances used in Jerusalem from the 10th to 18th century. A bibliography, list of abbreviations and an index conclude the book.

Acknowledgments

It is a pleasure to acknowledge all those who assisted me in this study and its publication.

Librarians and curators throughout Israel (Bar-Ilan University, Haifa University, the National Library, Hebrew University, Jerusalem) and Britain (Wellcome Institute Library, The British Library) assisted me in finding the sources for this study, as well as the relevant literature. Special thanks are offered to Dr. Allan Nigel, curator of the Eastern collection at the Wellcome Institute Library for his significant contribution, friendly attitude and helpful remarks and ideas.

A special thanks for supplying a working space, academic atmosphere, encouragements and other means of support is sent to the Wellcome Trust Centre for the History of Medicine at UCL College London and its staff and particular to Sally Bragg, Alan Shiel, Debra Scallan, Prof. Harold Cook, Prof. Vivian Nutton and Dr. Tilli Tansey.

The following specialists assisted me in researching the sources, collecting the data and identifying the substances: Dr. Zohar Amar (Department of Land of Israel Studies, Bar Ilan University, Israel); Dr. Yaron Perry (Department of Eretz Israel Studies, University of Haifa, Israel) and Arik Moussaieff (Department of Pharmacology, Hebrew University, Jerusalem, Israel).

At an early stage of writing, Dr. Zohar Amar (Department of Land of Israel Studies, Bar Ilan University, Israel) read a big portion of the draft of this work and made helpful suggestions with encouraging and precautionary criticisms.

It is a pleasure to thank and mention some of my teachers and supervisors, who helped me to establish and guide my academic career: Dr. Joseph Drori, Dr. Ivon Friedman, Prof. Joshua Schwartz (Department of Land of Israel Studies, Bar Ilan University, Israel) and Prof. Eran Dolev (Ichilov Medical Center and Tel-Aviv Medical School, Tel-Aviv University, Israel).

I thank the anonymous readers of this work and of the previous studies which were published by me and in cooperation with other colleagues, before the publication of the book. Their scholarly remarks were very helpful.

Several individuals have been of notable assistance to me and to the publication of this book: Orna Gilboa assisted me with the editorial work of the Hebrew previous works and version and Murray Rosovsky with the English editing. Special thanks and appreciation is given to Rebecca Toueg who assisted me with the English translation.

This study could not have been published without the generous support of grants and scholarships of the following organizations and institutes: British Council Chevening award for Post-Doctoral research and a grant of the Research Authority, University of Haifa.

Finally, I thank my wife Michal and my children Hagar, Amitay, Abigail and Ilay for their patience, understanding and cooperation.

Introduction
The History of Medicine in Jerusalem

This book deals mainly with natural curative substances used by the residents of Jerusalem throughout the ages, focusing particularly upon the medieval period. However, in order that the reader might obtain the fullest and most comprehensive picture possible, this chapter presents a brief review of the medical situation in the city on the basis of historical records. The state of medical science may be examined from a number of aspects during the course of history: medicine and its methods, physicians and healers, and medical institutions. Curative substances, which are the main topic of this book, will be discussed in the following chapters.

The curative methods which were practiced by medical savants until the advent of modern medicine were basically theories developed by Greek scientists and doctors. Some of these medical theories used by Romans, Arabs and Europeans have survived till today in the framework of traditional and folk medicine practiced in the Middle East and in the Muslim countries of Asia and Africa. The Romans advanced the field of medical science mainly in the organisational sphere: the development of sanitary facilities such as sewage systems, baths, waterworks, public health laws and the establishment of military medicine which led, among other things, to the institutionalised development and formation of the hospital.

The Byzantines (324-640 CE) established Roman medical institutions and services, and set them up in the areas under their rule. After the initial rejection of classical medicine because of its paganistic aspects, the Byzantines sanctioned the principles of Graeco-Roman medicine once Christianity was sufficiently established.[1] After Christianity became the official religion, the Church assumed responsibility for the care of the sick and made it an aim to provide social services for the general public by establishing an infrastructure of well-developed public medicine. In this way the Church reinforced its standing and influence over the local population and harmonised the relationship between religious and governmental authorities. Within the framework of the Byzantine Empire, the Church had a decisive impact upon the development and formation of the medical system in Palestine during the period of Byzantine rule and the period of Muslim rule which followed.[2]

The increasing influence of the monastic movement over Church, society and government became a major factor in the widespread activities of the medical system. One of the main focal points of monasticism was the Judean Desert, a solitary area yet close to Jerusalem. Medical establishments developed during the Byzantine period particularly in the east, in the region of Asia Minor, Syria and Palestine, owing to the increase of their Christian populations.[3]

Some of the monks were engaged in the practice of conventional medicine as well as in miracle cures. Writings by abbot monks describe cases of miracle cures such as those of Theodosios (430-529 CE) who was portrayed as the physician of the poor, blind and lame,[4] and Abtimios who miraculously healed many sick people including the son of a Saracen tribal chief whose entire tribe converted to Christianity as a result of the cure.[5]

One of the frequently applied curative methods involving religious elements that were practiced in Jerusalem area was the use of holy oil extracted from relics (bone remains of holy men).[6] It should be noted that in spite of the value attributed to these curative methods by historical sources, information may be obtained about the activities of eminent physicians engaged in the practice of medicine in the Jerusalem area, and monks played an important role in the spread of conventional medicine. During the Byzantine period, a few hospitals were also set up in the Jerusalem and the Judean Desert areas as part of a network of charitable institutions for welfare and hospitality.[7]

1 Allan, pp. 450-451.

2 Ashkenazi, Curing, p. 43.

3 Miller, pp. 68-71.

4 Theodosios, pp. 34-35.

5 Life of Abtimios, in Schwartz, pp. 18-23.

6 Life of Sabbes 45, in Schwartz, p. 136.

7 Ashkenazi, Curing; Antonini Placentini 24, p. 142; Wilkinson, pp. 84,137,162.

The Muslims (640-1099 CE) who ruled Palestine until the Crusader conquest, did not bring about any revolutionary changes in habitation or culture. The period of the Umayyad Caliphate (660-750 CE) is characterised by a continuation of the previous style of government and by the persistence of both material and spiritual cultures.[8] This trend of events, which preserved the basic aspects and institutions of Byzantine medicine in Jerusalem and regional areas, extended even into the period of the early Abassid Caliphs (750-850 CE). During this period, hundreds of Greek, Roman and Syrian medical documents were translated by Christian and Jewish translators who formed the connecting link between the different cultures.

Historical sources dating from the Umayyad and Abassid periods do not record the existence of physicians in Palestine in general or Jerusalem in particular. The causes for this apparently lie in the diminished Muslim population and the disconnection between the recorders of historical events and the local physicians. Information about physicians begin to appear from the tenth century in spite of the fact that during this period, according to the Jerusalem geographer al-Muqaddasi, medical science in Palestine was still under Christian control.[9] Among the five Jerusalem physicians mentioned by the historian Ibn Abi Usaybia, two of them were Christians: Joseph al-Nazrani and Anba Zakhriay Ibn Thuaba who was one of the teachers of the well-known Muslim physician in Jerusalem, al-Tamimi.[10] Among the Jewish physicians in the city, the Cairo Geniza mentions the head of the Jewish community in Jerusalem who was also a doctor.[11] It was al-Tamimi and his writings that became an example of the local medical tradition which had developed in the region and was adopted by the Muslims. His book offers information about curative substances, their extraction process and applications in the Jerusalem and surrounding areas, and frequently quotes the Greek, Roman and Byzantine medical savants.[12]

With the establishment of the Kingdom of Jerusalem (1099 CE), the Crusaders ruled Palestine for about two hundred years (until 1291 CE). Jerusalem was under their continuous control for 88 years (until 1187 CE). The abundant sources, which describe the city in this period naturally refer as well to the medical standards, methods and institutions. The medical situation in Jerusalem during the Crusader siege was extremely grave for the besieged because of the congestion in the city and the poor hygienic conditions, insufficient water supply, summer heat and starvation. These factors, most of which also affected the besiegers, must have caused the outbreak of disease that spread rapidly and worsened with the massacre of the besieged after the conquest of the city.

The period of Crusader rule was marked by fierce battles and the influx of thousands of Christian pilgrims and wayfarers. This made it necessary to establish medical institutions to treat battle wounds, plague victims and exhausted pilgrims. Most of the medical information is derived from letters written by pilgrims such as John of Wartzburg (1065 CE) who describes the hospital of St. John of Jerusalem (Order of the Knights Hospitallers) in which fifty patients out of the two thousand hospitalised there died every day.[13] There are also descriptions by the Crusader leaders of their illnesses, as well as weapon wounds, deliberate poisonings, cholera, leprosy and other severe maladies. Various sources describe the method of treatment, the patients' belongings, the food provisions, the duties of the medical staff, the funding of the hospital and its maintenance and even the principles of medical ethics.[14]

Saladin's conquest of Jerusalem (1187 CE) restored the city's Moslem character. He expelled the Crusaders, overlaid their traces and set his own seal upon it. The Eastern Christians remained in the city, and Moslems and Jews were encouraged to settle in it. The demographic changes that resulted had an enormous influence upon the status of medicine there. A highly important change was the establishment of a hospital mentioned in the sources as al-Bimarastan al-Tsalahi. According to the sources, after having fulfilled the precept of making a pilgrimage to Mecca, Saladin returned to Jerusalem, "established its prestige, transformed the church which had been built in the street of the Holy Sepulchre into a hospital, and transferred medical drugs and potions to it."[15]

During the Ayyubid Caliphate (1187-1250 CE) the rulers of Jerusalem, acting as they had done in other cities, set up hospitals, engaged court physicians for themselves and sometimes for their official subordinates, and turned medical science into a thriving and well-developed discipline in Syria and Palestine.[16] Extensive information regarding the activities of the physicians during this period can be found in the writings of two eminent authors, Ibn al-Qifti (1171-1248) and Ibn Abi Usaybia (1203-1270) who belonged to families closely connected to the government and who recorded the history of medical practitioners until their own time. From various historical sources[17] there emerges a picture which shows that while the control of Palestine was split between the Franks and the Muslims, the physicians remained neutral; they sometimes served both sides and were used as intermediaries, occasionally even undergoing religious conversion to accord with their official position.[18]

The Mamluk period (1260-1517) marks a turning point in the status of medical science in the region of the Near East and in areas under Muslim domination. A continuous process of decline began in scientific studies in contradistinction with the cultural revival and florescence in the West. From this

8 Amar, Grapes, pp. 249-252.

9 al-Muqaddasi, p. 183.

10 Ibn Abi Usaybia, p. 545.

11 Goitein, Society, p. 257.

12 The writer thanks Z. Amar and Y. Seri for the information. The descriptions by al-Tamimi of the Palestine residents and an analysis of his sources will be presented soon in a scholarly publication.

13 PPTS, Vol. 5, p. 44.

14 Amar & Lev, Jerusalem, pp. 28-52.

15 al-'Asali, Ma'ahid, p. 294, according to al-Nuwayri these took place in 1192.

16 Klein-Franke, p. 105.

17 Ibn al-Qifti; Ibn Abi Usaybia.

18 Amar & Lev, Jerusalem, pp. 53-57, 59-62.

time onward there are no prominent Muslim physicians in Jerusalem and there is also a noticeable lack of any original medical treatises. Ibn Khaldun, a contemporary of that period, was impressed by this fact and noted it in his book *Introductions to Historical Science* written c.1377 CE: " In contemporary Muslim cities, the [craft of medicine] seems to have deteriorated, because the civilization [population] has decreased and shrunk. [Medicine] is a craft required only by sedentary culture and luxury..."[19]

The process of cultural decline, corresponding with the policy of the Mamluk government in Palestine which was considered by them as an area of secondary importance, severely damaged the status and level of medicine in the region. The Mamluks constructed a large number of religious edifices in Jerusalem but did little to develop the city's infrastructure except for isolated instances of sabils (public water fountains), bathhouses and the repairing of aquaducts. In contrast with the Ayyubid period, there is no documentary evidence of medical study in Jerusalem during the period of Mamluk rule, nor of the position of a chief physician in the city.

The distance of Jerusalem from the ruling centres led to the exodus of experienced doctors to Egypt. The few doctors and pharmacists remaining in the city were not professional according to the testimony of pilgrims and visitors in Jerusalem. Letters written by Christian travellers from Europe indicate that the level of medical services provided by churches and monasteries in addition to their guest hospitality had fallen very low. The extensive Mamluk historiography written from the Egyptian point of view almost completely ignores the subject of Jerusalem hospitals and the appointment of doctors to positions in the city. It appears that the silence of Egyptian sources is additional proof of the inferior status of Palestine in general and of Jerusalem in particular within the Mamluk Empire.[20]

The inhabitants of Palestine rallied after the Ottoman conquest. The vigorous government with its new and efficient management, launched into the building of sacred and secular constructions which naturally improved the health and sanitation level in the city. This wave of construction, repairs and renovations also affected the medical institutions. The al-Bimarastan Hospital is mentioned once more, and in spite of the fact that its location is unclear, it was apparently the continuation or reconstruction of the al-Bimarastan al-Tsalahi institution.

A historical survey has revealed the activities of over fifty persons who held the title of physician in the city of Jerusalem from the time of the Ottoman conquest until the end of the 18th century. Some were natives of the city, some arrived at an advanced age to be buried in it, and a few worked in the city for a number of years. There were also several physicians among the Christian pilgrims and wayfarers in addition to the European monk physicians and pharmacists who were sent by the Franciscans to serve in Jerusalem. Public physicians during the Ottoman period belonged to a higher social class and were sometimes distinguished by their special garb, and may even have been allowed to wear a sword in their belts.

The medical expertise of the physicians practicing in Jerusalem during this period was variable. Some were "qualified, expert or specialist" doctors who had studied medicine at recognised institutions. Others received their training from qualified and authorised physicians or through working in hospitals. Licenses were granted by the authorities and indicated the area of specialisation. Physicians arriving from Europe, many of whom were Jews, were graduates of various universities mainly in Italy. All were members of a professional society headed by the "Chief Physician of Jerusalem" who supervised their training, level of knowledge and practical experience.

A secondary type of physician was the "folk" doctor who was not explicitly listed in government records. A large number of these were women who engaged in eye healing. On average, there were three Jewish physicians in every generation in Jerusalem and an indefinite number of Muslim and Christian physicians. It should be noted that a Jerusalem physician did not exclusively treat members of his own community but served the whole population.

Medical services in Jerusalem may be classified into three categories:

Public Medical Services – (General Hospital). This institution mainly served the Moslem population, although it was intended for the general public. Physicians of all the ethnic communities served in this hospital.

Community Medical Services – (Community Clinics or Hospitals for Ethnic Groups). For religious reasons, Christians and Jews preferred to use the medical services of their own communities recognised by the Ottoman authorities.

Private Medical Services – Many patients in the city who could afford it, used the services of private physicians. Generally, a shop was rented where patients could be received and treated. As is the practice today, some of these physicians were also employed in the public health system.[21]

Side by side with conventional medicine, there was also a widespread use in Jerusalem of amulets and curative remedies - a use that was recognised by the doctors in cases where they had no medical solutions to offer through conventional methods.[22] There were many witch doctors in Jerusalem, including women who engaged in witchcraft. Qualified physicians such as Rabbi Refael Mordecai Malki and his grandson, Rabbi David de Silva, wrote harsh words against them.[23] We should note, however, that Rabbi Refael Malki also strongly criticised qualified physicians in Jerusalem and the medical standards in the city.[24] A similar picture is given by the traveller Volney who visited Palestine in 1785.[25]

[19] Ibn Khaldun, VI:24, pp. 149-150

[20] Amar & Lev, Jerusalem, pp. 63-67.

[21] Ibid., pp. 75-83.

[22] Nahmias.

[23] Malki, pp. 26-27.

[24] Ibid., p. 73.

[25] Volney, p. 260.

Hygienic and sanitary levels in Jerusalem were low, causing the spread of infectious diseases and the outbreak of plagues which claimed many victims among the population.[26] They resulted from bad living conditions, crowded quarters, undrained sewage, garbage piled in the streets and stray dogs allowed to roam freely. Sources dating from this period blamed the health situation on the city climate, its drinking water and the food supply for the inhabitants.[27] The only solution for the needs of personal hygiene was in fact the public bathhouses (the hamam). Records state that Jerusalem in the 17th century had six bathhouses among which one was called the medical bathhouse (al-Shifa).[28]

The forerunners of European medicine in Jerusalem were the Jewish physicians and the medical staff in Franciscan institutions who had been educated in Europe, especially in Italy. European medicine was reflected in European medical literature utilised by the local physicians as well as in the names of diseases and medications in Spanish, Portuguese, Italian and Latin listed in local publications. The Franciscan dispensary in Jerusalem with its rich library, its medical staff and the variety of medications it stocked, also contributed to the infiltration of modern medicine from Europe.[29] The 19th century is characterised by the introduction of modern medicine into Jerusalem: the arrival of European doctors, the building of clinics, dispensaries and hospitals. This period will be reviewed briefly in the final chapters of this book.

[26] Arce, pp. 86-95.

[27] Malki, pp. 58-59, 60, 77; Yaari, Igrot, p. 137.

[28] Amar, Preservation, pp. 214-217.

[29] Amar & Lev, Jerusalem, pp. 93-96.

PART A

Chapter I
Historical Definition and Sources

The next few chapters present information derived from historical sources dealing with the medical use of natural substances in Medieval and Ottoman Jerusalem. Among the medical substances listed below, only those that are clearly defined and intended for medicinal use are mentioned. The definition of the term "natural medicinal substances" is not a simple matter at all because man has made use of a large variety of substances both as traditional or "folk" medicine (which is not the subject here) and in the framework of scholarly or "scientific" medicine of the Medieval and Ottoman periods.

The simplistic definition of natural medicinal substances is as follows: All the substances that originate from plants, minerals or living creatures and their products (e.g. honey, cheese) which were used as medication or which were a component of a medical compound. Although the sources do not provide any clear definition, a clearer picture of the concept can be seen after an intensive study of medical treatises written during the Middle Ages and the Ottoman period, which make many references to this region, such as the works of Ibn al-Baytar and Daud al-Antaki and in modern research into the subject.[1] In ancient medical treatises there are many entries in which descriptions are given of medicinal substances used in the Arab world. Some of them mention the uses made of these substances in the Levant in general and in specific regions in Palestine such as Jerusalem and its environs in particular.

The scientific term closest in meaning to natural medicinal substances is the Latin term *Materia Medica* which is still used today among physicians and pharmacists throughout the world, although it now mainly includes medications of chemical origin. So far, no Materia Medica for the general region of Palestine or specifically of Jerusalem has been discovered, nor perhaps was any ever written. Furthermore, there are very few historical sources such as the writings of the Jerusalem physician al-Tamimi, Rabbi Refael Mordecai Malki and Rabbi David de-Silva, which gave a direct description of the medicinal substances in use in Jerusalem.

[1] Lev, Materials.

Other medicinal substances, mainly medicinal herbs familiar to the region which were in daily use in Palestine and sometimes even in Jerusalem till the present day, do not appear in this listing because they are not mentioned in the sources in connection with Jerusalem.

The importance of this study lies in the documentary record of an ancient medical culture which is gradually dying out and disappearing. A rapid rate of transformations has occurred in the use of natural substances in medicine over the past two centuries during which far-reaching changes were made in the field of medicine and pharmacology throughout the world. Modern medicine has almost completely discarded the use of natural substances and shifted towards the massive use of chemical substances produced in industrial laboratories. This swift transition has dissociated modern man from ancient medical traditions which had passed down from generation to generation and which possessed clear, regional characteristics. This dissociation increased dependence upon modern doctors and chemists, yet at the same time, indirectly caused a return to natural, alternative medicine which utilises natural substances - a return which has now become an international phenomenon.

A wave of interest in natural medicine has swept across the world during the past two decades, and natural medicine has acquired a place of honour at the side of modern medicine. The documentation in this study and in similar research works will assist in understanding the sources of natural and traditional medicine and provide knowledge of the medical uses of natural substances in earlier times. It will help to focus research upon those substances which had once been used medically but have "disappeared" from the inventory of medicinal substances known today.

Scope of this Study

This study deals with the city of Jerusalem but includes the area of Greater Jerusalem as well as its agricultural hinterland, and in some cases even the city of Jericho (when explicitly referred to by the source as part of the Jerusalem district). It focuses on the period between the 10th and 18th centuries. The military expedition of Napoleon (1799) represents the beginning of the process in which there is a growing influence of Europe on Palestine and on Jerusalem in particular. The Franciscan medical and pharmacological activities, the later 19th century activities and traditional substances sold and used in Jerusalem until the present day are dealt with in Part I.

Sources for this Study

This study is based upon historical research deriving from a wide and varied range of information sources, first and foremost from medical literature. Other sources include historical annals, geographical literature, travelogues and various commercial documents. One of the main issues in which the author was concerned was the identification of the medicinal substances mentioned in the sources, since many of these different types of documents were written in a variety of languages and dialects. A significant portion of the written sources do not deal with medicine and most of the information is scattered throughout it at random. This information was located, translated and processed, and forms the basis for the list of medicinal substances in Jerusalem and their uses.

The sources for this study can be divided into two main groups: Primary Sources and Secondary Sources (i.e. supplementary material) which are presented and described below. The examples cited have been selected on the basis of their most salient characteristics since some of the information sources constitute both primary and secondary sources at the same time.

Primary Sources

This group comprises those sources which explicitly indicate the medicinal substances in connection with Jerusalem. Some of them describe the uses of those medicinal substances while others indicate their cultivation or marketing in Jerusalem. Certain references are made only to the names of substances and their appellations in the dialect of Jerusalemites and of the Palestine region as a whole.

a. *Medical Literature*

Medical literature is characteristic of many cultures in the region for the past 4000 years. However, most of the medical treatises which concern Palestine and Jerusalem were written during the Middle Ages. Hundreds of medical works of the medieval period survived in the Islamic East. Some were Graeco-Roman writings in translation and some were independent compositions by writers of that period. Occasionally one may find a reference to certain medicinal substances originating in the region or in Jerusalem as well as other substances imported into Palestine and Jerusalem.

Among the physicians who made explicit references to the use of medicinal substances in Jerusalem and in the Palestine region, mention should be made of the Jerusalem doctor al-Tamimi[2] and the Frankish eye doctor Benevenutus Grassus[3] who mentioned numerous "Jerusalem" medications in his book. However, Benevenutus is a problematic source because his biographical record is not entirely clear and because he does not explicitly indicate the uses of the medicinal substances in Jerusalem. He merely mentions the name of the medicine and notes that it is a "Jerusalem" medication.

Among the many medical treatises which were written during the Ayyubid period, it is worth mentioning the works of the Andalusian herbalist Abu al-'Abas al-Nabati[4] who visited the region during that time. His writings are quoted by his outstanding pupil Ibn al-Baytar[5] who was active in the region in the service of the Ayyubid rulers and who also mentions a few medications that were then in use in Jerusalem.

An Ottoman physician who should be mentioned is Daud al-Antaki[6] who, like his predecessors, also described many medicinal substances from the region of Greater Syria, including the area of Jerusalem and its environs, and his work contains a summary of the classical medical literature of the Middle Ages. Among the Jewish physicians who were active in Jerusalem and whose works were preserved, it is worth mentioning the Jerusalem doctor, Rabbi Refael Malki[7] and Rabbi David de Silva.[8]

b. *The Cairo Genizah*

Another type of primary source is the documentary material which is to be found in the Cairo Genizah. This includes a variety of literary material (mainly legalistic), documents relating to Jewish communal activities in Fustat, and private correspondence. Of special importance for this study are the documents of Jewish merchants dating from the 11th century.[9] In these sources lie a wealth of information concerning the trade in medicinal substances and their uses in the Mediterranean society of the region in general and of Jerusalem in particular.[10]

c. *Archives and Document Collections*

Some of the information is based on various archival documents which deal with a wide range of subjects. What is common among them from the viewpoint of the researcher is that their information is real, authentic and trustworthy. This group includes legal documents which were discovered in

2 al-Tamimi; Amar, Traditions; Amar & Seri.

3 Benevenutus; Kedar.

4 Amar, Herbalist.

5 Ibn al-Baytar al-Jami; Amar, al-Baytar.

6 al-Antaki; Plessner. A comprehensive study on the contribution of this important physician to information regarding medicinal substances in the Levant will be published in the near future.

7 Malki.

8 Amar de Silva.

9 These were published mainly by the research scholars S.D. Goitein and M. Gil.

10 Isaacs.

the archives of the Moslem Waqf (Islamic Sacred Trust). These documents, discovered and partially studied in recent years, contain information about the use of natural medicinal substances in Jerusalem.[11] This type of documentation also includes documentary collections from the Crusader period in which the archives of the military orders and of Church institutions are to be found.[12]

d. *Travelogues*

This literary genre began to develop during the Byzantine period but became widespread during the Middle Ages. Hundreds of travel books and correspondence were written by people of different cultural backgrounds.[13] The travelogues of Syria and Palestine contain actual historical data with references to minerals and herbal condiments and medications which were grown in the countryside and sold in the marketplaces, including those of Jerusalem. This information is derived from the books written by travellers beginning from the 13th century with the transition to "Palestinography".[14]

e. *Geographical Literature*

This literary genre is well known in Islamic literature and developed under the influence of Greek classical literature from the 10th century onward. The literature is usually arranged according to the different regions of the world, and the information it contains regarding medicinal substances appears sporadically. For example, one might mention the list of seedlings and products that al-Muqaddasi brought and which gives much information about Jerusalem. The Jerusalem geographer, al-Muqaddasi, is considered a reliable and important source because he knew the city at first-hand.[15]

Secondary Sources

This group includes sources which generally do not explicitly mention medicinal substances in direct connection with Jerusalem. Yet these works throw light upon the medicinal substances in the Near East during the Middle Ages and mention their names and medical uses which provide important assistance in their identification. Among the Hebrew works which are worth noting are those of Assaph Harofe[16] in spite of the fact that it is a matter of dispute where and when they were composed (ranging from the 6th to the 10th centuries).

The secondary sources also include the medical lexicons which reflect an increasing expansion in the field of medicine during the Middle Ages. These lexicons dealt with elucidating the names of medications and identifying the terms of the medicinal substances in the various dialects commonly spoken among the population of that period.[17] Since it frequently happened that a medication had various names and terms of identification, these lexicons were essential for those engaged in medical practice. Among the lexicons it is worth noting those of al-Ghafiqi[18] and of Maimonides who also mentions a few names of medications in Jerusalem.[19]

It should be emphasised that the basic information for the list of substances was supplied by certain important physicians who were active in the region of Jerusalem, mainly during the Middle Ages and the Ottoman period. Among them were al-Tamimi, Abu al-'Abas al-Nabati, Ibn al-Baytar, Benevenutus Grassus, Daud al-Antaki, Rabbi Refael Malki and Rabbi David de Silva. Each of them represents medicine and medicinal substances of a different period. Other sources supply information on the rest of the materials and add to our knowledge of those already mentioned to complete the picture of those periods for which no medical literature is extant.

Scientific Identification of Medicinal Substances

One of the main problems that faced the author of this study was the positive identification of the medicinal substances mentioned in the literary sources. For example, in the Arabic literary sources, there is a large variety of local dialects corresponding to the writers' country of origin and therefore the names of plants and animals that these sources contain are of limited usage and are not documented in the lexicons. This poses severe methodological problems such as the use of the same name for two different substances making identification difficult. There are different descriptions in separate sources for the same substance or, alternatively, identical descriptions of the form and usage of two plants with different names.

This study makes use of modern scientific methods of identification that are acceptable in the field of historical geography as well as the accepted method for identifying plants in the Bible and in rabbinical literature.[20] Also employed were the methods used during the Middle Ages for identifying plants and agricultural cultivation in Palestine[21] by means of which the medicinal substance of "al-Sham"[22] (Greater Syria) was identified.

The technique for identifying plants, animals and minerals was based on an amalgamation of scientific fields such as textual analysis, habitat adjustments, philology, comparisons with rabbinical texts and with historical and medical sources from adjacent regions and countries,[23] botanical

11 For example: Little; Lutfi; Cohen, Economy; Cohen, 18th Century.

12 For example: Bresc; Hospitalier.

13 For example: PPTS; Ya'ari, Igrot; Ya'ari, Travels.

14 Grabois; Gucci.

15 al-Muqaddasi.

16 Assaph.

17 For example: Maimonides, Glossaire.

18 al-Ghafiqi.

19 Maimonides, Glossaire.

20 Feliks, World.

21 Amar, Production.

22 Lev, Materials.

23 For example: Hooper; al-Rawi & Chaakravarty.

dictionaries,[24] and modern encyclopedias for the life sciences and medicine[25]. In the historical study of each substance and its medical uses, the author has followed the methodological approach put forward by the researcher J.M.Riddle[26] which deals with the identification of ancient medicinal substances and maintains that the scientific sources should be isolated in order to evaluate their importance and that sources dealing with traditional medicine should not be entirely overlooked.

For purposes of this historical study, use has been made mainly of texts which were translated and printed in a scientific manner because of the range of the research, the reliability of information and the possibility of deriving serious substantial conclusions from material which has been studied or printed. However, account has been taken of possible inaccuracies associated with translation or with difficulties in the identification of substances mainly due to the development of modern research since these studies were conducted.[27]

The medicinal substances which were found in the sources and which have been positively identified, as well as information about their use in the framework of medical practice in Jerusalem will be presented in the following chapters. These substances have been classified according to their origins: animals, minerals and plants. Other substances which were sometimes used as remedies and recorded in the sources as being found in Jerusalem, but with no direct reference to medicine, are mentioned briefly with reference to these sources.[28]

To sum up: the list of medicinal substances presented here reflects the medical and pharmacological information connected with Jerusalem and mentioned in the sources, and it constitutes a preliminary inventory of the subject. However, it should be remembered that this information is derived from all the available sources at the disposal of the author at the time of research. It may be possible to enlarge the scope of this listing when new sources are discovered.

24 For example: Issa.

25 For example: Ghaleb; Kamal, Encyc.

26 Riddle, Dioscorides.

27 In spite of this, the problematic terms and the names of substances was also checked at source.

28 Regarding the use of these substances in Levantine medicine, see the relevant terms in Lev, Materials.

Chapter II
Animal Origins of Medicinal Substances

Introduction

Since ancient times animals and products derived from different organs of their bodies have constituted part of the inventory of medicinal substances used in various cultures. Some of the animals are creatures of the wild which were sometimes hunted especially for this purpose such as the adder, while others were domestic animals and their products such as cows and chickens which were easily available to man in his natural habitat and were also used for food. The more rare and expensive of these substances were the body parts of animals such as the testicles of the beaver which were imported from distant lands along the trade routes. Sometimes various sources describe the use of human products such as mothers' milk, urine and semen which are commonly used in traditional medicine as well.

In Ancient Egypt, medical use was made of substances derived from animals such as bee honey, bat organs, ambergris from the sperm whale, and the glands of the musk deer.[1] In Mesopotamia (Assyria) medical lists were found which contained descriptions of the medical uses of substances such as wax and animal fat[2] and in Ancient China substances such as the glands of the musk deer were used.[3] Animals and their body parts were used even in classical medicine. Hippocrates mentions the used of six kinds of animals and their products including sea sponges, horns, eggs and milk.[4] Dioscorides describes the use of about 168 body parts and products of animals. Animals comprise 10% of the inventory of medicinal substances that appear in his book.[5] The Jewish Sages also mention animals and their products that were used as cures such as: snake, fish, honey, milk, cheese, eggs and body parts of animals and fowl such as: spleen, heart, lung, liver and stomach.[6] Ancient Arabic medicine - 'al-Tibb al-Nabawi' indicates the use of chicken eggs, cow cheese and bee honey.[7] The physician al-Kindi describes the medicinal use of substances including some from animal sources: coral, squid, medical skink, pigeon, lizard, crab, mouse, pearl, and animal parts such as: beaver testicles, gall, and cattle fat, fish stone, rhino and goat horns, and animal products such as: honey, wax, milk, eggs. All these comprise about 7% of all the substances.[8]

The accounts of travelers during the Middle Ages are an additional source of information about animals used for medicinal purposes. For example, Geoffrey of Unseefe (12th century) described the use of theriac against various kinds of insect bites while Jacques de Vitry describes the beaver who "bites off its own testicles with its teeth and throws them to the pursuing hunters" who make use of them for medicinal purposes. Jacques de Vitry mentions a pharmacist in Acre who raised various animals and used their excrement to prepare medications. Felix Fabri (15th century) described the hunting of the adder, which provided one of the components for theriac. Thomas Shaw (18th century) tells of the striped lizard found on the coast of Syria and used for the arousal of sexual desire.[9]

These animals are also used in present day traditional medicine. For instance, in Iraq twelve kinds of animals are described as medicinal sources including sea sponge, cow, camel, bee, fish, squid, sheep, nacre and silkworm, and they constitute 5% of all the substances mentioned.[10] In a survey conducted in Syria during the 1970's it was found that 2% - 8% of the substances in the possession of medicine vendors in the markets were of animal origin.[11] Similar data is also derived from surveys conducted in eastern countries. In Pakistan, for instance, 31 organic substances were listed (animal parts and products) which constitute 9% of all the

1 Bryan.

2 Thompson, Texts; Hakim, p. vii.

3 Gordon, Medicine, pp. 355-390; Kermers & Urdang, pp. 3-5.

4 Riddle, Tradition, p. 60.

5 Riddle, Dioscorides, pp. 146-167.

6 Perelman, Vol. I, pp. 50-98.

7 Ibn al-Qayyim, pp. 7-9.

8 al-Kindi. Similar data can be found in Maimonides, Glossaire.

9 Bodenheimer, II, pp. 187-246.

10 Hooper, pp. 189-193.

11 Ali et al.

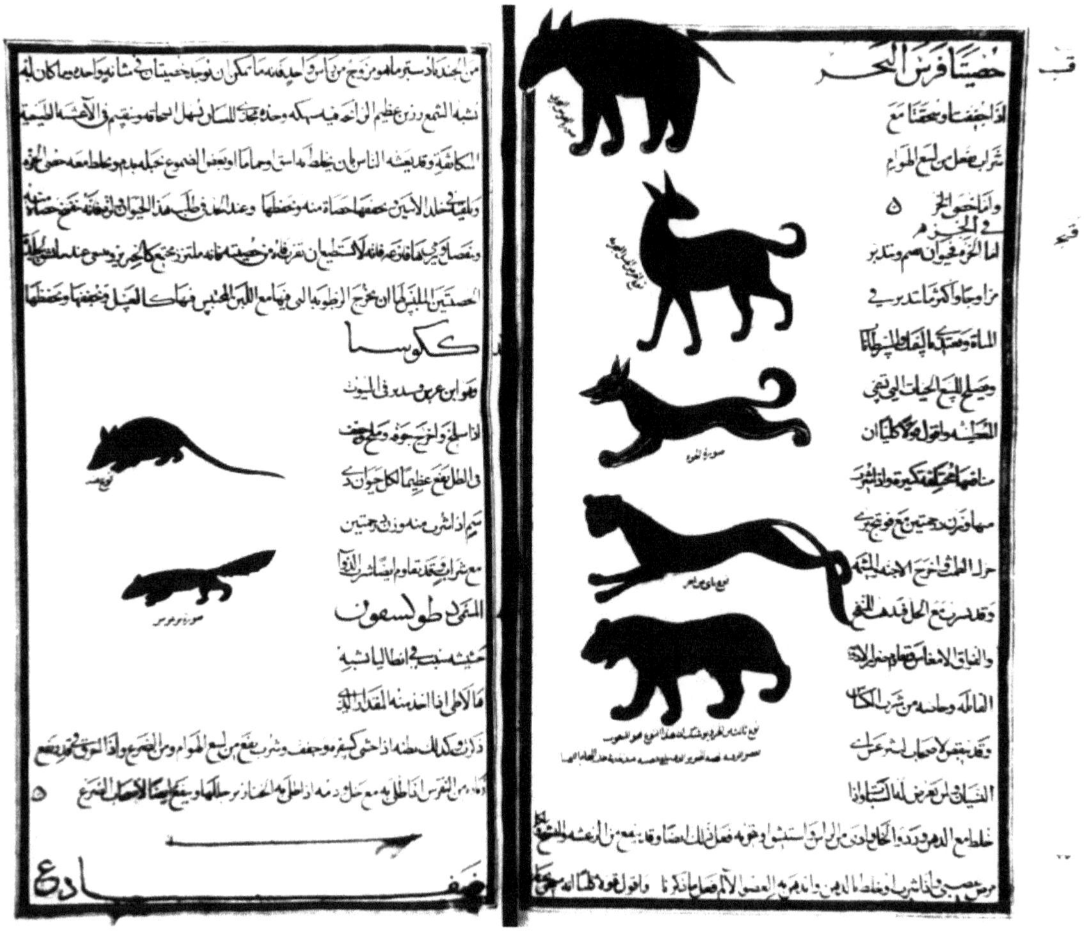

Figure 1 - Different Animals Used in Medieval Moslem Medicine

medicinal substances in the inventory of traditional medicines. Examination and research show that these substances are similar to those which were used as remedies throughout human history, irrespective of geographical borders, and include: sea sponge, bee honey and beeswax, squid, medical skink, lizard, silkworm, crab, spider, amber, pearl, nacre, hedgehog and earthworm.[12]

In a research study that examined the use of medicinal substances in the Levant during the Middle Ages, it was found that 9.5% of all the medicinal substances were of animal origins.[13] The primary purpose of some animal products, which were used as remedies was for food. The study also examined the reciprocal relationship of substances such as milk, cheese and honey as food products and their use as medicinal remedies.[14]

Animals and their Organs Used in Jerusalem Medicine

Research reveals evidence for the medicinal uses of twenty-three animals in Jerusalem from early times to the 18th century. These animals, their parts and the historical sources which mentioned them, are presented in Table 1. We decided to enlarge the scale of the data given for five specimens. The entries include sources that demonstrate the use of animals and their organs in scholarly medicine in Jerusalem during the Middle Ages and further information about names and uses in different periods including traditional uses in the present day. The twenty-three animals found in the historical sources comprise 10.5% of all the medicinal substances located so far.

Adder

Scientific name: *Echis coloratus*
Hebrew: Afea   Arabic: Afa'a

Description:
A poisonous reptile of the viper species. It is 80 cm. long and weighs 180 grams. Its natural habitat is the desert, mainly in the eastern and southern parts of Israel, from Mount Gilboa in the north to the mountains of Sinai in the south. Its venom is dangerous to mankind and may be deadly. Its bite mechanism is highly sophisticated to ensure the effective penetration of the poison concentrated in the large glands inside its cheeks. The poison contains substances causing hemorrhage and neurotoxic reactions.[15]

[12] Ali & Mahdihassan, Animal; Vohora & Khan, pp. 110-111; Fernie.

[13] Lev, Materials, p. 324.

[14] O'Hara.

[15] Plants & Animals, V, 152-153, 165.

Table 1 - List of animal's origin substances in 10th-18th century Jerusalem.

Scientific Name	Common Name	Extract/Product	Selected Sources
Ammoperdix heyi	*Desert partridge*	*Meet*	*DS*
Anser anser	*Goose*	*Oil*	*DS*
Apis mellifica	Bee	Honey	GN, BN, DS, RM
Avicula margarittifera	*Pearl*	*Pearl*	*FR, DS*
Bos Taurus	Cow	Milk, Cheese, Butter	DS, FR
Canis lupus	Wolf	Oil	FR
Capra hircus mambrica	Goat	Cheese and body parts	DS
Castor fiber	Beaver	Testicles	BN, FR
Echis coloratus	Adder, Ter	Body	JV, FR, FF, FS
Gallus gallus domesticus	Hen	Egg parts	DS, FR
Gazella sp.	Gazelle	Horn	DS
Homo sapience	Human	Boon, Stone	FR
Leiurus quinquestriatus hebraeus	Scorpion	Body	FR
Lumbricus sp.	Earthworm	Body	DS
Lytta vesicatoria	Spanish fly	Body	BD, FR
Moschus moschiferus	Musk Deer	Rectal gland	GN, FR, DS
Ovis	*Lamb*	*Body parts*	*DS*
Physeter catodom	Sperm Whale (Amberigris)	Intestine secretion	FR, BD, TA
Sepia officinalis	Cuttle Fish	Skeleton	FR
Tubipora musica or Corallium rubrum	Coral	Coral parts	FR, DS
Unidentified	Kermes	Insect body	FR
Unidentified	*Fish*	*Meet*	*DS, FR*
Vulpes sp.	*Fox*	*Oil*	*FR*

Sources
BD – al-Badri
BN – Benevenutus
DS – David de Silva
FF – Felix Fabri
FR- Franciscans
FS - Frescobaldi
GN – Genizah
JV – Jacques de Vitry
RM – Refael Malki
TA – al-Tamimi

History:
For centuries snakes and healing have been closely associated in different religions and cultures around the world. The image of Serapis, an Egyptian god and his temple, the Serapion, are linked with the snake. The Bible describes the brazen serpent made by Moses at God's command (Numbers 21:1-6) which was raised up on a pole so that whoever was bitten by a poisonous snake could gaze at it and be cured. Asclepius, the Greek god of healing, whose temple was used in Roman times also as a hospital, was associated with the snake image.[16]

The adder is mentioned in the Bible and the Talmud in connection with its longevity. The Jewish Sages described the Roman use of the snake as an antidote to snake poisoning, and there is a halachic ruling with regard to its medicinal uses. The adder is a frequent subject in scientific and sacred literature and in Arabic poetry.[17]

[16] Maimonides, Poisons, pp. 24-75; Margalit; Levkowitz

[17] EI, "Afa'a" entry.

Medicinal Uses in Jerusalem:
The medicinal uses of the adder were well-known, especially in medieval times. Many scholars and pilgrims describe in detail the capture and preparation of the adder for medicinal purposes, and it is often referred to as the 'Dead Sea Monster.'[18] Its flesh was used mainly to prepare theriac - a remedy to cure poisoning from bites and stings, and for a wide variety of other diseases.[19]

Jacques de Vitry, Bishop of Acre (13th century) reported in one of his books that the adder lives in the deserts surrounding Jericho, and that its meat combined with certain other substances, is used in the preparation of the famous remedy theriac for treating all kinds of poison except that of the adder itself.[20] The traveler Ernoul, who visited the Holy Land in 1231, wrote about a certain field in the vicinity of Jericho where adders were captured and sold to pharmacists in the

[18] For further details see: Nissenbaum, Monster.

[19] See entry for Theriac in Chapter V.

[20] PPTS, X, p. 676; Bodenheimer, II, pp.203-204.

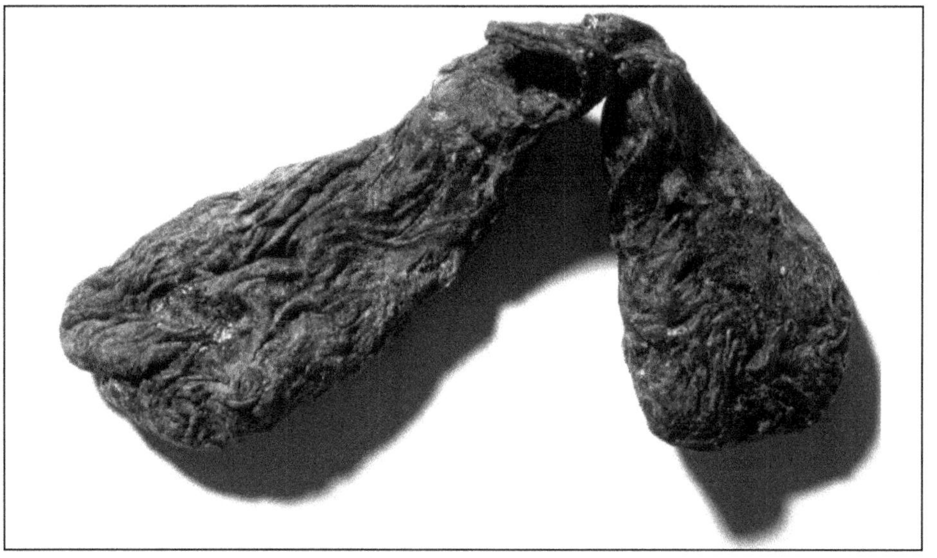

Figure 2 - Castor Testicles (*Castor fiber*)

cities who prepared treacle (theriac) from them.[21] Ludolph von Suchem who came to the Holy Land in 1340 describes the adder (Tyrus) of the Judaean desert and lists its medicinal uses.[22] Similarly, the three Italian travellers, Frescobaldi, Gucci and Sigoli who visited the Holy Land in 1384 described the ruins of Jericho and the snake hunted there for the preparation of theriac.[23]

The Adder as Medication in the Levant:
Felix Fabri informs us that the Mamluk ruler forbade the entry of foreigners to the desert regions for fear that "the noble, poisonous adder would be captured, stolen and become extinct." He mentions that the ruler recognised the importance of the adder for the famous antidote, theriac, which was produced from it and which is the origin for its name - Tyr or Ter. Fabri relates how the poorer people disobeyed the ruler's command and "sell the snake to Christian traders in Damascus and Beirut and even in Alexandria and Cairo."[24] Francisco Suriano also writes about the medicinal uses of the adder.[25]

Medicinal Uses in the Medieval Period:
Maimonides recommended eating adder meat as a "wonder remedy" for leprosy. The skin of the adder ground with honey was a highly valued medication for alopecia.[26]

Ibn al-Baytar reviewed the medicinal uses of the adder in classical medical literature and reported on certain cases which proved the remedial qualities of snake meat for the treatment of skin diseases such as leprosy, and for frailty and other illnesses.[27]

[21] Ibid., IV, p. 69.

[22] Ibid., XII, p. 136.

[23] Frescobaldi, p. 42.

[24] PPTS, II, pp. 151-153.

[25] Suriano, p. 255.

[26] Maimonides, Aphorisms, 9:108; 21: 53, 55; 22:2. Cf. al-Ghafiqi, No. 113.

[27] Ibn al-Baytar, al-Jami, 1:46-48; Leclerc, No. 120; al-Antaki, pp. 52-53.

Traditional Medicine:
The Bedouins of the Sinai desert use the adder to treat impotency, and among the Negev Bedouins the slough is commonly used to treat allergies and to expel the fear of snakes.[28] Yemenite Jews used adder meat as an antidote for snake bites.[29] In Pakistan, snake venom is used as a remedy for chronic aches and for diseases such as leprosy, skin diseases, heart trouble and nervous ailments.[30]

Modern Medicine:
Due to the large number of adder bites in Israel, a special modern antidote was developed. In spite of increasing cases of snake's bite in recent years, only one case of death has occurred since the establishment of the State.[31]

Beaver

Scientific name: *Castor fiber*
Hebrew: Boneh   Arabi: Jundibadastar[32]

Description:
The common beaver is a rodent which lives in North America and the northern parts of the old world mainly, in ponds surrounded by forests. It has an oil gland for lubricating its flat tail, which is covered with scales and used as a paddle for swimming. The dry secretion accumulated on the foreskin of the beaver's penis or its testicles was used as a medicinal substance.[33] According to Levey, medicinal use was made of this secretion and not of the testicles themselves. But since the lumps of dried

[28] Levey, Bedouins, p. 86; Abu-Rabia, p. 24.

[29] Reiani, No. 158.

[30] Vohora & Khan, p. 39.

[31] Plants & Animals, V, pp. 152-153, 165.

[32] Maimonides, Glossaire, No. 79. Cf. Leclerc, nos. 805, 1792, 1957; Kamal, Encyc., p. 797, No. 361; Ghaleb, p. 274, No. 5713; p. 284, No. 6013.

[33] Plants & Animals, VII, pp. 168-170.

secretion were sold in pairs, it was falsely assumed that these were beaver testicles.[34]

Identification:
According to Maimonides' description given in the first person, it appears that he knew the animal, its behavior and habits. Although we might deduce from this that he actually saw a beaver in its natural habitat, the fact is that he had spent most of his life in Spain, Morocco and Egypt where beavers cannot be found. We therefore think that he probably saw an otter - an animal that lives in Europe, North Africa and Asia (including the Middle East). Since the modern Arabic name for the otter is 'kalba al-mai'[35] which belongs to the weasel family (Maimonides calls it 'sammur') we may therefore assume that in these regions physicians made use of otter testicles for medicinal purposes though the original use was of the beaver testicles.

The otter - *Lutra seistanica* - is a species of weasel that preys on other animals. In Israel it can be found in rivers, ponds and water canals in the valleys.[36]

History:
Dioscorides mentions the '*kastoros orchis*' and its medicinal applications. He specifically wrote about its use in treating the bites of snakes, scorpions and other poisonous creatures, as well as to expel the placenta, induce sneezing and as an emmenagogue and an abortive.[37]

Beaver Testicles as a Medicinal Substance in Jerusalem:
Benevenutus, the Jerusalem eye-doctor, mentions the use of 'castoreum' as a component in the famous 'Jerusalem Electuary' which was used to treat cataracts.[38] Although its connection with Jerusalem appears indirectly in only one single historical source, it is mentioned here because it was widely used in the Middle Ages.

Medicinal Uses of in the Medieval Period:
al-Kindi reported about the use of the 'jundubadastur' as a component in an ointment for the nose and the head, in a clyster, as a remedy to cure insanity and in other ointments.[39] Maimonides asserted that the 'qastorin' was a component in a remedy for external use to treat the bites of snakes and other poisonous creatures, in a clyster to treat stomach pains and fever, and as a remedy to strengthen the body and the heart.[40] Daud al-Antaki, in the entry 'jundibadastar' described a small, wild animal covered with black hair used for medicinal applications such as headaches and earaches, to treat diseases of the liver and spleen, leprosy and pus in the eyes. It was also a component in theriac (treacle) as an antidote for poisonous animal bites.[41]

Traditional Medicine Uses:
Regarding present day uses of the common beaver in traditional and popular medicine, beaver testicles are rarely sold in the markets of Egypt, Syria and Jordan as their price is considerably high. It is used as a stimulant, a solvent for the production of traditional remedies, as an emmenagogue, and for the treatment of hysteria.[42] In Pakistan it is used to treat paralysis, arthritis, opium poisoning, scorpion bites, frailty and to improve the eyesight.[43]

Bee

Scientific name: ***Apis mellifica***

Description:
The honey bee is a social insect that has been cultivated for thousands of years. By nature the honey bee nests in closed spaces with narrow entrances in which the bee workers build a honeycomb made out of wax. The honeycomb is used for breeding the young and storing the honey. The workers produce the honey, which becomes concentrated due to evaporation while stored in the honeycomb. Many bee and beehive products have been used for medicine: honey, wax, honey water, queen food, pollen and bee sting poison.[44]

Honey

Hebrew: Devash Arabic: Asal

Description:
Honey is made of flower nectar which is collected by the worker bees in their crop where some chemical processes occur due to enzyme activity. In this way the honey becomes richer in monosugars as compared with the nectar. The taste and color of the honey depends on the plant from which the nectar was collected.[45]

History:
The ancient Egyptians used honey to treat eye diseases and so did the ancient Babylonians.[46] In the Bible, honey is mentioned in various contexts and we might even find a medicinal one mentioned in a biblical verse (Proverbs 24:13). The Jewish Sages in the Talmud asserted its medicinal uses as well. Pliny, who dedicated a whole chapter to the description of ointments, claimed that honey was an important

34 al-Kindi, p. 254, No. 66.

35 Plants & Animals, VII, pp. 167-170.

36 Ibid., pp. 18, 22, 36, 38.

37 Dioscorides, II.26.

38 Benevenutus, p. 37. On the problematics of this source see the Introduction.

39 al-Kindi, Nos. 1, 15, 147, 205. Cf. al-Ghafiqi, No. 228; al-Biruni, 1:112-113.

40 Maimonides, Poisons, pp. 103, 117; Maimonides, Regimen, 2:6; 4:8; Maimonides, Aphorisms, 9:92; 22:16; Maimonides, Answers 3:19.

41 al-Antaki, p.109. Cf. Ibn al-Baytar, al-Jami, 1:171-172; Leclerc, No. 516.

42 al-Kindi, p. 254, No. 66.

43 Vohora & Khan, p. 39.

44 Plants & Animals, III: 368-371; XII: 268-271; Putsiynakova, pp. 15-23.

45 Ibid., XII: 270.

46 Levey, Chemistry, pp. 86, 94, 104, 571.

component in each of them.[47] Dioscorides reported about several medicinal uses of the "mell."[48]

Identification:
In ancient times as well as in the Middle Ages, honey was a general name which included bee honey ('asal' in Arabic and 'devash' in Hebrew) and other kinds of honey made of grapes, carobs,[49] or dates. The latter was called 'dibs' in Arabic.[50] All kinds of sweet liquids were used for medicinal purposes.[51]

Honey as a Medicinal Substance in Jerusalem:
Benevenutus wrote that honey was an important component of a syrup named 'Jerusalem Electuary' which was used to treat cataract.[52] Refael Malki asserted that ordinary honey was a component in a medicinal syrup used by the Jews of Jerusalem. In another place he wrote that rose honey was a component in a general remedy for the poor.[53] Moses Poriat of Prague described the various kinds of products in the Jerusalem market in the 17th century and asserted that honey ('asal') was eight times more expensive than carob honey ('harob dibs').[54]

Honey as a Medicine in the Levant:
From a letter found in the Genizah which the writer, Natan ha-Cohen from Ashkelon sent to Ola ha-Levi in Fustat (1100 CE), we learn that bee honey was exported from the Land of Israel to Egypt.[55] Honey was also mentioned by al-'Uthmani as a component in a remedy that increases sexual desire and which also included 'samakah sayda' (triton) found in the Sidon region.[56] Hayim Vital described the use of honey for treating mouth diseases.[57]

Medicinal Uses of Honey in the Medieval Period:
al-Kindi reported that 'asal' was used as a component in toothpaste[58] and in other medicinal remedies. Even though honey was used intensively in Islamic regions during medieval times, it was sometimes considered as a remedy basis rather than a medicinal substance.[59]

Shabtai Donolo described medicinal uses of honey as well, though he recommended that its origin be double-checked. He claimed that honey was an important basis for liquid medications (syrups).[60] Maimonides informs us about a wide range of uses for honey in the medieval Levant: as a component in many remedies to treat symptoms such as rheumatism,[61] chest and lung pains, over secretion of sweat and saliva and as a dietetic food. Honey was included in remedies to treat burns, as a component in different clysters,[62] and in theriac. For treating bee or wasp stings - Maimonides recommended the drink of oximell (honey with vinegar).[63]

In his 'Asal' entry, Ibn al-Baytar described the use of honey in many remedies, including some to cure intestinal diseases and stomach disorders,[64] Daud al-Antaki asserted in his 'Dibs' entry that this name was given to the thick juice of both grapes and dates. Once they were cooked and were no longer fluid they were called 'rab' (jam).[65]

Some uses of Honey in Traditional and Popular Medicine:
It seems that the hygroscopic qualities of honey are the main reason for its extensive use throughout history, mainly for the treatment of wounds, burns and in surgical operations. In popular medicine as well as in homeopathic remedies, honey is used, for example, as a light purgative and as a remedy for intestinal ulcers.[66] Yemenite Jews used honey as a component in remedies for treating eye inflammations, colds, throat pain, insanity, high temperatures, weak sight and for improving sexual potency.[67] Honey was an important substance in many traditional remedies of Babylonian Jewry.[68]

Medicinal Qualities of Honey and Modern Medicinal Uses:
Honey was considered as a hot and dry substance used to purify liquids and to cleanse wounds.[69] Modern research reveals that it contains 80% sugar, mainly grape sugar (glucose), fruit sugar (fructose), monoglucose, organic acids, vitamins, enzymes and minerals such as: potassium, iron, phosphate, magnesium, copper and calcium.[70] Honey has been found to be a disinfectant which fights germs, fungi and pathogens. Eating honey increases the quantities of hydrogen dioxide (H_2O_2) in the human body, and it is a strong oxidizer which destroys harmful microorganisms.[71]

Conclusions:
The use of honey has always been widespread in the Holy Land and the Levant as a nutritious food. Its use in medicine

47 Plinius, XII: 54; Donolo, p. 12.

48 Dioscorides, II: 101.

49 On the use of carobs in making 'rab' (jam) and sweets in Shechem (Nablus) and in the region of 'al-Sham' see: Ibn Battuta, pp. 128-129.

50 These kinds of honey were traded in Palestine and the surrounding regions and are mentioned, for instance, in: Ashtor, Trade, p. 280; Prawer, Colonial, p. 443. Regarding honey derived from plant life, see detailed account in: Amar, Industrial, pp. 54-58.

51 Maimonides, Regimen, I:12; Ibid., p. 41, n. 126.

52 Benevenutus, p. 37.

53 Malki, pp. 63, 66.

54 Ya'ari, Travels, p. 280.

55 Gil, III: 588.

56 'Uthmani, p. 481.

57 Benajahu, p. 110.

58 al-Kindi, p. 108, No. 96.

59 Ibid., p. 304, No. 200.

60 Donolo, pp. 9, 11, 17-18.

61 Maimonides quotes this from al-Tamimi; Maimonides, Aphorisms, 22:57.

62 Ibid., 16:8, 45; 20: 42; 221: 17-18, 61. Cf. al-Biruni, 1:225.

63 Maimonides, Poisons, pp. 109, 124.

64 Ibn al-Baytar al-Jami, III: 121-123; Leclerc, No. 1542.

65 al-Antaki, pp. 150-151.

66 Plants & Animals, 12:270.

67 Reiani, No. 151/152.

68 For detailed references see: Ben-Yakov, p. 705.

69 Maimonides, Aphorisms, 21:75; 23:100.

70 Plants & Animals, 12:270.

71 Ibid.

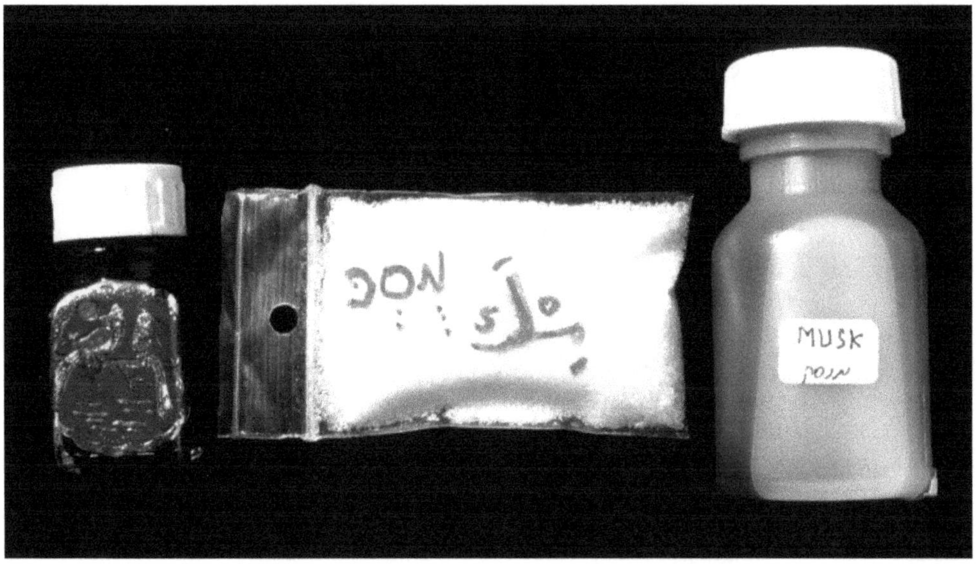

Figure 3 - Musk Deer (*Muschus moschiferus*)

began in early times and probably reached its climax in the Middle Ages, and these uses have continued until the present day. Some evidence of the medicinal uses of honey and other sweet liquids in Crusader and Ottoman Jerusalem have been presented here, while other sources describe the trade and medicinal uses in the medieval Levant.

Musk Deer

Scientific name: *Moschus moschiferus*
Hebrew: Ayal ha-musk Arabic: Misk[72]

Description:
Musk is a substance which is used as a perfume and medicine, and originates in the anal glands of the musk deer which lives in the mountains of Central Asia (the Himalayan Mountains and Tibet). The gland is found among the male of the species and is situated between the anus and the penis. It weighs 30-50 grams and is filled with liquid during the mating season. The substance in its crude state is dark brown in colour, but after a time it turns black. It is marketed either as a liquid or a solid substance.[73]

History:
Musk has been used in ancient eastern cultures. In Jewish sources it is mentioned in two Talmudic tractates in connection with a blessing to be pronounced on using it. In Christian sources the name first appears in Hieronymus (4th cent. CE). It is also mentioned in the Koran, and is cited by many Jewish and European physicians.[74] During the Middle Ages, musk was used as an important spice and was imported overland from Asia.[75]

[72] Maimonides, Glossaire, No. 290.

[73] Chizik, pp. 29-30; Shapira, Musk, p. 95

[74] For a complete historical survey see Ibid., pp. 95-101.

[75] Prawer, Jerusalem, pp. 402.

Medicinal Uses in Jerusalem:
al-Tamimi describes the preparation of the 'nad' (perfume made of musk and ambergris) which the mother of the Abassid Caliph, al-Muqtadar (908-932 CE) used to make and offer every Friday as incense on the Temple Mount rock in Jerusalem (Beit al-Maqdis). He added that: "The head of the Temple servants used to give my father some of this 'nad' and my father would melt it in 'ben' (oil of the fruit of the ben tree) and produce 'ghalia' (perfume mixture) from it, which is unequalled for its good scent."[76] al-Tamimi also offers a detailed formula for preparing the perfume or scent called 'ajun al-misk'.[77] A glass jar of perfume and musk was mentioned in a Karaite *ketuba* in Jerusalem dated 1028 CE.[78] Muschio was mentioned by David de Silva as a substance, which helps to strengthen the sick, treat "cold" illness and heart weakness.[79]

Musk in the Levant:
Musk (mousquelliat) was traded in Acre during Crusader times.[80]

Medical Uses During the Medieval Period:
al-Kindi reported the use of 'phar' as an ointment against baldness, and for pus-infected wounds.[81] Maimonides quotes al-Tamimi who claims that 'misk' was a component in a medication against headache and eye ache and as a medicine for treating diarrhea. Musk was also a component in a medication called "great atriphal" to strengthen the limbs and heart, to prolong old age, to enhance the senses and sexual potency. Tibetan musk was used as a component in "a vendor's powder to cause instant sleep."[82]

[76] Amar & Seri, p. 51; al-Nuwayri, 12, p. 64

[77] Amar & Seri, p. 51; al-Nuwayri, 12, p. 90.

[78] Gil, p. 557, No. 305.

[79] Amar, de Silva, p. 127.

[80] Assises, 2, p. 174.

[81] al-Kindi, Nos. 16, 56, 93, 147.

[82] Maimonides, Aphorisms, 3:11; 4:11; 9:30; 14:49; 21:75; Maimonides, Sexual, 18:3.

Ibn al-Baytar in his entry 'musk' describes the animal, its habitat, methods for hunting it and the means for producing the medicinal substance. Musk is described as a hot and dry drug to counter body odour or sweat and bad breath, to strengthen the heart and brain, to warm internal organs, to promote the sexual appetite and strengthen the male sexual organs. Musk also alleviates headache, cleanses the eyes and is used as a medication against diarrhea, as well as being a component in aperients and against hemorrhoids and flatulence.[83]

Traditional Medicine:
The 'phar' is a type of musk used in India as a drug for arousal and a stimulant, and also as a medicine against spasms. Tamil doctors use the substance as an anti-spasmodic in children and also to counteract dysentery and typhoid fever. Today very little use is made of this substance.[84] It is still used in traditional medicine in Pakistan and can still be obtained from medicine vendors in the markets.[85]

Modern Medicine:
Musk is a hot and dry drug, delicate and penetrating, containing oil, gum and protein. The beaver's testicles *(castrum)* were used as a substitute.[86] An experiment conducted in the 1960's proved that musk oil is a disinfectant.[87]

Conclusion and Summary:
Musk is considered an important aromatic substance in the production of perfumes and is sold in a special container made of silk and lead because of its strong odour.[88]

Musk oil is one of the most well-known and valuable medicinal substances of animal origin that has ever been used in medical history. Its medicinal use is mentioned in a wide variety of sources in different cultures both in the east and west. In our region musk is mentioned only in a commercial connection (11th-13th cent. CE), but since its medical use was so widespread during the Middle Ages in many different countries and is referred to in a large number of medical correspondences, it has been included in the list of medicinal substances in this study.

Sperm Whale (Ambergris)

Scientific Name: *Physeter catodom*
Hebrew: 'Inbar Arabic: Anbar

Identification:
Muntner, the editor of Maimonides' *Regimen Sanitatis,* mistakenly identified ambergris with the "liquidambar orientalis" but noted that in the late Middle Ages this was the name given to the gray or black substance "found in the intestines of the whale and in its bladder which is spilt into the sea and is washed ashore."

Ambergris contains a perfumed cholesterol substance which was used for strengthening the bones and for increasing sexual potency.[89] The scholar Ben Ya'akov defined ambergris as "a perfume of exceptionally good scent produced from the aural excretions of sick whales which floats on the surface of the water and is gathered on the shore." This substance was also used for medical purposes.[90] The research scholar Levey identified "anbar as-sandalani" with a substance found on the seashores of India, China, Madagascar, Somalia and even Morocco.[91]

Description and History:
Ambergris is a perfumed substance with a sweet scent similar to musk. It is flammable and burns with a bright flame. It is highly valued in the east and serves as a perfume and a medicinal substance. Ambergris floats on the surface of tropical seas or is found cast upon the shore in large lumps which weigh up to five kilograms. It originates apparently from the bile secretions of the sperm whale.[92] Dioscorides claims that ambergris (*lungourion*) is suitable as a medicine for treating stomach and intestinal problems.[93]

Medicine in Jerusalem:
al-Tamimi, in his book *Tib al-'Arus* (the bride's perfume) describes the preparation of the 'nad' (a perfume made of musk and ambergris) which was made by the mother of the Abassid Caliph, al-Muqtadar (908-932 CE) and was offered as incense on the rock of the Temple Mount in Jerusalem every Friday. al-Tamimi adds that: "the headman of the servants used to give my father some of this 'nad ' and he used to melt it in "ben" (oil of the fruit of the ben tree) and thus produce "ghalia"(a perfumed mixture) which was of an incomparable scent."[94]

Ambergris in the Levant:
The scholar al-Mas'udi (10th cent.) notes that ambergris is to be found on the shores of 'al-Sham' cities.[95] Ambergris was one of the perfumes which were an important part of the east-west trade during the Crusader period. It originated in the east and used to be sent over to Europe through the ports of the Holy Land by Italian ships.[96]

Medical Uses During the Medieval Period:
According to al-Kindi, ambergris was a component in the medication for sore throat as well as being a perfume.[97]

83 Ibn al-Baytar, al-Jami, 4, p. 155; Leclerc, No. 2127. Cf. al-Antaki, pp. 297-298. See also: Levey, Ibn Masawayh, pp. 398-399.

84 al-Kindi, p. 310, No. 217.

85 Vohora & Khan, p. 38.

86 In detail: Chizik, p. 30; Shapira, Musk, p. 95; Levey, Masawayh, p. 399.

87 Mishra et al.

88 Chizik, p. 30.

89 Maimonides, Regimen, p. 115.

90 Ben-Yakov, p. 565.

91 al-Kindi, p. 307, No. 209.

92 EI, "Ambergris" entry.

93 Dioscorides, II, 100.

94 Amar & Seri, p. 51; al-Nuwayri, 12, p. 64.

95 al-Mas'udi, I, p. 366.

96 Prawer, Jerusalem, p. 402..

97 al-Kindi, No. 77.

Maimonides reports that it is a substance that strengthens body and spirit by its good scent and that it was a component in a formula for heart medicine which he quotes in the name of Ibn Sina. Ambergris was considered a hot and dry drug.[98]

Ibn al-Baytar in his 'Ambergris' entry quotes various doctors in connection with this substance:

- Abu Hassan asserted that the substance was an excretion of aquatic creatures found in the sea and this is eaten by other creatures which regurgitate it. The substance is oily, floats on the surface and has a perfume. It is used to strengthen the heart and brain and to cure semi-paralysis of the body and face.
- Ibn Sina contradicts this theory of its origins and detailed the various types and their special qualities: beneficial for the aged, for the brain, for the senses and for the heart.
- Other physicians described its uses as a palliative for pains of the stomach, head and back, to counteract colds and to cure nervous diseases.
- al-Tamimi is also quoted for having recommended the use of this substance for bandaging joints in cases of joint pains. When ambergris is melted with plant oil it is also used for curing mental diseases and paralysis.[99]

al-Qazwini reported that the substance reaches the shore and is sometimes found in the belly of sea fish. Among its medicinal qualities are: fortifying the mind, senses and heart. Used internally in minimal doses, it is beneficial to the aged (because of its warm coloring), but in larger doses it is harmful to the body and can be fatal.[100]

Traditional Medicine:
The Jews of Iraq made medical use of ambergris to treat scabies, to strengthen pregnant women and for the general fortifying of the body, especially the head, liver, stomach, eyes and heart.[101]

Summary and Conclusion:
Ambergris is one of the most exotic medical substances because of its origins (secretions of the sperm whale) and the way it is collected (on seashores). Its uniqueness caused it to be used as a component in many and varied kinds of medications. Yet, owing to its scarcity, it price was costly, it was in very high demand in eastern markets and it was also exported to Europe.

[98] Maimonides, Aphorisms, 21:75; Maimonides, Regimen, 2:20; Maimonides, Answers, 3:19.

[99] Ibn al-Baytar, al Jami, 3, pp. 134-135; Leclerc, No. 1587. Cf. al-Antaki, pp. 239-240.

[100] al-Qazwini, pp. 214-215.

[101] Ben-Yakov, Nos. 112, 138, 351-352, 361.

Chapter III
Mineral and Metal Origins of Medicinal Substances

Introduction

Various minerals, metals and stones formed part of the natural medicinal substances in early times and in many different cultures. Some of these substances were easily available to man in his natural habitat, others were collected in close vicinity to him, a few were mined and processed by industrial methods, and the more expensive ones were brought over the trade routes from near or distant lands.

It is known, historically, that in ancient Egypt minerals and metals were used such as potassium nitrate, asphalt, iron, copper sulphate, salt, magnesium, sodium carbonate, lead and white lead.[1] In medical listings discovered in Mesopotamia (7th century BCE), 120 kinds of metals, stones and minerals were identified as having been used for remedies, including alum and bitumen (asphalt).[2] Even in ancient Chinese medicine they made use of minerals and metals such as: alum, iron, sulphur and mercury.[3]

Classical medicine also made use of minerals and metals. Hippocrates mentions 400 medicinal substances among which nine minerals and six metals were identified.[4]

Dioscorides described the use of about 96 kinds of metals, minerals and stones including: asphalt, zinc, antimony, iron, sulphur, kinds of clay, salt, copper, sodium, lead, calcium, and carbon which comprised 10% of the basic medicinal substances used by this important physician. Other minerals as well which were actually poisons, such as mercury and arsenic, were used as remedies.[5] Even the Jewish Sages mentioned certain minerals that were used as remedies such as lime, lead, and kohl[6] while in neo-Aramean (Syrian) medicine there is mention of substances such as potassium powder, glass and white lead.[7]

In Arabic medicine, minerals and metals form a small but important component of the basic materials in medicinal substances. For example, the physician al-Kindi describes the use of 300 substances, 27 of which were minerals and metals comprising about 10% of all the substances.[8] Maimonides noted the use of approximately 42 kinds of minerals, stones and metals.[9] The research scholar, S. Hamarneh, estimates that in the 10th century the use of chemicals and minerals in Arabic medicine reached its peak as a result of the combined information derived from the writings of classical physicians, eastern medical knowledge and well-developed trade relations among the various parts of the Islamic Empire and its interconnections with other countries. This surge in medical information is reflected in the many references to minerals and chemicals found in the writings of physicians such as al-Razi, al-Majusi and al-Zahrawi who practised medicine in Cordoba in the Western Caliphate.[10]

A similar situation and the use of identical substances was preserved in the traditional medicine of the region. Traditional medicine in Iraq, for example, describes 17 minerals and metals which were used including: alum, antimon, arsenic, sulphur, clay, fossils, copper, salts, sodium carbonate, and lead.[11] In a survey conducted in 1970 in Syria of shops selling medications, it was found that 5% - 20% of the medicinal substances were minerals and metals. In the sources for

1 Bryan.

2 Thompson, Texts; Hakim, p. vii. On substances and the chemical industry see: Levey, Chemistry.

3 Gordon, Medicine, pp. 355-390.

4 Riddle, Tradition, p. 60

5 Riddle, Dioscorides, pp. 146-167.

6 Perelman, I:50-98.

7 Budge, Pt.II. For details see: Bodenheimer, pp. 128-134.

8 al-Kindi. On the production and use of chemical substances in Iran and Iraq in the 10th century see: Stapleton.

9 Maimonides, Glossaire. Cf. Stapleton, pp. 317-324.

10 Hamarneh, Chemical.

11 Hooper, pp. 189-193.

medicinal substances among the Jews of Iraq, the use of about nine types of similar substances are described[12] while a study of traditional medicinal substances from natural sources which was conducted in the 1960's in Pakistan, the use of 43 minerals and metals were noted.[13]

Minerals and Metals used in Jerusalem Medicine

Research reveals evidence for the medicinal uses of 14 minerals in Jerusalem from early times to the 18th century. The minerals and the historical sources which mentioned them are presented in Table 2. We decided to enlarge the scale of the data given for six specimens. The entries include sources that demonstrate the use of minerals and metals relating to their medicinal use in Jerusalem during the Middle Ages and more information about names and uses in different periods as well as traditional uses in the present day. Statistically, the minerals and metals comprise 6.7 % of the list of medicinal substances similar to those found in the list of traditional medicines in the region, and are not unlike the data given in the listings of other substances in classical and medieval times.

Table 2 – List of mineral substances used in 10th-18th century Jerusalem

Name	Selective References
Alum	HR, DS
Amonia	DS
Arsenic Sulfide	DS
Asphalt	TA, GN, IB, FH
Jews' Stone (Cidaris sp.)	AN
Earth (Clay)	DS
Kohl (Antimony, Galena)	GN
Mercury	DS
Salt (Halite)	GN, TA, DS
Sulphur	TA, GN
Tartrate	DS
Thermal (mineral) water	DS
Vitriol sp.	DS
Zinc	BN, DS

Sources

AN – Daud al-Antaki
BN – Benevenutus
DS – David de Silva
FH – Frederick Hasselquist
GN – Genizah
HR – Haram Documents
IB - Ibn al-Baytar
RM – Refael Malki
TA - al-Tamimi

[12] Ben-Yakov, pp. 433-438. Cf. The list of medicinal substances of the Yemenite Jews in Reiani, Nos. 172-182.

[13] Ali et al. For another study that describes the identity of the substances and their uses and has contributed to the identification and collection of information see: Ali & Mahdihassan, Mineral.

Alum

Scientific name: ***Stypteria***
Hebrew: Alom Arabic: Shab, Alum[14]

Description:
Alum is a composition of different salts of metals with crystallization water. The prototype of this group of materials is natural alum saltpetre. Alum is a natural astringent and therefore has been used throughout history in the tannery industry, as an aftershave and to stop bleeding.[15]

History:
In ancient Babylonia, white as well as black alum was used in chemical technologies and in medicine. The black kind was manufactured by exposing the alum to plant decoction.[16] White alum has been used to wash the mouth and the nose, stop bleedings and treat skin diseases, scabies, gonorrhea, dysentery and eye inflammations. Disocorides described different types of *stypteria* and their medicinal uses which were similar to the uses in ancient Babylonia. Dioscorides added the uses of the alum in treating leprosy, infected gums and ear disorders.[17] The main centre for manufacturing the alum in the Middle Ages was in the deserts of Egypt, from which a high quality alum was manufactured and sold by the Bedouins. This production was a state monopoly in the 12th and 13th centuries and according to the historical sources, the alum was distributed all over the Middle East and Europe.[18]

Medicinal Uses in Jerusalem:
'Shab asfar' (dark alum) was mentioned in the 'Haram' Archives as a substance which was sold in drug seller stands in the market of Jerusalem during the Mamluk period.[19] Even though it was used in different industries, it is clear that it was sold for cosmetic and medicinal uses. 'Alumi' was mentioned by David de Silva, as an astringent and a substance for the treatment of several eye ailments.[20]

Alum in the Levant:
In a list describing the taxation at the port of Acre (13th cent.), alum is mentioned as a substance which was transported to Europe via the Levant.[21] Alum was mentioned in the list of taxation by the city of Venice (1233 CE).[22] It seems as though alum was an important commodity and a medicinal substance in the medieval Levant.

Medicinal Uses in the Medieval Period:
al-Kindi claimed that the Yemenite alum 'shab yamani' was a component in a remedy to treat toothache and in

[14] Maimonides, Glossaire, No. 368.

[15] HE, IV, pp. 487-488.

[16] Levey, Chemical, pp. 158-164.

[17] Dioscorides, V. 123.

[18] In detail: Ashtor, Levant, p. 35, Notes 29-30.

[19] Lutfi, p. 292.

[20] Amar, de Silva. P. 112.

[21] Assises, p. 174.

[22] Venice Laws, p. 285.

toothpaste.[23] He also reported the medicinal use of yellow alum which was probably unpurified alum.[24] Maimonides asserted that the Yemenite alum was the main component in a remedy which "causes sexual desire among men" and was also used for "shaving without hazard."[25] al-Qazwini mentions the alum stone 'hajar alum' as a remedy to treat bleedings, wounds, tooth pains and as an astringent.[26] Ibn al-Baytar added that the alum was used to clear and purify water and wine.[27] Daud al-Antaki wrote that the 'shab' is a component in treating eyes, ears, skin and tooth ailments. It was also used as a deodorant, to strengthen the stomach and as a contraceptive.[28]

Traditional Medicine:
Babylonian and Yemenite Jewry, like other inhabitants of Middle Eastern countries have traditionally used alum for the treatment of eye diseases and inflammation, strengthening the sight, gums and teeth, curing wounds and preventing bleedings. The substance was also used to cure skin ailments, combat lice, strengthen hair roots, treat burns, heart pains, cough and tuberculosis.[29]

General Uses:
Alum is used in Iran and Iraq for the manufacture of colours, paper and tannery, and was also used as a shaving stone.[30]

Asphalt (Pitch, Bitumen, Tar)

Scientific name: *Pix*
Hebrew: Asfalt Arabic: Zipht[31]

Description:
A resinous mineral, solid or semi-solid, which consists of a mixture of hydrocarbon created naturally, probably due to a solidification or oxidising process. Asphalt sometimes erupts from the earth along the shores of the Dead Sea, from springs in 'Nahal Hemar' in the Judean Desert and all along the Mediterranean coast. Asphalt has been extensively used by several ancient cultures in the old world. It was an important and expensive commodity and was used in agriculture, industry and medicine.[32]

History:
Deposits of asphalt were discovered at the Neolithic site of Gilgal (9000 BCE) and in Bayda (South Jordan). According to the remains found in the ancient city of Arad, asphalt continued to be used throughout the Chalcolithic period as well. But the main ancient use of asphalt was as the key material in the mummification process, which was prevalent in ancient Egypt. Mummification was considered as part of medicine, and was performed by highly trained physicians. It began to be practiced in Egypt during the Iron Age and continued well into the Byzantine period.[33] Asphalt is mentioned in the Bible several times and with different names: 'kufer' in the Noah's Ark story, 'himar' and 'zefet' in the story of the baby Moses and his 'ark,' and 'zefet' in the destruction of Sodom and Gomorrah, as well as in the prophetic books.[34] Asphalt has also been used for building in Mesopotamia.[35]

Classical sources mention asphalt and the way it was commercially gathered. Dioscorides described *asphaltos* and asserted that the substance, which was brought from Judea was of the best quality.[36] Josephus Flavius wrote that asphalt cures the body and it was blended with many remedies.[37] The Jewish Sages mention 'kofra' and 'zefet' in connection with various uses.[38] In Arabic literature asphalt of the Dead Sea was known as 'kafar al-Yahud' (asphalt of the Jews). During the medieval period it was considered the best of its kind. During the Crusaders rule of the Levant, Dead Sea asphalt was used for industrial and medicinal uses and might have been exported as well. According to travellers' accounts, many of the inhabitants of the Dead Sea region gained their livelihood by gathering and trading in asphalt.[39]

Medicinal Uses in Jerusalem:
al-Tamimi described the use of asphalt from the Dead Sea as one of the components in theriac.[40] Some letters found in the Genizah (1061-2 CE) deal with asphalt. One letter is by Israel Ben Nathan from Jerusalem who asked Naharai Ben Nissim from Fustat (Old Cairo) to send him asphalt from Alexandria "since it is impossible to find it in Jerusalem." In another letter Israel Ben Nathan explains that he needed the substance to "cure his little daughter's eye."[41]

Asphalt in the Levant:
During the Crusader period, 'kafar' of the Dead Sea was used for similar needs, and may have also been exported.[42] Ibn al-Baytar wrote in his 'Kafar' entry that this was the 'kafar al-Yahud' mentioned by al-Tamimi in his Murshad. Ibn al-Baytar added that its origin is from "The sea of Judea, which is the Dead Sea in Palestine, near Jerusalem and in the 'Ghur' not

23 al-Kindi, Nos. 78, 103.

24 Ibid., No. 105. See also: p. 292, No. 165.

25 Maimonides, Sexual, 10; 16:2.

26 al-Qazwini, p. 200.

27 Ibn al-Baytar, al-Jami, III, p. 53-54; Leclerc, No. 1279.

28 al-Antaki, p. 209.

29 Reiani, No. 182; Ben-Yakov, p. 609. Further references on p. 696.

30 HE, III, p. 488; Hooper, p. 189.

31 Maimonides, Glossaire, No. 138; al-Kindi, pp. 319-320, No. 243.

32 HE, V, pp. 49-50; Mazor, pp. 363-364; Kaplan, Asphalt; Kaplan, Bitumen; Nissenbaum, Utilization; Nissenbaum, Dead Sea; Nissenbaum, Asphalt.

33 Connan et al.

34 Summary in: Kaplan, Bitumen, pp. 81-82.

35 Summary of sources in: Kaplan, Asphalt, pp. 230-234. Cf. Nissenbaum, Utilization.

36 Dioscorides, I. 99

37 Josephus, JW, IV:8:3.

38 Summary in: Kaplan, Bitumen, pp. 81-82.

39 In detail: Raz, p. 188; Kaplan, Asphalt, pp. 235-236.

40 al-Tamimi, pp. 29-30.

41 Gil, p. 163, No. 479; p. 165, No. 480; p. 175, No. 482.

42 Prawer, Colonial, p. 471.

far away from Jericho."[43] Similar descriptions were given in the entry 'Kafar al-Yahud.' Daud al-Antaki asserted in his entry 'Hamar' that in al-Sham (Greater Syria) they call it 'kafar al-Yahud.'[44]

The Franciscan monk, Roger, who was a physician and pharmacist, described the medicinal use of asphalt[45] while he was serving in the East. Frederick Hasselquist wrote about his personal observations of asphalt gathering at the Dead Sea by Arabs, its export to Egypt and its distribution there. He also mentions its similarities to mummy.[46]

Medicinal Uses in the Medieval Period:
According to al-Kindi, the 'kir' was an important component in some remedies for the treatment of hemorrhoids, wounds, and swollen lips.[47] Shabtai Donolo claimed that asphalt was one of the medicinal substances which melts while heated and becomes glued to the hands.[48] Maimonides asserted that 'zefet' was a key component in a bandage for the treatment of "pains in the nerve."[49] According to his writings, asphalt was one of the components of theriac.[50] al-Qazwini suggested that 'zift' was used to treat symptoms and diseases such as skin diseases, arthritis, cough, muscle pains etc.[51]

Traditional Medicine:
Babylonian Jews used asphalt to cure eye diseases, back pains, heart disorders and to make bandages for wounds.[52] In Egypt, asphalt was used as an expectorant and for the treatment of ulcers and wounds.[53]

General Uses:
Asphalt was one of the unique minerals of the Holy Land which was used throughout antiquity as a basis for medicinal remedies.[54] It seems that one of the Arabic names for asphalt – 'kafar al-Yahud' – is evidence of its origins in the Land of Israel. A wide variety of historical sources described the production of asphalt mainly in the area of the Dead Sea, its international trade and its different uses, mainly for medicine and mummification. Among the medicinal uses of asphalt is its external treatment of eye and skin diseases and as a component in some remedies for the curing of wounds. Asphalt was one of the important constituents of medieval theriac,[55] an ointment to treat cattle skin diseases and to protect medicinal substances from pests.[56]

According to the wide range of historical sources, it seems that different kinds of asphalt were traded in the Levant under various names and of many origins. Though Israel, and mainly the Dead Sea area, was the central source for asphalt production in the ancient world, the letter from the Genizah which tells of the appeal made in Jerusalem to obtain asphalt from Egypt might suggest that even though the writer lived near the main sources for asphalt, he need a special kind of asphalt which was collected on the sea shores of Egypt for medicinal treatment.

Jews' Stone (Lapis Judaicus)

Scientific name: ***Cidaris sp.***
Hebrew: Kipod yam meoban Arabic: Hajar al-yahud, Zaiton bani isra'il[57]

Identification:
The identification of this substance was possible due to the detailed description in the classical and medieval historical sources. Daud al-Antaki, for example, described the 'hajar al-yahud' as a: "soft-rounded stone, curved with lines."[58] Helpful information was obtained through the synonyms mentioned by medieval physicians and scholars such as Maimonides,[59] as well as that derived from the ethnographic and linguistic research by early modern scientists who have examined the origins and identification of natural medicinal substances which are still sold today in the markets of Pakistan.[60]

Description and History:
Jews' stone is the petrified spine and skeleton of the sea-urchin, an animal with a radial shape, hard external skeleton, rounded or elliptical. It feeds mainly on algae and small sea creatures, and is active at night in shallow waters. The petrified skeleton and spine of the Cidaris species can be found in Jurassic marine geological layers in Middle East countries such as Lebanon and Israel. The small, oval-shaped fossils (2 x 3.5 cm) contain 95% chalk (carbonated calcium).[61] Dioscorides described the *ioudaikos lithos* as: "beautiful shaped stone, grown in Judea" and among its medicinal applications he mentions the dissolving of renal stones.[62]

Medicinal Uses in Jerusalem:
Daud al-Antaki who described the fossil, gave us the synonym 'zaiton bani Isra'il' and claimed that this stone was formed in Jerusalem and in the mountains of 'al-Sham' (Greater Syria).[63]

43 Ibn al-Baytar, al-Jami, IV, p. 75; Leclerc, No. 1956. On 'hemar' see: Ibid., No. 705.

44 al-Antaki, p. 132.

45 Roger, p. 219.

46 Hasselquist, pp. 284-285.

47 al-Kindi, Nos. 76, 122. Cf. Ibn Sina, p. 306; al-Biruni.

48 Donolo, pp. 14, 18.

49 Maimonides, Aphorisms, 9:115. Regarding its medical properties, see: Ibid., 21:75, 88.

50 Maimonides, Sexual, pp. 105-107.

51 al-Qazwini, p. 214. Cf. Ibn al-Baytar, al-Jami, IV, pp. 26-27; Leclerc, No. 1818; al-Antaki, p. 261.

52 Ben-Yakov, pp. 162, 165, 171-172, 175, 184, 226, 234, 348,-349.

53 Ducros, p. 178.

54 HE, V, pp. 49-50.

55 In connection with this see: Berman.

56 Amar, Substances, p. 54.

57 Maimonides, Glossaire, No. 164.

58 al-Antaki, p. 118. Cf. Dioscorides V. 155.

59 Maimonides, Glossaire, No.164.

60 Ali & Mahdihassan, Animal, pp. 70-72; Kamal, Encyc., p. 800, No. 409.

61 Plants & Animals, IV, pp. 59, 170; Hooper, pp. 194-195; Mazor, pp. 170-171.

62 Dioscorides, V.155.

63 al-Antaki, p. 118.

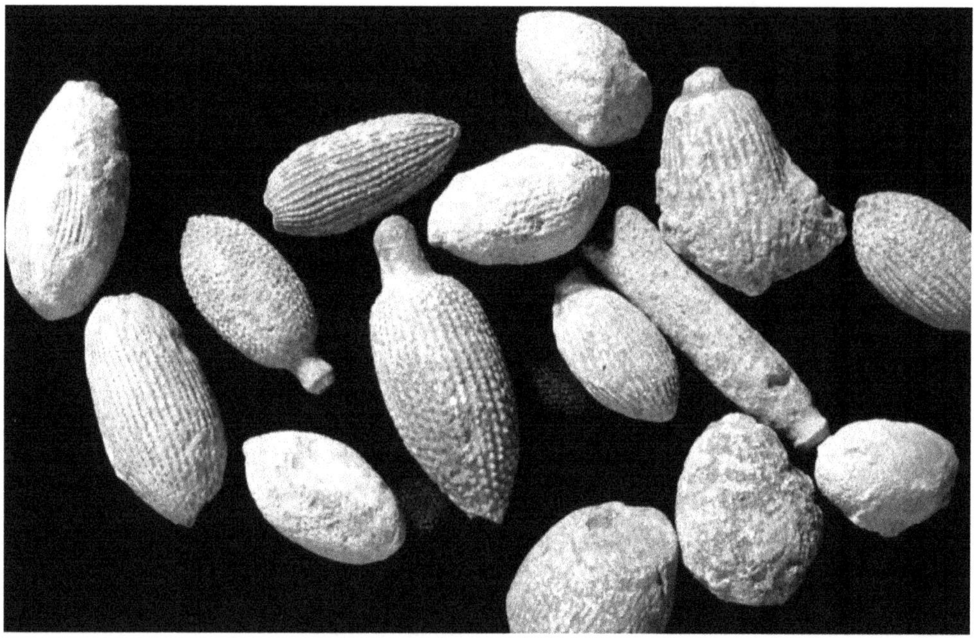

Figure 4- Jews' Stone (Cidaris sp.)

Jews' Stone in the Levant:
al-Biruni wrote that 'hajar al-yahud' is a nut-shaped stone which has curved parallel lines and is found only in Palestine.[64] Ibn al-Baytar described 'hajar al-yahud' as a white acorn with curved parallel lines, and added that the stone, which was without taste, was soluble in water and was prescribed for dissolving stones in the bladder. Ibn al-Baytar also reported that he had collected the stones in the mountains of Beirut in 'al-Sham' from whence it was usually brought to Damascus.[65]

Medicinal Uses in the Medieval Period:
Maimonides asserted that the 'hajar al-yahud' was used in a plaster to treat bites and stings besides its general use as a diuretic and to dissolve stones in the renal tracts.[66] Daud al-Antaki claimed that powder made out of the 'hajar al-yahud' prevented the formation of kidney and bladder stones and also dissolved them. He called it a warm and dry drug and added that the powder cured wounds and was a component in an ointment for softening hard skin.[67]

Traditional Medicine:
Cidaris fossils are common medicinal substances which have been sold in Middle Eastern and Asian markets including Iran, Iraq, Persia and Northern India. Most of the fossils are imported until the present day from Lebanon. Their traditional uses includes the external treatment of wounds and they are prescribed internally to cure swellings and diarrhea. Babylonian Jews as well as the Arabs in Israel have used the fossils to clear obstructions in the renal tracts.[68]

64 al-Biruni, p. 121.

65 Ibn al-Baytar, al-Jami, II, p. 5; Leclerc, No. 601.

66 Maimonides, Poisons, p. 101; Maimonides, Aphorisms, 21:65.

67 al-Antaki, p. 118; Cf. Ibn al-Baytar, al-Jami, II, p. 5; Leclerc, No. 601.

68 Hooper, p. 195; Ben Yakov, p. 324; Ali & Mahdihassan, Animal, pp. 70-72, Lev & Amar.

Conclusions:
The petrified sea-urchin is a unique example of the use of fossils for medicine. The fossils, which had been considered until the present day as a mineral, retained its ancient historical uses throughout the ages. Their main use was in clearing stones from the kidney, bladder and renal tracts.

The origin of the fossils has always been the Lebanese mountains due to the ancient rock formations exposed there. However, these stones have been called 'ioudaikos lithos,' 'hajar al-yahud' or 'zaiton bani Isra'il' which hint at the connection to the ancient Jewish regions of Judea, and this link is strengthened by the description of Daud al-Antaki of the fossil formations in the Jerusalem mountains. The term 'Jerusalem' is probably used here, as in many other cases, in order to magnify its medicinal value, because these fossils cannot be found in this region. Cidaris fossils can be found in the Jurassic layers at the foothills of Mount Hermon, in the mountains of Lebanon and in the Negev.

Kohl

Arabic: Kuhl, Ithmid[69]

Kohl is a fine powder associated with the darkening of eyelids, and it was also used for remedial purposes. There were at least two main substances which were termed 'kohl' and 'ithmid': galena and antimony.

Galena

Scientific name: *Plumbum sulphidum* (PbS)
Hebrew and Arabic: Galena

69 Maimonides, Glossaire, No. 27.

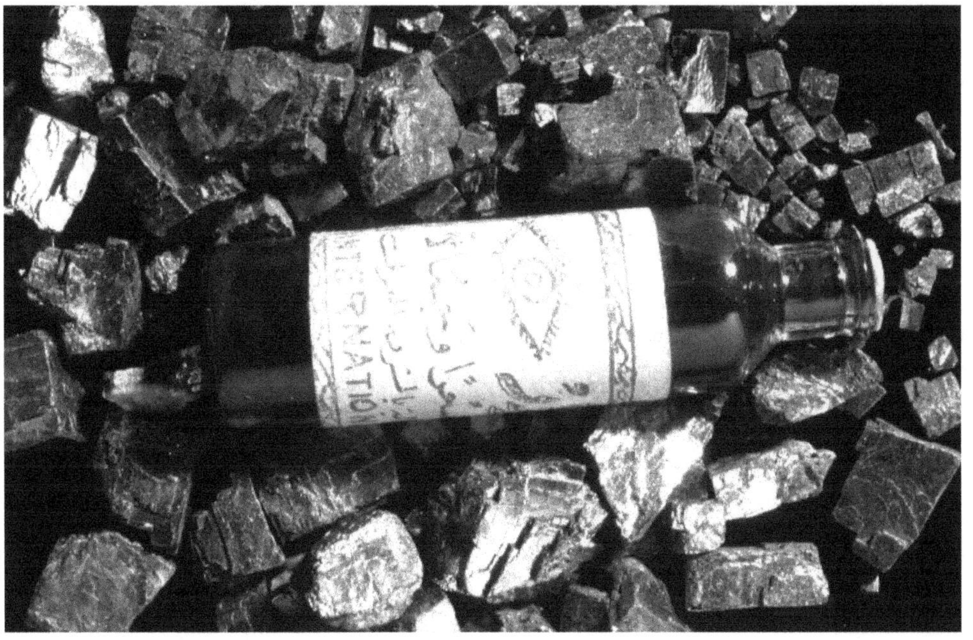

Figure 5 - Kohl

Description:
Galena is a mineral, which is a composite of sulphate and lead containing up to 86.5% of lead. It is the most important source of lead in the world, and sometimes it is even a source of silver (up to 2%). In nature it appears as grey cubic crystals which have a shiny metal colour. In Israel there are ancient galena mines in Mount Hermon.[70]

Antimony

Scientific name: *Stibium (Sb)*
Hebrew and Arabic: Antimon

Description:
Antimony is a metallic substance of crystalline texture. From the days of ancient Egypt (3000 BCE) until the present, its black colour has made it suitable for painting and darkening the eyelids. For cosmetic and medicinal purposes, natural antimony sulphide (Sb2S3) made of stibnite powder has been commonly used. The historical origins of stibnite was Iran and Arabia, and it was sometimes referred to as 'mestem' (Disocorides and Pliny called this substance stibium).[71]

History:
'Pukh' or eye-shadow, was mentioned in the Bible in connection with Queen Jezebel in the Book of Kings (II, 9:30) and is also referred to in Jeremiah (4:40). A similar mention is made in Ezekiel (23:40) which was translated in the Vulgate as stibium.[72]

The Jewish Sages refer to kohl as ' kahla' or 'pukh' and often mention its cosmetic and medicinal uses.[73] According to Dioscorides, the *stimmi* (antimony) was a drying drug, which was used to stop bleedings, clean wounds and heal eye diseases. *Molubdaina* (galena) had similar uses.[74]

Medicinal Uses in Jerusalem:
In a letter found in the Genizah (dated 1040 CE), Abraham Ben Shmu'el from Ramla asked Shlomo Ben Yehuda from Jerusalem for "some kuhl to clear the white colour from my little daughter's eye."[75] In another letter (dated 1064) from Abun Ben Tsedaka (Jerusalem) to Naharai Ben Nissim (Fustat), the kohl trade in Jerusalem is described.[76]

Medicinal Uses in the Medieval Period:
According to Maimonides, antimony was a cold and dry substance [77] and was used only externally. al-Biruni reported on the use of 'ithmid' (antimon) as a cure for eye diseases and mentions it toxicity.[78] al-Qazwini asserted in his entry 'Antimon' that it is the 'ithmid' which was described by Aristotle as a "substance well known throughout the East." al-Qazwini added that 'antimon' is as beneficial to the eye as 'kuhl' in removing defective tissues, strengthening the eye nerves and treating inflammations and pains, mainly among the elderly.[79] In late medieval Europe, antimony was used to induce vomiting, but since it was a strong drug and had toxic effects, this use slowly declined.[80]

Traditional Medicine:
Yemenite Jews have been using 'ithmid' or 'kuhl' externally to treat the wounds of the body and eyes, stop nose bleeds

70 HE, XXVII, pp. 761-762.

71 Ibid., III, pp. 472-473. For further information about this substance and its uses in Europe during the Middle Ages see Ibid., pp. 473-476; EI, p. 536.

72 HE, III, p. 472; EI, p. 536.

73 On the history of antimony and its uses see: Gordon, Medieval, p. 664.

74 Dioscorides, V. 99-100.

75 Gil, I, p. 421, No. 230.

76 Ibid., II, p. 234, No. 500.

77 Maimonides, Aphorisms, 21:87.

78 al-Biruni, II, p. 70.

79 al-Qazwini, p. 186; Ibn al-Baytar, al-Jami, I, pp. 12-13; Leclerc, No. 18. Cf. Ibn al-Baytar, al-Jami, IV, p. 53; Leclerc, No. 1898; al-Antaki, pp. 37-38.

80 HE, III, pp. 475-476.

and cure eye inflammations. As an internal use, 'kuhl' has been a component in remedies to strengthen the heart and treat tuberculosis.[81] Babylonian Jews have used 'kuhl' to treat different eye diseases.[82]

In many Middle Eastern countries 'kuhl' is used as eye shadow and as a cure for eye diseases.[83]

Modern Medicine:
Antimony has been used in modern medicine as a chemotherapy drug for the treatment of tropical diseases caused by worms and parasites, such as bilharzia.[84]

Sulphur

Scientific name: *Sulfur* (S)
Hebrew: Gofrit Arabic: Kabrit

Description:
Sulphur is a mineral with the atomic weight of 16. During the course of geological history sulphur deposits have accumulated in the regions of hot and shallow lakes and were discovered in several areas of this region mainly in the Jordan Valley and in the Negev.[85]

History:
Sulphur was well-known in most ancient cultures. In ancient Egypt it was used in the preparation of colours and in cosmetic materials.[86] In ancient Babylon its smoke was used as a disinfectant and it also served in the treatment of diseases and scratches.[87]

It is mentioned in the Bible as an incendiary substance in the destruction of Sodom and Gomorrah (Gen.19:24) and is also referred to in the account of the Torah giving on Mount Sinai (Deut. 29:24). The Greeks and Romans were familiar with the techniques of sulphur burning and the use of its smoke as a disinfectant. Dioscorides describes the use of *theion* to treat asthma, leprosy, scorpion stings, skin diseases and problems in hearing and staunching the flow of blood (hemorrhages)[88] while Pliny describes the medicinal use of sulphur in treating various skin diseases. Roman and Byzantine armies also made use of sulphur as a combustible substance and it was later used in the production of gunpowder.[89]

Sulphur in the Levant:
al-Tamimi writes about sulphur which was produced in the Dead Sea area and describes its trade and uses. He especially mentions "white sulphur" which he says: "originates from the shores of the Dead Sea which lies between Tsoar and Jericho in the land of Palestine and is in the vicinity of Jerusalem."[90] The geographer, al-Muqaddasi reports that sulphur was produced in the Jordan Valley.[91] The trade in sulphur is mentioned in an 11th century court document from Tsoar which was discovered in the Cairo Genizah.[92] Hayim Vital notes that "crushed white sulphur" was a component in a medication for treating asthma.[93]

Medicinal Uses in the Medieval Period:
al-Kindi describes the use of yellow sulphur which was a component in medications for skin diseases and mental illnesses.[94] Maimonides reports that sulphur "which is non-combustible" was used as an external medication for 'crushed' bodily injuries and for washing and drying the body. It was also used to treat bites, scorpion stings, and snake's bites, and its smoke was used to repel poisonous creatures.[95] al-Qazwini describes the formation of sulphur and quotes Aristotle who names three colour-types of sulphur: red, white and yellow. He also describes its medicinal uses: to treat paralysis, migraine, wounds, inflammations, leprosy, skin diseases, joint inflammation, colds, bites, to dispel lice and snakes, to whiten the hair and for swellings.[96]

Traditional Medicine:
Among the Jews of Iraq the 'kabrid' (sulphur) was a component in remedies for skin diseases and for bee stings, and yellow sulphur was used for treating scorpion stings, skin dryness and hair growth for baldness. The use of black sulphur smoke is also mentioned for dispelling crawling insects entering the ear and to treat chillblains.[97]

In Iran and Iraq, sulphur was used as a component in ointments to treat skin diseases and syphilis. In Egypt it was used to treat stomach ulcers, skin diseases and herpes.[98]

Modern Medicine:
Chemical derivatives of sulphur were used as an emetic, as a component in shaving creams, in ointments for skin diseases and for warts. Since early times, the sulphur in hot springs had also served as medical treatment especially for rheumatism. The substance was also tried successfully against leprosy.[99]

---

81 Reiani, No. 175.

82 Ben-Yakov, pp. 162-163, 170, 173.

83 Hooper, p. 189; Lev & Amar.

84 HE, III, p. 476.

85 HE, XI, p. 151; Challenger.

86 HE, V, p. 149.

87 al-Kindi, p. 322, No. 252.

88 Dioscorides, V.124.

89 HE, XI, pp. 149-150.

90 al-Tamimi, p. 20a. For greater detail see: Amar & Seri, p. 31.

91 al-Muqaddasi, p. 184.

92 Goitein, Jewry, p. 200.

93 Benajahu, p. 97.

94 al-Kindi, Nos. 20, 47, 205.

95 Maimonides, Aphorisms, 15:33; 19:6; Maimonides, Poisons, pp. 101, 118, 128, 135. In connection with its medicinal qualities see: Maimonides, Aphorisms, 21:89.

96 al-Qazwini, pp. 213-214. Cf. Ibn al-Baytar, al Jami, III, pp. 49-50; Leclerc, No. 1880; al-Antaki, pp. 266-267.

97 Ben-Yakov, pp. 77, 96-97, 109, 259, 285, 342, 364.

98 Hooper, p. 193; Ducros, p. 196.

99 HE, XI, p. 155; Cawston.

Conclusions:
Sulphur is a mineral, which is widely found in this region, especially in the Jordan Valley and around the Dead Sea, and it is easily gathered and processed. The use of sulphur was commonly accepted since early times and was mainly used for treating skin diseases, wounds, and toxic poisonings. Its uses in modern times is described in many and varied sources.

Zinc

Scientific Name: ***Zincum-oxidat***
Hebrew: Avatz Arabic: Tutya[100]

Description:
Zinc is found in nature as a hard, bluish-white metallic element (Zn, No.30). It appears in nature as calamite ($ZnCO3$) and sulphide (ZnS) from which it is manufactured by industrial processes such as smelting and refining.[101] Modern scholars agree that the medieval 'tutya' in its narrow sense means zinc at different stages of oxidation. Though the term includes other oxodized metals,[102] we agree with this statement.

History:
Zinc has been medicinally used since early times in various ancient civilizations including the Babylonian[103] and the Roman. The Greek physician Dioscorides described the medicinal uses of *diphruges* as a cure for skin diseases, wounds and tumors. Those uses were due to its drying and cooling qualities.[104]

Medicinal Uses in Jerusalem:
The Frankish physician, Benevenutus, described a Jerusalemite remedy for the treatment of the eyes. Among the different substances, he mentioned white wine and 'tutya' and in a different remedy he reported about "Alexandrine tutya", rose leaves and white wine as a cure for other eye diseases.[105] We have no doubt that the 'tutya' was in extensive used in Jerusalem as it was in the Levant according to our historical sources. 'Tuzia' and 'tutya' were mentioned by David de Silva as an external medicinal substance for the treatment of eye diseases.[106]

Zinc in the Levant:
The Jerusalem Muslim physician, al-Tamimi (10th cent.) reported that the 'tutya' was collected on sea shores near Tyre, Beirut and other cities along the coast of Lebanon. He stated that this kind of 'tutya' was inferior to the 'mahmudi' kind brought from the Maghreb (North Africa).[107] A most significant testimony of 'tutya' as a cure for the eye was found in the Genizah letter dated 1060 CE. The writer, Yosef Ben-Yeshua of Tripoli mentions zinc as an eye treatment.[108]

Rabbi Hayim Vital of Safed (16th-17th cent.) informs us of an internal use of 'tutya hindaba' for curing hemorrhoids. He added a warning against high dosage, which have a harmful effect on the patient. A powder of 'tutya zinc' was one of the substances in his remedy for syphilis.[109]

Medicinal Uses in the Medieval Period:
al-Kindi, a Muslim physician, (10th cent.) wrote that zinc is used in many remedies for the treatment of eye diseases, mainly to reduce humidity, to clear cataracts and improve the eyesight.[110] Both Maimonides and al-Biruni were of the opinion that zinc should be used to cure external cancerous sores.[111] The 13th century scholar, al-Qazwini, reported about different kinds of zinc (white, yellow and green) and emphasized that their origin was the Indian Ocean and its shores (Yemen for example). One of the practical medicinal uses of zinc was to eliminate bad smells (sweat and urine).[112]

Traditional Medicine:
Yemenite Jews have been using zinc sulphate ($ZnSO4$), which they name "tutya" to treat eye diseases, cancerous wounds, and wounds of the sexual organs.[113] Babylonian Jews have used zinc for external uses such as the treatment of cutaneous leishmaniasis, eye diseases and swollen lips.[114]

Summary and Conclusions

Analysis of the minerals and metals described above shows that the list can be subdivided as follows:

Metals – Zinc is the only metal produced by a process of mining, manufacture and refining.

Minerals – Asphalt is a natural substance without metallic components and mummy (rissasphalt) is a side product of asphalt.

Metallic Salts – These are compounds of substances found in nature or produced by a relatively simple process. Among them are: kohl (galena or lead sulphate) and alum (potassium sulphate).

Stones – The fossilized spine of the sea-urchin (Jews' stone) was once considered a mineral.

---

100 Maimonides, Glossaire, No. 382.

101 HE, I, p. 24.

102 al-Kindi, p. 250, No. 55. Regarding the names of substances during medieval times, see: Maimonides, Glossaire, Nos. 342, 382.

103 al-Kindi, p. 250, No. 55.

104 Dioscorides, V.120.

105 Benevenutus, pp. 19, 42. Regarding the problematics of the source see Introduction.

106 Amar, de Silva, p. 142.

107 al-Tamimi, p. 102, a-b.

108 Gil, p. 216, no. 426b.

109 Benajahu, p. 102, 111.

110 al-Kindi, Nos. 151, 157-159, 163, 165, 168, 174, 178. Cf. Ibn al-Baytar, al-Jami, I. pp. 143-145; Leclerc, No. 437. Cf. also al-Antaki, pp. 98-99; al-Biruni, II, pp. 22-23.

111 Maimonides, Aphorisms, 9:30, 111; 16:55; al-Biruni I, pp, 95-96.

112 al-Qazwini, p. 188.

113 Reiani, No. 176.

114 Ben-Yakov, pp. 87, 178, 280.

From the geographical aspect it appears that half of the minerals were mined and manufactured in the region, such as asphalt, earth, lead sulphate, Jews' stone. sulphur, salt and thermal water. Geologically speaking, these substances are connected with the Red Sea rift – asphalt is found in the Dead Sea, lead sulphate on Mount Hermon, and according to the sources, Jews' stone is to be found in the Judean hills and in the Jurassic rocks which abound in Southern Lebanon and the Galilee. Substances such as zinc and alum (potassium sulphate) were imported from neighboring countries where they were mined or manufactured. The Land of Israel was the main source in the region for asphalt and Jews' stone which were exported from there in the past as well as in the present to the entire eastern region.

Chapter IV
Plant Origins of Medicinal Substances

Introduction

Plants have been used as medicinal substance since prehistoric times.[1] When man discovered the nutritious quality of food plants he also found that other plants and sometimes the food plants themselves had medicinal value. However, very little residual evidence has been found of medicinal plants in archaeological excavations throughout the world.[2] Various sources describe the use of natural substances for healing in ancient civilisations. From these we learn that plants were the main source for the production of remedies. A large amount of information on ancient Chinese medicine (beginning with the third millennium BCE) has been compiled into a book in Chinese called *Tsao Pen* which contains thousands of medical prescriptions[3] most of them being of plant origin and based on well-known plants such as canabis (hashish) and rhubarb.

The Ebers Papyrus contains 877 medicines and prescriptions, mostly of plant origin such as: aloe, barley (beer), castor (oil), cedar, centaury, cumin, elder, fennel, fig, flax, frankincense, garlic, grapevine (wine and vinegar), henbane, juniper, lentisk, mandrake, myrrh, olive (oil), onion, poppy seed, saffron, tarragon and yeast.[4] Actually, the greater majority of medicinal substances mentioned in other sources from early times were from the plant world.[5]

The researcher, Moldenke, notes that 133 out of 244 kinds of plants mentioned in the Bible were agricultural crops which were cultivated for economic purposes: for industrial uses in general and for cosmetic and medicinal production in particular.[6] Other scholars have identified 25-30 of them which served as remedies.[7] Among the more important plants are: colocynth, marjoram, balsam, onion, mandrake, cumin, tarragon, prickly saltwort, black cumin, mother die and fig.[8]

The medical sources of Mesopotamia also refer to medicinal plants such as: cassia, date, dogwood, fig, giant fennel, myrtle, pear, prickly saltwort and willow, which are mentioned in medical documents in Nippur (21st cent. BCE).[9] The Code of Hammurabi, King of Babylon (18th cent. BCE) contains descriptions concerning the use of medicinal plants such as cassia, henbane, liquorice and mint.[10] Hippocrates the Greek mentions 400 medicinal substances, most of them (90%) being plants,[11] and according to legend, Theophrastus, Aristotle's pupil, inherited Aristotle's plant garden which contained many varieties of plants from all over the world. Theophrastus who dedicated his life to plant research, wrote many books in which he prominently described medicinal plants. The most important of his works was the *The History of Plants*[12] in which 500 medications are listed.[13]

During his travels, Dioscorides, who was a physician in Nero Caesar's army, collected many specimens of plants and examined their medicianl virtues. His famous work, *De Materia Medica* [14] describes more than 600 kinds of plants among which are: acacia, aconite, almond, aloe, balsam, buckthorn, cumin, dill, grapevine (vinegar and wine), liquorice, mandrake, mint, mother die, olive (oil), poppy seed, rose (oil) and tarragon.

Pliny the Elder, a contemporary of Dioscorides, was the author of *Historia Naturalis*[15] which contained eight volumes dealing

1 Palevitz, p. 264

2 Yaniv, p. 20

3 On Chinese medicine in detail, see:Gordon, Medicine, pp. 355-390. On pharmacology, see: Kermers & Urdang, pp. 3-5.

4 Bryan. The identification of the various substances was made by the editor and translator of the book. On healing through ancient Egyptian medicines, see: Nunn, pp. 136-162; Estes; Stetter, p. 107-122.

5 Low ; Feldman; Feliks, World; Moldenke.

6 Moldenke, p. 152. Amar identified 120 kinds of plants, some of which can be defined as medicinal plants. See: Amar, Substances, p. 51.

7 Harrison; Duke; Preuss; Zayyda; Muntner; Ulman; Shoshan; Palmer; Rosner. On pharmacology in this period, see: Hamarneh, Origins, pp. 17-21.

8 Yaniv, p. 21; Jacob; Ulman, 26, p. 194.

9 In detail: Kramer.

10 Yaniv, p. 20.

11 Riddle, Tradition, pp. 47-61.

12 Theophrastus.

13 Kremers & Urdang, pp. 14-27.

14 Dioscorides. On the Land of Israel aspects see also: Zilberstein.

15 Plinius.

with medicinal plants. It is interesting to note that the original source of some of these substances indicated by physicians of the classical world is the Levant, and include: balsam from Judea, elephant's ear and tamarisk grown in abundance in Syria, onion and henna from Ashkelon, giant fennel from Syria and storax ointment produced in this region.[16]

The research scholar I. Low lists 400 kinds of plants mentioned in the Talmud,[17] 70 of which are defined as medicinal plants. Among the medicinal plants mentioned by the Jewish Sages are: asparagus, black cumin, cabbage, cumin, dodder, garlic, grapevine (wine and vinegar), lavender, leek, marrow (squash), olive (oil), onion, pepper, pine gum (resin), radish, rose (oil) and watercress.

The medical tradition formulated during the early Islamic period indicates the use of plants such as: black cumin, cedar, citron, date (both fruit and kernel), eggplant, fig, garlic, henna, onion, rice and watermelon.[18]

Plants used in Jerusalem Medicine

A hundred and seventy-four plants were traced and identified as medicinal plants, which were used in Jerusalem from early times to the 18th century. These are 80.2% ,of the total number of medicinal substances found in the historical sources. The plants, their common names and the historical sources that mentioned them in connection with Jerusalem, are presented in Table 3. The data for fifty seven of these plants are described in the entries following this Table.

Agaric

Scientific name: *Agaricus sp.* (Agaricaceae)
Hebrew: Paku'a Arabic: 'Arikon, Gharikon

Description:
Mushroom belonging to the basic fungi species with cap and stem (sometimes double-stemmed). The sides of its overlapping cap are free and unattached to the stem. Its spores are smooth and brown in colour. In Israel there are 18 types, mostly edible. The main types of Agaric grown in Israel are:

A. Common Agaric (*Agaricus campester*) - widespread, edible and commercially cultivated type.
B. Field Agaric (*Agaricus arvensis*) - commonly found, large and edible.
C. Cultivated Agaric (*Agaric bisporus*) - agriculturally grown.[19]

Identification:
''Arikon' was once a general term for all mushrooms originating from Agarica - the name of a region in Southern Russia. Today it is especially identified with the type Agaricus albus from which the acid 'agarisin,' which acts upon the flow of faeces and sweat,[20] is produced. It seems reasonable to accept this definition.

History:
Dioscorides thought that the *agaricon* was a plant used for the treatment of the liver and spleen, to cure asthma, dysentery and epilepsy, and to counteract the effect of poisons.[21]

Medicinal Uses in Jerusalem:
According to Refael Malki the 'agarico' was a component in a general medicine in Jerusalem. In another place there is mention of a "white and spongy male agaricon" which was a component in a general medicine for poor people to treat colds and headaches.[22] 'Agaricon' was also mentioned by David de Silva as substance for the treatment of internal diseases, poisons, leprosy, aches and sciatica.[23]

Agaric in the Levant:
Hayim Vital says that the 'garicon' was an important component in a medicine for treating and curing asthma. It is stated there that the agaric was a component in a pill to cure sciatica.[24] Another description of the use of edible mushrooms in al-Sham is given by Ibn Wahshiya in the entry 'Atlab.'[25]

Medicinal Uses in the Medieval Period:
al-Kindi used the ''arikon' in a medication for treating malaria, for problems of the intestines and liver and for jaundice, and he also used it to prepare a special liquid for transfusions.[26] According to Maimonides, the 'agarico' was reliable for its cleansing qualities and was mostly used as a drug which was dependable for its results in treatment. It was also a cleansing substance for phlegm and a component in the "big" theriac. Agaric is listed among the hot and dry drugs.[27] Ibn al-Baytar states that the 'arikon' was good for the nerves and was used as a diuretic. He also quotes Ibn Sina who recommends it for treating epilepsy and malaria.[28] Saladino d'Ascoli defined agaric as a useful medicine. He says that the plant grew near trees, and that it was a medicine for all kinds of internal obstructions.[29]

Traditional Medicine and General Uses:
Various types of agaric are edible and are generally called 'champignons' (mushrooms). Their agricultural cultivation

16 Regarding this see also: Amar, Substances, pp. 54-55.

17 Low, Perelman, I, pp. 50-98.

18 Ibn al-Qayyim.

19 Description in :Plants & Animals, IX, p. 141; XII, p. 84; Zohary, p. 115.

20 Identification, comments and addenda by Muntner in Maimonides, Regimen, p. 88. Cf. Low I, p. 43.

21 Dioscorides, III.1.

22 Malki, pp. 65, 67.

23 Amar, de Silva, p. 112.

24 Benajahu, pp. 97, 104.

25 Ibn Wahshiya, I, p. 101.

26 al-Kindi, Nos. 113, 211, 214. Cf. al-Biruni, I, p. 244.

27 Maimonides, Regimen, 2:11; Maimonides, Aphorisms, 13:13; 21:33, 69; Maimonides, Poisons, p. 112.

28 Ibn al-Baytar, al Jami, III, pp. 146-148; Leclerc, No. 1622. Cf. al-Antaki, p. 243.

29 Saladino, p. 85.

Table 3 - List of the Medicinal Plants used in Jerusalem during the 10th-18th century

Scientific Name	Common Name	Selective References
Acacia arabica	Gum Arabic	RM
Achillea sp.	Yarrow	IB, AN, TA
Acorus calamus	Sweet Sedge	DS
Agaricus sp.	Agaric	RM, DS
Ajuga sp.	Bugle	TA
Alcea sp.	Hollyhock	DS
Allium cepa	Onion	DS
Allium porrum	Leek	DS
Allium sativum	Garlic	TA, DS
Allium sp.	Garlic	TA
Aloe sp.	Aloe	GN, BN, RM, DS
Amygdalus communis = Prunus amygdalus	Almond	GN, DS, RM
Anastatica hierochuntica	Rose of Jericho	IB
Anchusa sp.	Borage	RM
Anethum graveolens	Dill	DS
Apium graveolens	Celery	RM, DS
Aquilaria agallocha	Indian Aloe-tree	DS
Arbutus andrachne	Eastern Strawberry Tree	IB
Artemisia absinthium	Absinet	DS
Artemisia sp.	Wormwood	DS
Asparagus officinalis	Asparagus	DS
Asphodelus aestivus (ramosus)	Tall Asphodel	NA, IB
Astragalus gummifer	Tragacanth	RM
Astragalus sarcocolla	Sarcocolla	GN
Balanites aegyptiaca	Jericho Balsam	IB, TA
Boswellia carteri	Frankincense	BN, DS
Brassica campestris	Bird Rape	DS
Brassica oleracea	Cabbage	DS
Calicotome villosa	Spiny Broom	IB, TA
Caltiris quadrivalvis	Flixweed	DS
Carthamus tinctorius	Safflower	LU
Castanea sativa	Chestnut	DS
Cassia fistula	Purging Cassia	GN
Cassia (Senna) sp.	Cassia	RM, HR
Cicer arietinum	Chickpea	DS
Celtic australis	European Nettle Tree	MD
Chiliadenus iphionoides	Varthemia	IB
Cichorium intybus	Chicory	RM, DS
Cinchona sp.	Quinin	EH, DS
Cinnamomum camphora	Camphor	DS
Cinnamomum zeylanicum	Cinnamon	GN, RM, DS
Citrullus colocynthis	Colocynth	RM
Citrullus vulgaris	Watermelon	DS
Citrus aurantium	Siville Orange (Sour Orange)	RM
Citrus limon	Lemon	DS
Citrus medica	Sweet Lime	DS
Cocos nucifera	Coconut Palm	BN
Coffea arabica	Coffee	DS
Coix lachryma-jobi	Job's Tears	IB
Commiphora myrrha	Myrrh	RM
Commiphora opobalsamum	Balsam	FH
Convolvulus scammonia	Scammony	RM
Cordia myxa	Sebesten	GN
Coridothymus capitatus	Headed Thyme	IB, RM
Coronopus squamatus	Watercress	TA, IB, AN
Corylus avellana	Hazel Nut	DS
Crocus sativus	Saffron	BN, DS, RM
Cucumis melo	Common Melon	DS
Cucumis melo var.chate	Chate Melon	DS
Cucumis sativum	Cucumber	DS

Scientific Name	Common Name	Selective References
Cuminum cyminum	Cumin	DS
Curcuma longa	Turmeric	RM
Cuscuta epithymum	Dodder of Thyme	IB, TA
Cydonia oblonga	Quince	DS
Daemomorops draco	Dragon's Blood	DS
Daucus carota	Carrot	IB, TA
Eruca sativa	Garden Rocket	HR
Eryngium sp.	Sea Holly	NA, IB
Eugenia caryophyllata	Clove	GN, BN, RM, DS
Ferula sp.	Sagafino	DS
Ferula assa-foetida	Asafetida	DS
Ficus carica	Fig Tree	DS
Gentiana lutea	Yellow Gentian	DS
Glycyrrhiza glabra	Common Liquorice	LU
Guaiacum sanctum	Guaiacum	DS
Hedra helix	Common Ivy	DS
Helleborus niger	Christmas Rose	DS
Hordeum vulgare	Barley	DS
Hyssopus officinalis	Hyssop	AS, IB, IR, AN
Ipomoea turpethum	Turpeth	BN, RM
Jasminum sp.	Jasmine	TA
Juglans regia	Walnut	MU, LU, DS
Juniperus sp.	Juniper	DS
Juniperus sabina	Savine	DS
Kickxia sp.	Toadflax	IB, TA
Lactuca sativa	Lettuce	DS
Lagenaria vulgaris	Bottle-gourd	DS
Larix sp.	Larch	DS
Laurus nobilis	Laurel	DS
Lawsonia inermis {alba}	Henna	GN
Lens culinaris	Lentil	DS
Lepidium sativum	Garden Cress	TA, IB
Lilium candidum	Madonna Lily	RM
Linum usitatissimum	Flax	DS
Lupinus termis	Lupins	DS
Lycoperdon lividium	Deer Balls	AN, IB
Majorana hortensis	Sweet Marjoram	GN, RM, DS
Mandragora autumnalis	Autumn Mandrake	DS
Matricaria recutita (chamamilla)	Chamomile	DS
Melilotus albus	Sweet Clover	MA, IB
Mentha sp.	Mint	DS
Mentha pulegium	Water Mint	DS
Moringa peregrina	Ben Tree	TA
Morus sp.	Mulberry	DS
Myristica fragrans	Nutmeg	BN, RM, DS
Myrtus communis	Myrtle	DS
Nardostachys grandiflora (jatamansi)	Spikenard	DS
Nicotiana tabacum	Tobacco	DS
Nuphar lutea	Yellow Pond Lily	HR
Nymphaea alba	White Water Lily	HR
Ocimum basilicum	Basil	RM, DS
Olea europaea	Olive Tree	DS
Origanum syriacum	Wild Marjoram	GN, RM, DS
Oryza sativa	Rice	DS
Paeonia sp.	Coral Peony	DS
Papaver somniferum	Opium, Poppy Head	DS
Parietaria judaica	Wall Pellitory	DS
Petroselinum sativum	Parsley	DS
Phoenix dactylifera	Date	DS
Pimpinella anisum	Anise	GN, RM, DS
Pimpinella cretica	Cretan Anise	DS

Scientific Name	Common Name	Selective References
Pinus sp.	Pine	GN, DS
Piper sp.	Pepper	DS
Pistacia lentiscus	Lentisk	RM, DS
Pistacia vera	Pistachio	DS
Plantago sp.	Flea Wart	DS
Populus sp.	Poplar	DS
Portulaca oleracea	Purslane	RM
Potentilla tormientilla	Tormentil	DS
Prunus (Cerasus) sp.	Cherry	HR
Prunus domestica	Plum	RM, DS
Prunus persica	Peach	DS
Punica granatum	Pomegranate	DS
Pyrus communis	Pear	GN, DS
Pyrus malus = Malus sylvestris	Apple	DS
Quercus sp.	Oak	DS
Quercus sp.	Oak Gall	DS
Raphanus sativus	Radish	DS
Reseda alba	Mignonette	NA, IB
Rheum sp.	Rhubarb	RM
Rhus coriaria	Tanning Sumach	KH, LU, DS
Rosa canina	Dog Rose	BN, RM, TA, DS
Rosmarinus officinalis	Rosemary	DS
Rubia tinctorum	Common Madder	DS
Rumex acetosa	Garden Sorrel	DS
Ruta sp.	Rue	DS
Saccharum officinarum	Sugar Cane	DE, GN, RM, DS
Salix sp.	Willow	DS
Salvia sp.	Sage	DS
Sambucus ebulus	Dwarf Elder	DS
Sambucus nigra	Elder	DS
Santalum album	Sandalwood	DS
Sarcopoterium spinosum	Prickly Burnet	NA, BA, IB
Sassafras officinale	Sassafras	DS
Satureja thymbra	Savory of Crete	IB, RM
Seasamum indicum	Oriental Sesame	DS
Sinapis alba	Mustard	DS
Sisymbrium sp.	Hedge Mustard	IB, TA
Solanum melongena	Eggplant	DS
Solanum inacum	Dead Sea Apple	IB, AN
Spinacia oleracea	Spinach	DS
Styrax officinalis	Officinal Storax	IB
Tamarindus indica	Tamarinds	DS
Tamarix sp.	Tamarisk	DS
Terminalia sp.	Myrobalan	GN
Thea sp.	Tea	DS
Theobroma cacao	Cocoa	DS
Triticum sp.	Wheat, Flour, Braed	LU, DS
Valeriana celtica	Celtic Spikenard	DS
Vicia faba	Garden Bean	DS
Viola odorata	Sweet Violet	RM, DS
Vitis vinifera	Grape Vine	All sources
Zingiber officinale	Ginger	RM, DS
Ziziphus spina-christi	Christ Thorn Jujube	LU, EH

Sources

AN – Daud al-Antaki
AS – Ibn al-Khair al-Ashbili
BA – Baghdadi
BN – Benevenutus
DE – Delaville
DS – David de Silva
EH – Elazer Horn
FH – Frederick Hasselquist
GN – Genizah
HR – Haram Documents
IB – Ibn al-Baytar
IR – Ibn Rushd
KH – Khusraw, Nasir
LU – Lutfi
MA – Maimonides
MD – Mujir al-Din
MU – al-Muqadassi
NA – al-Nabati, Abu al-'Abas
RM – Refael Malki
TA – al-Tamimi

began in Europe in the 17th century. In Israel today the cultivated kind is grown.[30] Dried mushrooms are used in Iran for the internal treatment of worms. In India, the mushroom is used as a congealing agent to staunch blood, and in Egypt the plant was used in the past to suction blood and in bandaging wounds.[31]

Almond

Scientific name:
***Amygdalus communis = Prunus amygdalus* (Rosaceae)**
Hebrew: Shaked Arabic: Luz[32]

Description:
The almond tree grows wild and relatively tall (up to 8 metres) with long, tapering leaves. Its white and pink blossoms appear in the spring before the leaves buds, and its nuts are large and sweet. Two main species are known: the sweet almond (*Amygdalus communis* var. *dulcis*) used for food and industry, and the bitter almond (*Amygdalus communis* var. *amara*) containing amygdalin.[33]

History:
The almond tree has grown in Israel since early times. It is mentioned in the Bible several times, for example: When the sons of Jacob took down "the choice fruits of the land" to Egypt (Gen. 43:11), or when Aaron's rod blossomed and produced almonds (Num.17:23) as a sign from God. It is also often mentioned in the Mishna and Talmud.[34] Dioscorides noted the *amugdale* and indicated its medicinal uses as an emmenagogue, to relieve headaches, cure intestinal wounds, cough, inflammation, sunburn, skin diseases, to soften the stomach and eliminate stones. The gum of the tree and the oil derived from the nuts are also used for these purposes.[35]

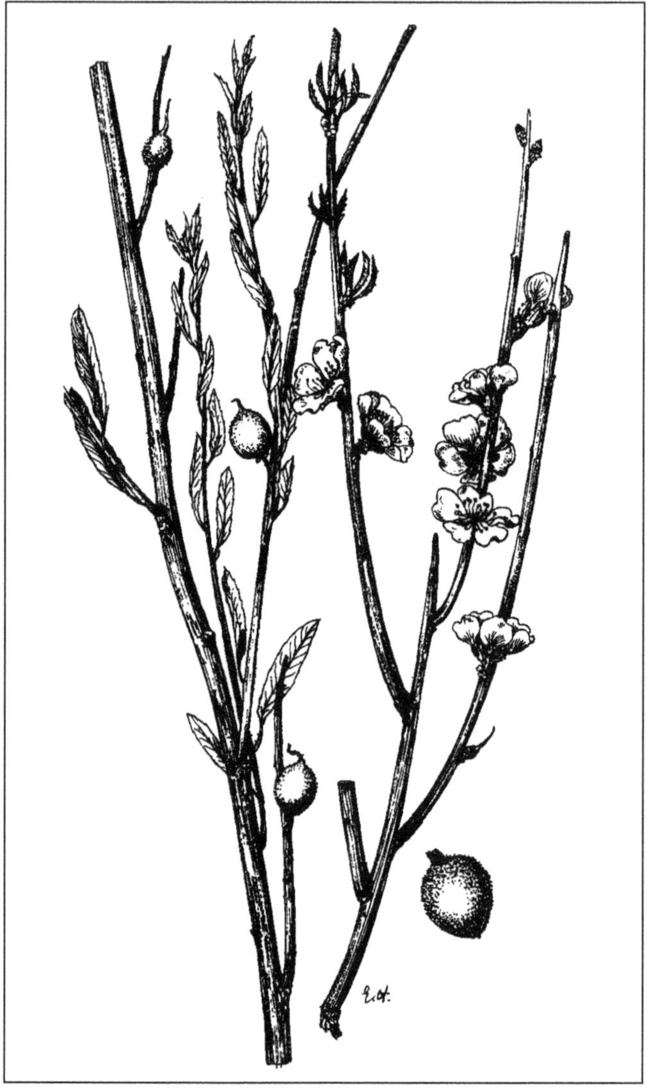

Figure 6 - Almond Tree (*Amygdalus communis*)

Medicinal Uses in Jerusalem:
In a letter dated 1065 from the Cairo Genizah sent by Abun Ben Zedaka of Jerusalem to Naharai Ben Nissim of Fustat, there is mention of 'zamgh luz' - merchandise bought for export.[36] In another letter, dated 1196 in Jerusalem, Abu Zakri, a physician of the Ayyubid Caliph, mentions the medication made of sugar and almonds, which was used as a remedy.[37] In his book, Refael Malki suggested abolishing the use of almonds, which was a widely used component of medicines for the city poor before his arrival in Jerusalem. Elsewhere he describes a medication concocted of almonds and sugar, which was called 'almindrada' or almond milk, and the method for its preparation. Malki claimed that this cathartic medication did more harm than cure. Almond oil, according to Malki, was used to preserve pills in glass jars.[38] Almond was mentioned by David de Silva as a nutritious food and the oil that was pressed out of the seeds was used to treat internal and external diseases and pains, mainly of the throat.[39]

Almonds in the Levant:
There is a considerable amount of evidence from medieval times that mention the agricultural cultivation of almonds in various parts of this region including Ashkelon, Transjordania, Jaffa, Safed, Acre, Jerusalem, Shechem and Baalbek.[40] In his book of religious law written in 1006 CE, Levi Ben Yefet, the Karaite, who was active in the Land of Israel, allowed the eating of "roasted almonds" on the Sabbath as a medication against diarrhea.[41] al-Dimashqi noted two kinds of almond: 'luz al-mar' (bitter almond) and 'luz al-hilwa' (sweet almond) in a list of 90 medicinal and useful plants that grow on Mount Lebanon and which can be profitably gathered as a means of livelihood.[42] Hayim Vital describes the use of the pounded

30 Uphof, pp. 16, 432; Hill, p. 292; Plants & Animals, XII, p. 84.

31 Hooper, p. 81; al-Kindi, p. 209; Ducros, pp. 156-157.

32 Dinsmore & Dalman, No. 658; Issa, Dictionary, p. 148, No. 15.

33 Plants & Animals, X, p. 137; XII, pp. 139-140; Hill, pp. 356-357.

34 Feliks, World, pp. 56-59; Goor, Fruits, pp. 288-290.

35 Dioscorides, I.176.

36 Gil, III, p. 245, No. 501.

37 Goitein, Jewry, p. 324.

38 Malki, pp. 45, 58, 66.

39 Amar, de Silva, p. 141.

40 Goor, Fruits, pp. 293-295.

41 Levi Ben Yefet, p. 47a.

42 al-Dimashqi, p. 200.

shells of the almond nut - 'lozim' - as a component in a medicine for clearing the renal tracts and to improve the appetite. Elsewhere he recommends using fresh "oil of sweet almonds" in the preparation of medicines for treating asthma.[43]

Medicinal Uses in the Medieval Period:
Assaph Harofe wrote that almond oil strengthens the heart, relieves stress, and heals the intestines. The oil of bitter almonds was beneficial in treating headaches, general pains, cough, breathing problems, lungs, kidney stones, liver ailments, renal obstructions, impotence and female menstruation.[44] Maimonides reported on the use of almonds in the context of the diet recommended to the Sultan. Elsewhere it is mentioned that almonds and almond oil were an emetic and a component in a medicine for purifying the blood and to fortify the spirit, as well as being a component in medicine called "the great atriphal" which strengthened the organs and delayed old age. Almonds were also used in bandaging bites by stray dogs.[45]

al-Biruni and Ibn al-Baytar in their 'Loz' entries described the almonds and listed similar medicinal uses.[46] Sweet almond oil - 'dahn al-luz al-hilwa' - is also mentioned as a cold and moist drug used as a remedy.[47] Elsewhere in the entry 'zamgh al-luz' (almond tree gum), Ibn al-Baytar claims that this was a medicinal substance which Dioscorides had used as a bitter, astringent drug. Its typical virtues were in pain relief, blood purification, curing of skin diseases, chronic cough, and dissolving kidney stones.[48]

Traditional Medicine and General Uses:
The almond nut is used as food and in the production of confectionary.[49] Arabs in Israel used almond juice to remove birthmarks.[50] Yemenite Jews used almonds externally to treat hemorrhages and internally to treat kidney stones, spleen, throat pains and cough.[51] Traditional medicine among the Jews of Iraq makes extensive use of the almond tree and its products to treat eye diseases, dysentery, earache, to relieve birth pangs and to increase mother's milk.[52] In Iran and Iraq, the species of bitter almonds is grown and the ointment made of the nuts is used to treat carbuncles.[53]

Even in Europe, traditional medicine uses the almond tree and its products.[54]

43 Benajahu, pp. 95-97, 111.

44 Assaph, 4, p. 399.

45 Maimonides, Answers, 4:20; Maimonides, Aphorisms, 13:44, 51; 20:77; 21:72; Maimonides, Regimen, 3:4, 9, 11; Maimonides, Poisons, p. 130. Cf. Ibn Sina, p. 354.

46 al-Biruni, I, p. 294; Ibn al-Baytar, al-Jami, IV, pp. 111-112; Leclerc, No. 2040. Cf. al-Antaki, p. 284.

47 Ibn al-Baytar, al-Jami, II, 111-112; Leclerc, No. 927.

48 Ibn al-Baytar, al-Jami, III, p. 86; Leclerc, No. 1412.

49 Plants & Animals, XII, p. 140; Uphof, p. 33.

50 Krispil, p. 1577.

51 Reiani, p. 43, No. 98.

52 References in: Ben-Yakov, p. 761. Cf. Krispil, p. 1577.

53 Hooper, p. 157.

54 Grieve, pp. 21-26.

Almond oil, for example, is used as a softening drug, for pain relief, and for calming the cough.[55]

Modern Medicine:
Bitter almonds contain a toxic substance - amygdalin - comprising 4% of the quantity. An additional constituent of bitter almonds, which is also toxic - blue acid - is present as 0.24%. It is known that eating 12 nuts can cause serious poisoning.[56]

Aloe

Scientific name: ***Aloe sp.*** **(Liliaceae)**
Hebrew: Aloy Arabic: Sabir, Sabra Mora, Asibar[57]

Description:
There are 250 species of aloe; most of them grow in tropical South Africa. Aloe is a perennial bush with large, succulent, rosette leaves (90-190 cm) with spiny edges and sharply pointed at the tips. The flowering stem is high and the colour of the flower is yellow. Domesticated plants grow near ancient villages and in gardens. Dry decoction of the succulent leaves of different species is the basis for the production of a black and shiny substance, its colour and quality depending upon the level of its refining.[58]

History:
The medicinal applications of the plant were known in ancient Babylon where it was used as a diuretic and a remedy for stomach disorders.[59] Dioscorides described the use of the *aloe* decoction which was brought from India to treat ailments of the intestine, blood, sputum, ulcer of the sex organ, headache and gum pains. In addition, Dioscorides describes the use aloe to treat wounds, as a purgative, anaesthetic, and the prevention of hair loss.[60] The Jewish Sages mention the 'alwin' which grows on the rooftops in the Land of Israel (Tosefta, *Shevi'it*, I, 12).[61]

Medicinal Uses in Jerusalem:
A letter found in the Genizah, dated 1045 CE, describes the purchase of relatively inexpensive aloe in Jerusalem and its transfer to Fustat.[62] Benevenutus claimed in his book that aloe was a component in a remedy called the "Jerusalemite pill" used for the treatment of cancer.[63] Rabbi Refael Malki wrote that aloe was a component in a general remedy used to treat headaches, gases and catarrh among the poorer members of the Jewish community of Jerusalem. Another pill, which also included aloe was used to treat headaches, gases, amnesia

55 Uphof, p. 33.

56 Chizik, p. 738; Palevitz, p. 269.

57 Maimonides, Glossaire, p. 90, No. 318; Malki, p. 66.

58 Zohary, p. 602; Plants & Animals, XII, p. 199.

59 al-Kindi, p. 297.

60 Disocorides, III.25.

61 On the history of aloe see: Haller, pp. 647-650.

62 Gil, No. 485.

63 Benevenutus, p. 33.

and tendon pains.[64] David de Silva mentioned the aloe, among other uses, as a vermifuge.[65]

Aloe in the Levant:
In a letter found in the Genizah, dated 1060 CE, which was sent by Yosef Ben Yeshu'a of Tripoli to Naharai Ben Nissim, 'tsabar asktry' is mentioned in connection with the trade of medicinal substances by the Jews of the Middle East.[66] Aloe is mentioned in a customs list of taxable materials traded in Acre under Crusader rule.[67]

Aloe was also exported from Egypt to Europe among other Eastern drugs and spices.[68] Evidence of the continuation of such exports in the 15th century is found in the accounting books of Italian trading businesses which describe the purchase of four packets of aloe as well as clove, scamonia, cotton and fabrics that were bought in Acre and shipped to Italy.[69] It seems that aloe was an important commodity in international medieval trade.[70] Hayim Vital reported the use of aloe - 'asibar' - as a treatment for hemorrhoids and sciatica. He also recommended the use of burnt aloe ash as part of the general treatment for mouth diseases.[71]

Medicinal Uses in the Medieval Period:
al-Kindi described the wide medicinal applications of aloe which was a component in toothpaste and in remedies for the treatment of eye diseases, insanity, epilepsy, excess sweat and abscesses.[72] Ibn Masawayh described different kinds of aloe, classified them according to their medicinal qualities and suggested the use of aloe to strengthen the stomach, nervous system and the liver.[73] Maimonides prescribed aloe from the island of Succotra as a component in a remedy for the treatment of hemorrhoids, stomach diseases, bleedings, wounds, and as a purgative.[74] Daud al-Antaki described aloe and some medicinal applications as "cleaning the brain", respiratory problems, chest pains, stomach disorders, skin disease, wounds, leprosy, and hemorrhoids.[75] It was also used as a carminative and to clear obstructions.

Traditional Medicine:
In Iran, *Aloe perryi* is used as a natural purgative[76] and *Aloe succotrina* is used in Egypt to clean wounds and to induce menstruation.[77] Yemenite Jews apply fresh aloe decoction to cure wounds in the mouth, eye, and nose, and for external bleeding. The dried fluid is used as a strong purgative, as a treatment for intestinal disorders, to prevent dizziness, to cure the swelling of sex and urinary organs and to cure rheumatism.[78] Similar applications are known among Babylonian Jewry,[79] the Arab minorities in Israel, and in European popular medicine.[80]

General Uses:
Aloe was considered a hot and dry drug[81] and it was recommended that it be preserved in a dry and protected place for up to ten years.[82] In Europe it was widely used as a component to add strength to ointments.[83] Modern research reveals that *Aloe sp.* contains several glycosides, mainly aloin.[84] It is used as a component in various cosmetic preparations[85] and medicinal drugs. Among its medicinal applications are: inducing menstruation, curing burns, expelling intestinal worms and as a purgative.[86]

Anise

Scientific name: *Pimpinella anisum* (Umbelliferae)
Hebrew: Kamnun ha-Anis **Arabic: Anison**[87]

Description:
Anise is an annual plant that originates from Asia Minor. It is tall (up to 80 cm.), hairy-stemmed and strong-scented, and has feathery leaves and white, umbrella-shaped blossoms with double-seeded fruits.[88]

History:
Anise is one of the most ancient seed-spices in the world, and aniseed has been found in the tombs of the Pharoahs. In early times it was cultivated in Egypt, Asia Minor and the Greek islands. During the Roman period its use became widespread and it was grown as an agricultural crop throughout the Empire, including the Mediterranean littoral, France and England. Today it is also grown in India, Africa, Spain and Italy.[89]

Dioscorides described the use of the plant *anison* for treating the bites and stings of poisonous creatures and to relieve headaches and earaches.[90]

64 Malki, p. 66.
65 Amar, de Silva, p. 113.
66 Gil, No. 496b.
67 Assises, p. 174.
68 Ashtor, Trade, p. 53.
69 Ibid., p. 299.
70 Prawer, History, p. 125.
71 Benajahu, pp. 100, 104, 110.
72 Cumulative references in: al-Kindi, p. 297; Ibn Sina, pp. 415-416.
73 Levey, Ibn Masawayh, p. 401.
74 Maimonides, Aphorisms, 9:46, 50; 13:13, 44, 47; 15:56; 17:38; 21:29; 22:63
75 al-Antaki, p. 222. Cf. al-Biruni, II, p. 8.
76 Hooper, p.83.
77 Ducros, p. 141.
78 Reiani, p. 9, No. 6.
79 Cumulative references in: Ben-Yakov, p. 748.
80 Grieve, pp. 26-28.
81 Maimonides, Aphorisms, 21:75
82 Saladino, p. 79.
83 Donolo, pp. 15, 19, 21.
84 Plants & Animals, XII, p. 85. Composition of the substances and their applications in: Morton, pp. 48-50; Shahnaz et al.; Haller, pp. 650-657.
85 Plants & Animals, XII, p. 85; Morton, p. 50; Uphof, p. 27.
86 Plants & Animals, XII, p. 85; Morton, p. 50; Uphof, p. 27; Haller.
87 Maimonides, Glossaire, p. 20, No. 19; Dinsmore & Dalman, No. 758; Issa, Dictionary, p. 140, No. 5.
88 Plants & Animals, XII, p. 93.
89 Loewenfeld & Back, p. 55.
90 Dioscorides, III.56.

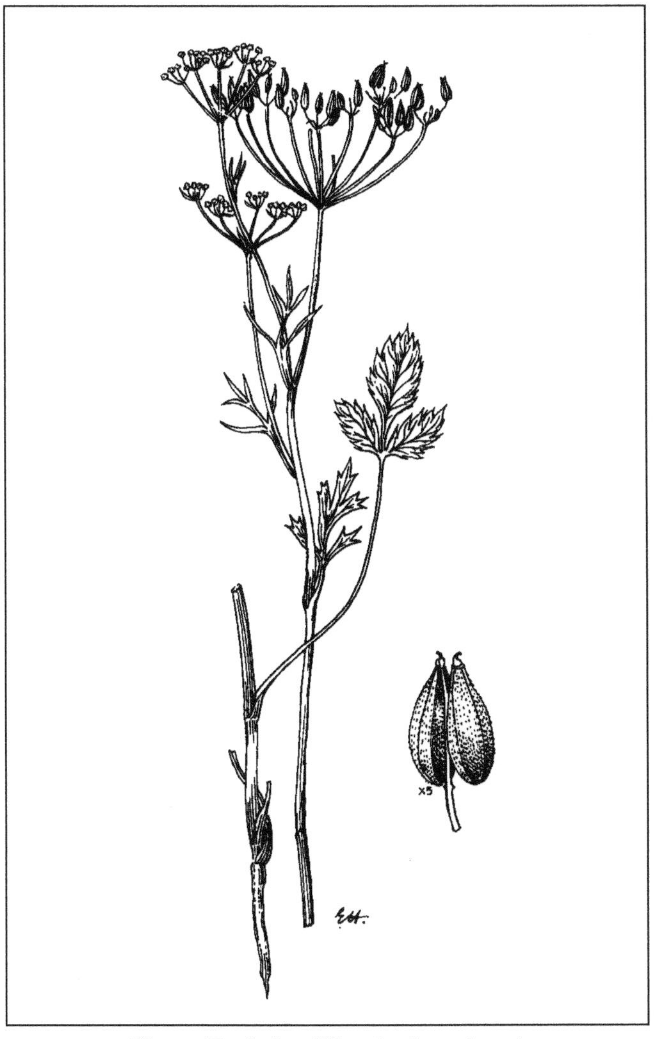

Figure 7 - Anise (*Pimpinella anisum*)

Medicinal Uses in Jerusalem:

In a Genizah letter dated 1060, Yisrael Ben Natan of Jerusalem asks Naharai Ben Nissim in Fustat to send him half a 'karat' of anison.[91] Refael Malki reports that the 'gabbaim' (treasurers) of synagogues in Jerusalem used to prepare various medicines for the city poor and that anison was one of the important components for a remedy to strengthen the heart and brain and another as a purgative.[92] David de Silva mentioned the 'anison' as a medicinal substance that opens obstructions in the urinary tracts and to expel worms in the stomach.[93]

Anise in the Levant:

In a commercial document dated 1233, anison (anis) is mentioned as a merchandise imported from the Levant to Europe.[94] Al-Ghazi, the Muslim scholar, reported on the growing of anison in Damascus and its uses as a constricting drug, diuretic, emmenagogue, fever abatement and headache relief.[95]

91 Gil, p. 142, No. 470.

92 Malki, pp. 62, 67, 88.

93 Amar, de Silva, p. 112.

94 Prawer, Colonial, p. 478; Venice Laws.

95 Hamarneh, Plants, p. 240.

Medicinal Uses in the Medieval Period:

According to al-Kindi, anison was a diuretic as well as a component in an ointment for treating the liver, in eye ointment and in a medication for treating stomach disorders.[96] Maimonides noted that anise was used as a constituent in a beverage for strengthening the heart, which was administered after an emetic. It was a component in the medicine "the great atriphal" which strengthens the heart and brain and also a component in a light purgative. Boiled anise was used as a susbstitute for wine in a medicine to treat poisoning and was also one of the components of theriac. Anise was considered a hot and dry drug.[97] al-Tamimi (as quoted by Maimonides) states that 'anison' arouses sexual desire and heals the womb. [98] According to al-Baytar in his entry 'anison' this substance was a purgative and the best kind was that which came from Crete and Egypt.[99] Daud al-Antaki in his entry 'anison' and describes its medical uses such as: reducing swellings, oedema, and gases, relieving headaches, and chest pains, treating difficulties in breathing and coughs, weakness of the kidney and spleen, dissolving renal stones, stopping excess tears, opening blockages, as well as for abortions and regulation of the heart beat.[100]

Traditional Medicine:

Israeli Arabs use aniseed to reduce gases especially in babies. Yemenite Jews use the 'yansoon' to regulate breathing, to increase appetite, to prevent constipation, to increase urine flow and to relieve stomach pains, headaches and colds.[101] The Jews of Iraq are accustomed to eating the roots and to use the seeds for remedies.[102] In Iran and Iraq 'anison' is used mainly as a component in a medication against cough[103] while in Egypt, the seeds of the anise are used as carminative, stimulant and an emmenagogue.[104] Similar uses are made of this plant in Europe as well.[105]

Medicinal Qualities:

The main essential oil derived from the fruit - ethnol - consitutes 1.5%-4% of its weight. Aniseed is used as aromatic stimulant to induce phlegm, sweat and gas emissions.[106]

General Uses:

The leaves are used as a seasoning for salads and the seed for baking and the production of alcoholic beverages.[107]

96 al-Kindi, Nos. 114, 162, 225. Cf. Ibn Sina, pp. 243-244.

97 Maimonides, Aphorisms, 13:6; 21:80; Maimonides, Regimen, 3:6, 11; Maimonides, Poisons, pp. 14, 93, 105, 107.

98 Maimonides, Aphorisms, 20:86.

99 Ibn al-Baytar, al-Jami, I, pp. 59-60; Leclerc, No. 159.

100 al-Antaki, p. 59. Cf. al-Biruni, I, p. 44.

101 Reiani, p. 39, No. 88.

102 Ben-Yakov, p. 506. Compare uses by other communities in Krispil, pp. 470-475.

103 Hooper, p. 147. In detail: al-Rawi & Chaakravarty, p. 74.

104 Ducros, p. 12.

105 Grieve, pp. 41-42.

106 Uphof, pp. 407-408; Reiani, p. 39, No. 88; Grieve, pp. 41-42; Plants & Animals, XII, p. 93. Regarding the contents of substances, see in detail: al-Rami & Chaakravarty, p. 74.

107 Loewenfeld & Back, p. 55; Uphof, pp. 407-408; Hill, p. 454.

Balsam

Scientific name: *Commiphora opobalsamum* (Burseraceae)
Hebrew: Afarsemon Arabic: Basham, Balzam, Balasan[108]

Description:
Balsam is a small tree (up to 3 metres) which grows in the desert areas of Arabia. It has horizontal and entangled branches, its bark is brown, the leaves small and shiny with tiny berries. Resin gum is obtained by making a gash in the trunk and it is brownish red in colour.[109]

History:
The use of balsam resin was common in the ancient Levant and all over the East. The resin of the balsam is identified with the biblical 'tsori' (balm) or 'bosem' (scent) as mentioned in the Song of Songs (5:1, 13; 6:2)[110] and it was also called 'shemen hamishha' (anointing oil). In Accadian it was called 'basmu' and was used medicinally by the Babylonians.[111] It seems that until King Solomon's rule, balsam resin was imported to the Levant from Africa and Arabia. Since that time it was cultivated in the gardens of Jericho and Ein Gedi. This fact was recorded by Josephus Flavius, and according to his contemporary sources of the Second Temple period, balsam trees were brought to the Holy Land by the Queen of Sheba.[112] On a broken piece of jar found in Masada (a fortress on the western shore of the of the Dead Sea) an inscription was found that said: "Mz ...Balsana" - which might be archaeological evidence for the use of balsam resin.[113]

Balsam resin is often mentioned in historical sources of the Second Temple period, in Jewish as well as in Roman and Hellenistic literature.[114] The Jewish Sages were proud of the balsam production in the Land of Israel and created a special blessing for the 'tsori gil'ad' (Balm of Gilead) and the ointment made out of it. They also mention 'tseloheyut apobalsun' (balsam bottle) and 'melaktei afarsemon' (balsam collectors) and describe some medicinal as well as cosmetic applications. Agricultural aspects of the balsam were researched and published by Feliks and Amar.[115] Pliny reports that balsam was the "most excellent of all perfumes, and nature had granted it to one country among all others, the land of Judea ..." He described its medicinal uses and the various ointments made from it, and even mentioned 20 prescriptions.[116] Dioscorides claimed that 'balsamon' - the scented balsam resin - was a drug used against poisons and toxins. It was a flammable substance, and it was used to thicken liquid medicines and also for the treatment of epilepsy, weakness, and dizziness.[117]

Medicinal Uses in Jerusalem:
In the travel records of the Bishop Wilblad who visited the Holy Land during the Umayyad period (circa 724), the following event is described:

> "While he was in Jerusalem, Bishop Wilblad bought himself a little 'balsamum' and placed it in a small bottle. He then took a 'cannam' (a hollow stick), put it into the bottle and filled it with 'petrae oleo' (petroleum). After cutting the stick down to the the height of the bottle neck, he corked it. When he and his entourage arrived at Tyre the people imprisoned them and searched their belongings to see if there was something hidden. Had anything been found they would have been condemmed to death. They only found the bottle of balsam, but did not know it was balsam because they could only smell the petroleum, so the travellers were left alone."[118]

From this source we learn that during the Umayyad period balsam oil was still obtainable in Jerusalem and it apparently came from the agricultural farms in the Jordan Valley. The story shows that even in this period balsam was one of the monopoly products and its distribution was zealously controlled by the Muslim authorities.[119]

Refael Malki described the history of 'balsamo' cultivation which he identified with the biblical 'tsori.' This essence which was brought from Mecca (Arabia) was used as a medication to strengthen memory, the brain, the digestive system and the stomach, and also to cure and close wounds. Because of its high price in Jerusalem during his time, Malki offered a prescription for a substitute medication.[120]

Balsam in the Levant:
From descriptions by various pilgrims it appears that in the area surrounding Jericho, balsam trees still grew even after the destruction of the Second Temple (70 CE).[121] Different reports from medieval times show that it grew in Egypt in a place called 'Ein Shams' (Heliopolis). Its resin was produced by making an incision in the bark, scraping the gum and collecting it with cotton wool.[122] With regard to its production in ancient times, see the research by Feliks.[123] A later dated description of balsam oil, its uses and trade in Egypt is given by Frederick Hasselquist who visited the region in 1750.[124]

---

[108] Maimonides, Glossaire, p. 92, No. 324. Updated list of Arabic names in: Issa, Dictionary, p. 55, No. 7.

[109] Description in :Uphof, p. 146; Feliks, World, pp. 256-258; Grieve, p. 78.

[110] Feliks, World, pp. 248, 256-258.

[111] al-Kindi, p. 245, No. 43.

[112] Josephus, JA, VIII, 6: 6.

[113] Yadin & Naveh, I, p. 47.

[114] For example: Low, I, pp. 299-304; Feliks, World, pp. 256-258.

[115] Amar, Production, pp. 49-52.

[116] Plinius, XII.54.

[117] Dioscorides, I.18.

[118] Tobler, Descriptions, p. 40. Petroleum was probably used because of its strong smell.

[119] In detail: Amar, Production, pp. 51-52.

[120] Malki, pp. 135-136.

[121] Tobler, Journey, p. 255. Cf. Petrus Dchono, Sandoli, II, pp.186-187.

[122] al-Qazwini, p. 218. On the cultivation of balsam in Egypt see: al-Biruni, I, pp. 73-75; Khusraw, p. 49; al-Idrisi, p. 326; al-Baghdadi, pp. 41-45; Ibn al-Baytar, al-Jami, I, p. 107; Borchard, p. 61. Additional sources in: Amar, Production, p. 52, n. 15.

[123] Feliks, Afarsemon; Feliks, World, pp. 256-258; Feliks, Balsam.

[124] Hasselquist, pp. 293-297.

Medicinal Uses in the Medieval Period:
Assaph Harofe reported on the use of 'balsamo' oil to treat diseases of many internal organs such as the spleen, kidneys, liver, womb and lung, and also to treat cough, tuberculosis, obstructions in the urinary tract, skin diseases, bites and stings.[125] According to al-Kindi, 'balsan' was a component in a clyster.[126] Even in Europe during the Middle Ages, balsam oil was an important component in medicines. Shabtai Donolo quotes Pliny who described in great detail the concoction of ointments from balsam oil.[127]

Maimonides notes that balsam bark was a component in a medication called 'the great atriphal' to strengthen various organs especially the heart and the senses, to delay aging and as an aid in coitus.[128] Elsewhere, mention is made of a plant used in a medication against "evil vapours of the stomach". Balsam was an important component in this medication, and balsam oil was also used to counteract poison.[129] In describing the preparation of medication against poisoning, it is explicitly stated that balsam oil, as compared with other components, was extremely hard to obtain because it was available only in Egypt.[130] Ibn Rushd reports that "the 'balshami' is 'afarsemon' ... the oil has many excellent qualities and its effects are marvellous" and among its uses are: pain relief, dissolving stones in the urinary tract, curing infertility and as a medicine against poisons.[131]

According to al-Qazwini, 'balsan' resembles the rue in its scent and leaves, but it tended to be white in colour. As to its medicinal qualities, he quotes Ibn Sina: "Its berries and leaves are effective against pains in the lung and thigh sinew, epilepsy, dizziness, infertility, snake bites, poisons in general and the scorpion in particular. It also removes the membrane to extract the embryo and placenta, and it eases difficulties in passing urine and dispels tremors.[132] Daud al-Antaki says that 'basham' strengthens the teeth, dries wounds, stops bleeding, tears and and sweat, increases menstruation and dispels gases. It also strengthens the body, nerves, stomach and hair.[133] Hasselquist notes that balsam is very effective in strengthening the weak stomach and curing wounds.[134]

Traditional Medicine:
Balsam oil (Mecca Balsam) is used as an incense and for the preparation of perfumes. Its world supply is limited and expensive.[135] In Iraq they use the fruit of the balsam tree called 'balsan' which is identified with 'afarsemon'. From this fruit, a substance is produced which serves as a drug to dispel gases, to relieve stomach aches and as a stimulant. In Iran it is used as a component in a medication to treat colds and tremors. In Arabia the resin of the tree is used to treat poisoning, stings and to cure wounds.[136]

Conclusion:
Balsam oil which is produced from the resin of the tree is listed among the earliest and well-known medicinal substances in the ancient world. Its cultivation and the production of the resin and oil was one of the most guarded secrets of the Arabs, the Jews of the Second Temple period, and of the different Arab rulers in the later centuries. Information regarding the medicinal uses of the plant can be derived from many and varied sources. Reliable evidence about the purchase of balsam oil in Jerusalem by the Bishop Wilblad at the beginning of the 8th century testifies to the fact that the region of Judea was a source for balsam oil either because they continued to grow balsam trees there or because the region served as a place of transit for its trade. In spite of the glorified aura which once surrounded balsam oil in ancient times, its production and medicinal uses have nearly ceased altogether.

Basil

Scientific name: *Ocimum basilicum* (Labiatae)
Hebrew: Reihan Arabic: Reihan[137]

Description:
The sweet or common basil is an annual plant, tall (60 cm.) with square stems, and branching spikes, white flowers and small, black seeds.[138]

History:
The term 'reihan' is used of scented plants in general and of the basil plant in particular. The scientific term 'basileus' means 'king' because of its unique perfume. Disocorides notes that *okimon* which is identified with basil is used for improving eyesight and treating depression, swellings and scorpion stings.[139]

Medicinal Uses in Jerusalem:
According to Refael Malki, 'reihan' was a component in a medicine for malaria.[140]

Basil in the Levant:
al-Muqaddasi describes the crops grown in Jericho and mentions basil in addition to the dates and bananas.[141] The

[125] Assaph, 4, p. 398.

[126] al-Kindi, No. 146.

[127] Donolo, pp. 12-13.

[128] Maimonides, Regimen, 3:11.

[129] Maimonides, Aphorisms, 9:46a; 22:52.

[130] Maimonides, Poisons, p. 108.

[131] Ibn Rushd, p. 157.

[132] al-Qazwini, p. 218. Cf. Ibn Sina, p. 265; al-Biruni, I, pp. 73-75; II, pp. 79-80; al-Ghafiqi, No. 117.

[133] al-Antaki, pp. 75-76. Cf. Ibn al-Baytar, al-Jami, I, pp. 107-109; Leclerc, No. 336.

[134] Hasselquist, pp. 293-297.

[135] Hill, p. 172; Uphof, p. 146.

[136] Hooper, p. 104; Uphof, p. 146; Feliks, World, p. 258.

[137] Maimonides, Glossaire, p. 27, No. 48; p. 100, No. 360; Issa, Dictionary, p. 126, No. 4; Dinsmore & Dalman, No. 1336; Leclerc, Nos. 94, 205, 511, 589, 593, 926, 1676, 1077; Serapion, p. 497, No. 73; Ducros, p. 64.

[138] Plants & Animals, XII, p. 96; Loewenfeld & Back, pp. 60-61.

[139] Dioscorides, II.171.

[140] Malki, p. 78.

[141] al-Muqaddasi, p. 175.

research scholar, Hamarneh, claims that basil grew in 'Ajlun and was part of the panoramic scenes of the childhood and medical practice of the physician Ibn al-Quff al-Karaki (13th century).[142] Ibn al-Baytar in his entry 'hamaham' describes the plant and listed its medicinal uses. He claimed, quoting Ishaq ibn 'Amran that the "wide-leaved 'al- habeq al-bustani' is called 'habaq nabati' in al-Sham, and has soft, green quadrangular stems, white flowers and seeds like that of the 'habaq' which is a hot and dry type."[143]

Ibn al-Qayyim al-Jawziyya notes that basil, which was highly preferred by the people of 'al-Sham' (Greater Syria) and Iraq, was called 'habaq.'[144] al-Ghazi describes the 'habaq' known in Greater Syria as basil and listed ten different kinds which were used as remedies.[145]

Medicinal Uses in the Medieval Period:
al-Kindi noted two kinds of basil: one was a component in a medication for the poor[146] and the other was a component in an ointment to treat rheumatism and as an eye ointment.[147] Shabtai Donolo listed the 'basilikon' among the plants used for remedies.[148] According to Maimonides, basil was easily digestible, gave strength to the spirit, and increased appetite. It was a component in a medicine "useful for coitus and for scenting the breath" and also in a medicine that relieved "deep distress and depression, and induces strong emotional desires."[149] Ibn al-Baytar, in his entry 'Reihan saliman' claims that basil was used among other things to treat erysipelas, stomach ulcers, and scorpion stings.[150] al-Qazwini reported that basil was effective in staunching nosebleeds, cleansing and improving eyesight, opening blockages in the urinary tract, and treating scorpion stings.[151] It was also used to treat hemorrhoids, dizziness and to reduce bad smells from the armpit.[152]

Traditional Medicine:
Yemenite Jews used the plant for decoration, as a perfume and for the treatment of various kinds of skin rashes, wounds and scabies (eczema).[153] The Jews of Iraq frequently used the plant as perfume, for sauces to increase appetite, to induce sleep, to bind wounds and strengthen the heart.[154] In Egypt, the plant was used as a diuretic, to calm the nerves, to treat heart and head disorders.[155] In Iran, the basil's seeds were used as a medication against influenza, gonorrhea, and dysentery, while the blossoms served as a carminative diuretic and stimulant.[156]

General Uses:
Fresh basil leaves, dried or ground, are used for seasoning salads and flavoring soups, sauces and meats. The essential oils made out the basil seeds constitutes 0.15% of the weight and serves as a component in many cosmetic preparations.[157]

Ben Tree

Scientific name: *Moringa peregrina* (Moringaceae)[158]
Hebrew: Moringa Arabic: Ban[159]

Description:
Tropical tree, which grows in the big valleys of Saini desert, southern Negev and the Judean desert. The tree is high (up to 8 meters), with white trunk and pink-whitish flowers. The fruits are long (up to 30 cm.) and rounded.[160]

Medicinal Uses in Jerusalem:
The ben tree (moringa) is a medicinal plant in Jerusalem. al-Tamimi describes the 'ban' as "partly growing in Egypt and a little is imported from the region 'shraa' [from the south-eastern shores of the Dead Sea] and the region of al-Balka [a region east of the Jordan River] and some of it grows on the banks of the Dead Sea between Tsoar and Jericho."[161] al-Tamimi writes in his essay on perfumes *Tib al- 'Arus* about various techniques for the production of moringa oil, including a prescription which he himself had invented. It is worth mentioning two Indian personalities, Abu Amran Mussa al-Yehudi known by the name of 'al-Bani' and Abu Said al-Yehudi al-Attar, who were experts in producing the oil.[162] In the literature in praise of Jerusalem, Abu Bakar Ben al-Harathi describes the lighting of oil lamps on the Temple Mount with 'ban' oil (moringa) and 'zanbak' oil (jasmin). The guards there asked him to give them a lamp so that they could anoint their bodies with the oil.[163]

The Ben Tree in the Levant:
al-Ghafiqi and Ibn al-Baytar in their entries for 'Ban' quote Dioscorides who writes about the locality of the tree and notes that it is found in 'Falastin' (especially in Petra) and is known there as 'batir.'[164]

---

142 Hamarneh, Plants, p. 245.

143 Ibn al-Baytar, al-Jami, II, p. 33; Leclerc, No. 704.

144 Ibn al-Qayyim, p. 362.

145 Hamarneh, Plants, p. 245.

146 al-Kindi, No. 178.

147 Ibid., Nos. 139, 212.

148 Donolo, p. 22, n. 283.

149 Maimonides, Aphorisms, 20:49; 21: 70, 75; Maimonides, Regimen, 2:20; Maimonides, Answers, 8; Maimonides, Sexual, Introduction, 3; 5:6; 16:2.

150 Ibn al-Baytar, al-Jami, II, p. 148; Leclerc, No. 1075.

151 al-Qazwini, p. 240. Cf. Ibn Sina, p. 274.

152 Ibid., p. 251.

153 Reiani, p. 35, No. 77.

154 Ben-Yakov, pp. 53, 55, 268, 315, 361.

155 Ducros, p. 112.

156 Hooper, p. 145; al-Rawi & Chaakravarty, p. 69.

157 Plants & Animals, XII, p. 96; Uphof. p. 365; Hill, p. 463.

158 Plants & Animals, X, p. 124.

159 Maimonides, Glossaire, No. 378; Ibn al-Baytar, al-Jami, I, pp. 79-81; Leclerc, No. 226; Dinsmore & Dalman, No. 406; Issa, Dictionary, p. 120, No. 18.

160 Plants & Animals, X, pp. 123-124.

161 Amar & Seri, p. 50; al-Nuwayri, XII, pp. 79-80, Cf. al-'Asali, p. 279.

162 Amar & Seri, p. 50; al-Nuwayri, XII, pp. 83, 89.

163 al-Wasti, p. 83.

164 al-Ghafiqi, No. 118; Ibn al-Baytar, al-Jami, I, pp. 79-81; Leclerc, No. 226.

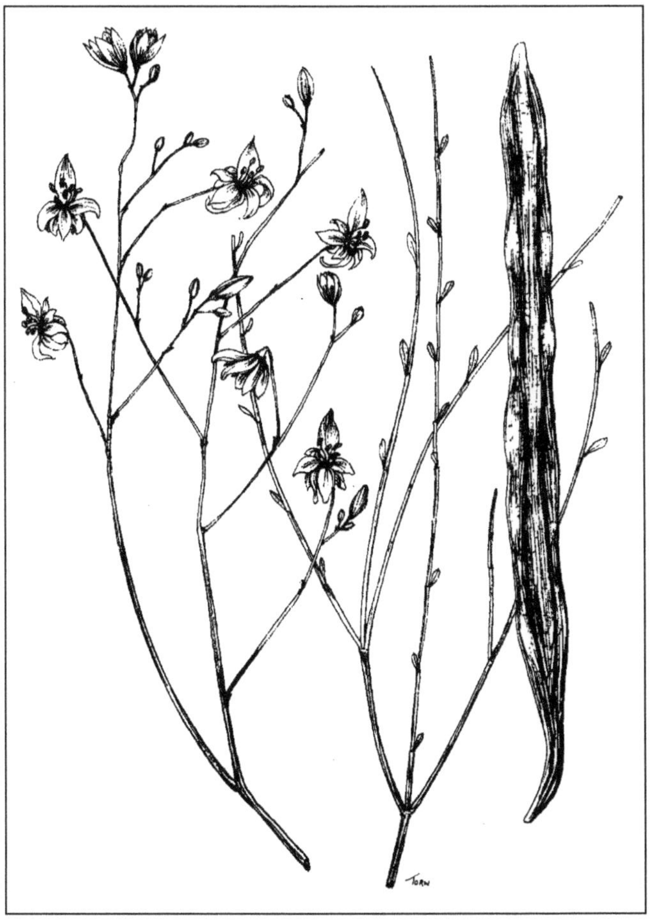

Figure 8 - Ben Tree (*Moringa peregrina*)

Medicinal Uses in the Medieval Period:
al-Kindi describes the use of the seeds to increase the growth of hair and beard, to strengthen the teeth and gums, to staunch nosebleeds and as a component in ointments.[165] Maimonides describes the use of 'ban oil' in a sleeping draught.[166] Elsewhere, Maimonides mentions the 'white and red ban' as a component in a medication called 'the great atriphal', which delays old age, strengthens the senses and increases sexual potency. In addition he recommended smearing 'al-ban oil' on the forehead in winter.[167] al-Qazwini describes the tree and its seeds, and quotes Ibn Sina who says that it is effective against leprosy, various skin diseases and toothache. A quotation from an anonymous physician describes its use against boils and nosebleeds.[168] Ibn al-Baytar quotes many physicians in connection with the medicinal uses of this plant such as: treatment of the spleen, rheumatism, skin problems as well as an emetic and purgative, to strengthen the gums and stop nosebleeds. The author also quotes Galen who describes the use of its stem extracts for diseases of the skin, liver and spleen, to induce vomiting and as a purgative. The seeds were used as an astringent.[169] Daud al-Antaki notes that the 'ban' was a hot and dry drug used against chills, swellings and excess sweat, for strengthening, for closing wounds, for skin diseases, cleansing of the intestines, curing the spleen, hemorrhoids, and increasing urine flow.[170] Hasselquist states that the moringa was scentless and suitable for the concoction of perfumes and of ointments which were applicable for the head and nose. He also stated that the plant grew in the Sinai desert and in Egypt.[171]

Traditional Medicine:
Oil produced from moringa seeds was used to lubricate watches.[172] Sinai Bedouins used the plant against lice on camels and for making tent poles.[173] In Egypt the oil from the seeds was used to anoint the body, and women ate the seeds to fatten themselves.[174]

Conclusions:
The ben tree is an impressive tree which grows in Israel, in desert oases and in many ravines in the Judean desert. It is no wonder that Arab desert dwellers knew the tree and recognised its medicinal qualities. Its medicinal uses were mainly from the oil derived from its seeds which was beneficial primarily for treating skin diseases and to cure internal ailments and for strengthening. Apparently these uses were very localised and we have no evidence of its trade or of its use beyond the borders of the Near East. In traditional medicine the medicinal use of the ben tree (moringa) was retained only in Egypt.

Borage

Scientific name: *Anchusa sp.* (Boraginacea)
Hebrew: Lashon ha-par Arabic: Lisan al-Thawr[175]

Description:
There are 50 species of borage, six of which grow in Israel. Half of them are annual and the other half are perennials. The plant leaves are elongated and covered with bristles, the flower has a corolla of joined petals, and its colours vary from violet to white. The berry contains four sections, which functions as a disseminating unit.[176]

History:
The Hebrew name derives from the Arabic one which compares the rough, bristly leaf to the cow's tongue. The scientific name is derived from the Greek and is linked with the production of red colouring. It is presumed that this colouring is produced from species that do not grow in this

[165] al-Kindi, Nos. 74, 141, 144, 220. For additional sources see: Ibid., p. 241, No. 32.

[166] Maimonides, Sexual, 18:2.

[167] Maimonides, Regimen, 3:11; 4:13.

[168] al-Qazwini, p. 218. Cf. Ibn Sina, p. 264.

[169] Ibn al-Baytar, al-Jami, I, pp. 79-81; Leclerc, No. 226.

[170] al-Antaki, p. 67.

[171] Hasselquist, p. 288.

[172] Zohary, p. 402.

[173] Levey, Bedouins, p. 80; EI, 'Ban' entry.

[174] Levey, Bedouins, p. 80; Osborn, p. 173.

[175] Maimonides, Glossaire, p. 66, No. 211; p. 103, No. 376; Issa, Dictionary, p. 15, Nos. 10, 12; Ibn al-Baytar, al-Jami, III, p. 69; Leclerc, No. 1344; Dinsmore & Dalman, Nos. 1172-1179. For further information regarding identification see: Amar, Ibn al-Baytar, p. 66, n.50.

[176] Plants & Animals, XI, p. 51.

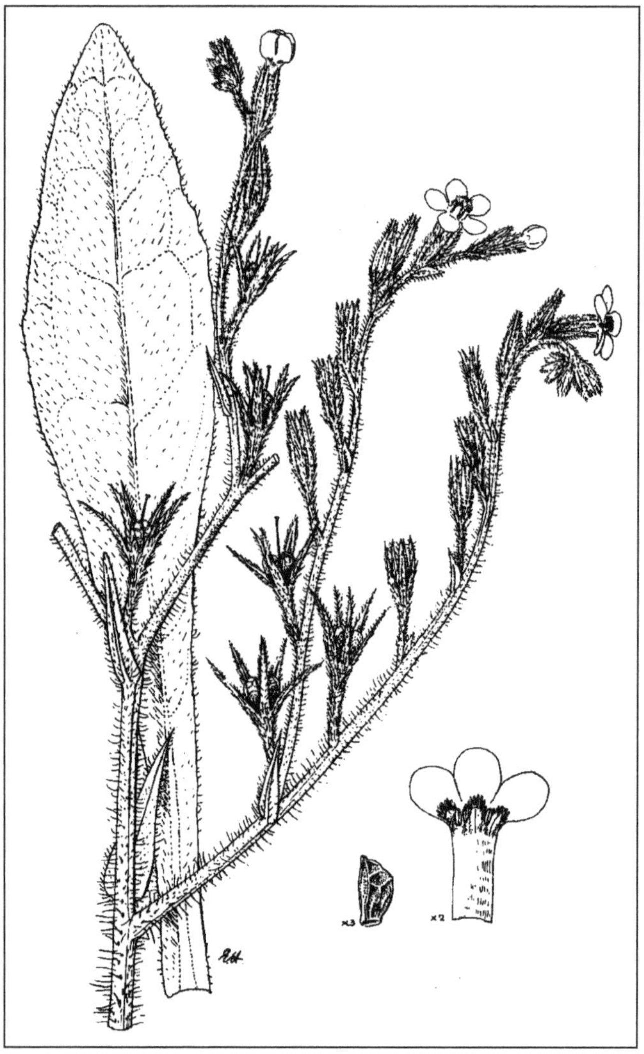

Figure 9 - Borage (*Anchusa italica*)

region.[177] Disocorides describes the *anchusa* and suggests using the leaves soaked in wine as an emetic and leaves soaked in olive oil as a cure for growths on the skin and for burns.[178]

Medicinal Uses in Jerusalem:
Refael Malki claims that liquid derived from the 'lishan-al-tor' was a medication in Jerusalem, but in his opinion this had no medicinal value.[179]

Borage in the Levant:
According to al-Israili the 'lasan al-tor' was brought to Egypt from al-Sham (Syria) and from Turkey, and a medicinal liquid was prepared from it.[180] Ibn al-Baytar wrote in his entry 'Hamaham' that this was the 'lisan al-thawr' of the people living in al-Sham and the East.[181]

Medicinal Uses in the Medieval Period:
According to Maimonides the 'lingua bobina' was a light drug and a component in an emetic as well as in other medicines including 'the great atriphal.'[182] Ibn al-Baytar in his entry 'shangar' quoted Galen who claimed that the root of the plant was bitter, astringent, cleansed the stomach, relieved pains of the kidney and spleen, and was applicable for internal use. Other physicians describe the external use as in bandages for wounds to reduce swellings and to disinfect the wound. The root was used for various skin diseases but was also applicable for internal use, and was an effective medicine for the stomach.[183] Daud al-Antaki stated in his entry 'lisan al-thawr' that the plant provided a drug for strengthening the eyesight and the sense, to ease the passage of excretions, and was effective against madness and melancholy. It also relieved pains of the mouth, teeth, chest, lungs, and cured coughs and heartburns, and was used as a component in medicinal stimulants for fainting fits and to treat jaundice.[184] In Europe various types of borage were used to treat stomach ulcers, burns, worms, stomach pains, diarrhea and high fever.[185]

Traditional Medicine:
Israeli Arabs use the bristly borage (*Anchusa strigosa*) to clot open wounds and for the general strengthening of the body. They use the root internally to reduce stomach pain and externally to treat temporary paralysis resulting from fear.[186] Persian Jews use the blossoms to make a beverage for strong stomach pains, diarrhea, high fever, jaundice, earache and also to strengthen the hair and the body.[187] In Iraq they use the blossoms of the Italian borage (*Anchusa italica*) and of the bristly borage called 'lisan al-thawr' as a component in a medicinal tea, as a strengthening drug for children, as a medication to reduce the pulse rate and as a diuretic (a substitute for the medicinal borage - *Anchusa officinalis*).[188]

Medicinal Qualities:
The blossoms of the medicinal borage, sometimes causes a quickening of the heartbeat and is used for treating chills. The stem is used as a drug for inducing sputum, lowering temperature, curing inflammations and nervous disorders. The root is used as a medicine to treat diarrhea and cure wounds.[189]

During the 1970's a pharmacological research study was conducted to examine the influence of borage root extract upon living creatures. The results showed that this extract repressed motor activity and caused various effects such as loss of muscle elasticity, lack of coordination, vomiting and diarrhea.[190]

---

177 Ibid.

178 Dioscorides, IV.23-25.

179 Malki, p. 77.

180 al-Israili, p. 282.

181 Ibn al-Baytar, al-Jami, II, p. 34; Leclerc, No. 708.

182 Maimonides, Aphorisms, 21:72; Maimonides, Regimen, 2:10; 3:4, 8, 9, 11.

183 Ibn al-Baytar, al-Jami, III, p. 69; Leclerc, No. 1344. Cf. Ibn Sina, p. 435; al-Biruni, I, p. 361.

184 al-Antaki, p. 281. Cf. Ibn Sina, p. 352; al-Biruni, I, p. 292.

185 Grieve, p. 120; Dafni, Edible, p. 79.

186 Palevitz et al, p. 100; Krispil, p. 622.

187 Krispil, p. 622.

188 al-Rawi & Chaakravarty, p. 13.

189 Steinmetz, pp. 88-89.

190 Shalmovitz, p. 69.

Carrot

Scientific name: *Daucas carota* (Umbelliferae)[191]
Hebrew: Gezer Arabic: Jazar[192]

Description:
The carrot is a widely cultivated vegetable plant (60-90 cm.), with branching stems, feathery leaves and an edible, firm and fleshy root. There are many varieties: the wild carrot is native to Europe and Asia, and the North American variety has long, tapering orange roots. One of these varieties which mentioned below is the parsnip.

History:
The carrot was an ancient agricultural crop in India, Asia Minor and even Switzerland. It is not mentioned in the Bible, Mishna or by the Jewish Sages under this name, but the Jerusalem Talmud refers to the 'astafnini' (Demai, 2:1; Ma'asarot, 2:4). The colour of the vegetable root (the edible part) used to be purple. The orange coloured species known today was cultivated in Holland during the 18th century.[193]

Classical physicians described the carrot *Staphulinos* and noted its medicinal uses.[194]

Medicinal Uses in Jerusalem:
al-Tamimi mentioned the 'daukwa' which can be identified with a cultivated subspecies of the carrot - *Daucas carota* as one of the vegetable plants that grew in the Jerusalem area. Among its main virtues listed by al-Tamimi was its beneficial effect against the bites of snakes and scorpions.[195] Ibn al-Baytar called it 'daukwas' and noted that one of its varieties was well known in al-Sham and Beit al-Muqadis (Jerusalem).[196]

Carrot in the Levant:
In his entry 'istaplin' Ibn al-Baytar states that this is the word for the 'jazar' (carrot) in the al-Sham dialect. [197] Daud al-Antaki called the seeds of the wild carrot by the name 'daukwa'[198] The name 'jazar' appears in the list of crops in Greater Syria during the Mamluk period.[199]

Medicinal Uses in the Medieval Period:
Assaph Harofe described the use of "a weed called 'daucos'" which had sweet roots and was used in opening obstructions in the urinary tract, for kidney pains, cough, and "for snake bites, and those who have blood in their urine or vomit blood."[200] al-Kindi claimed that carrot seeds relieved stomach disorders, dissolved stones in the kidneys the urinary tracts, and cured sexual addictions. According to him, the 'daukaws' (wild carrot) was used for treating hemorrhoids.[201] Maimonides reported that the carrot seed called 'fishtanga' was one of the many components in a medication called 'the great atriphal' which is used for strengthening the organs, especially the heart, to delay old age, to strengthen the senses and improve coitus. The carrot was listed among the hot and dry drugs.[202]

Ibn al-Baytar in his entry 'daukwas' quotes classical and contemporary physicians in describing its medicinal uses such as: for urine flow, emmenagogue, reducing stomach pains and cough, treating scorpion stings and preventing lustful desires.[203]

Daud al-Antaki in his entry 'Jazar' lists similar uses and adds that the plant improves the memory, cures jaundice and excess sweating.[204]

Traditional Medicine:
In Iraq, Egypt and Iran the carrot is used as a stimulant, carminative, purgative, diuretic, emmenagogue, and to arouse sexual desire and soothe the skin.[205]

Parsnip

Scientific name: *Pastinaca schekakul*

The parsnip is a biennial plant with a white root and is one of the carrot varieties that grew in the Land of Israel during medieval times.[206]

Parsnip in the Levant:
Ibn al-Baytar in his entry 'Jamjam' describes a type of carrot with roots similar in shape and size to those of the wild carrot and which was called 'shekakul' in al-Sham.[207] Rauwolf wrote that in Aleppo (Syria) the inhabitants ate carrots, which they called 'secacul' with roots that were gray-coloured on the outside but white on the inside and which tasted soft and sweet.[208]

Medicinal Uses in the Medieval Period:
According to Maimonides, the 'schekakul' was a moist drug and a component of 'the great atriphal.' Elsewhere it is

---

191 Plants & Animals, XII, pp. 78-79

192 Maimonides, Glossaire, Nos. 73, 94, 223; al-Razi, 20, pp. 456-458; Issa, Dictionary, p. 69, No.4.

193 Plants & Animals, XII, pp. 78-79; Low, III, p. 449; Feliks, Yerushalmi.

194 Dioscorides, II.59.

195 Amar & Seri, p. 18; al-Tamimi, pp. 21b-22a.

196 Ibn al-Baytar, al-Jami, II , p. 119; Leclerc, No. 970.

197 Ibn al-Baytar, al-Jami, I, p. 39; Leclerc, No. 96; al-Antaki, p. 50.

198 al-Antaki, p. 159.

199 al-Qalakshandi. 87; al-'Umari, p. 25.

200 Assaph, IV, p. 409.

201 al-Kindi, No.s 207, 221, 226.

202 Maimonides, Regimen, 3:11; Maimonides, Aphorisms, 21:80. Cf. al-Ghafiqi, No. 207.

203 Ibn al-Baytar, al-Jami, II, p. 119; Leclerc, No. 970.

204 al-Antaki, pp. 105-106. Cf. Ibn Sina, p. 287; al-Biruni, I, pp. 108-109.

205 Ducros, p. 21; Hooper, p. 112; al-Rawi & Chaakravarty, pp. 36-37 where the contents of active substances are given. See also: Ben-Yakov, p. 326.

206 Issa, Dictionary, p. 135, No. 17; Discussion of identity in: Amar, Production, p. 71. On the cultivated species *Pastinaca sativa* see: Uphof, p. 391. Medicinal uses in: Grieve, pp. 615-617.

207 Ibn al-Baytar, al-Jami, I, p. 169; Leclerc, No. 514. Cf. Maimonides, Glossaire, No. 361; al-Antaki, pp. 216-217.

208 Rauwolf, p. 74.

mentioned as an ingredient in a "beneficial powder for coitus."[209]

Conclusion:
Today the carrot is an agricultural crop grown for food, although in the past the garden carrot and varieties of wild carrot similar to it were used as medicinal substances. Many sources describe these medicinal uses in this region and in neighboring countries during the Middle Ages. The carrot is one example among many in this study of a food plant which was also used for medicinal purposes, but these uses now remain only vestigially in traditional medicine.

Cassia

Scientific name: *Cassia {Senna} sp.* (Leguminosae)[210]
Hebrew: Kassia   Arabic: Sana

Various types of cassia are used as remedies in the Near and Far East.[211]

Description:
Cassia, also called senna, is an annual or herbaceous perennial plant, shrub or tree of the genus *Cassia*. There are about 400 species, mostly tropical, but a few are found in temperate regions. Many are popular ornamentals because of their rapid growth, pinnate leaves, and yellow or rose flowers, which often grow in large clusters. The fruit is a pod. Senna, the dried leaves of many species, provides an extract used as a cathartic.[212]

History:
Its uses as a medicinal plant began in the 9th or 10th century. It was brought to Europe by Muslim physicians and was used throughout the Middle East and Europe as a cathartic substance.[213] Frederick Hasselquist reported that Egyptian farmers collected this plant and sold it to Jewish licensed dealers who exported it to Europe, mainly to Marseilles and Venice, for medicinal use.[214]

Medicinal Uses in Jerusalem:
The 'sini' (senna) is mentioned in a medical work by Refael Malki. According to him, the plant was a component in a general syrup which was concocted by synagogue 'gabbaim' (treasurers) in Jerusalem during the 17th century.[215] A legal document dated 1711 says that senna leaves were used in Jerusalem for medical purposes.[216] In this case, an Arab husband gave his pregnant wife some senna leaves contrary to the instructions of the physician, Salmon ben ha-Yehudi. This medicine was mistakenly administered instead of chicory or yellow pond-lily juice and it caused the miscarriage of the child and the death of the woman.

Medicinal Uses in the Medieval Period:
According to Assaph Harofe the Indian Senna was a cathartic drug, a remedy for the eyes and for women's illnesses.[217] al-Kindi claimed that Meccan senna was a component in a medicine from which an infusion was prepared.[218] Maimonides listed many uses for senna, mainly as a remedy for the intestines. The 'sini' was a hot and dry drug.[219] Ibn al-Baytar, quoting other sources, says that senna was a medicine well known among the dwellers of the Hejaz and was used to cure epilepsy, to treat smallpox and as a purgative.[220]

Traditional Medicine:
The leaves and fruit of various types of cassia are used all over the world in traditional medicine as a cathartic substance.[221] Desert cassia (*Cassia italica*) is used by Bedouins in Sinai and Egypt as a purgative.[222] The leaves of the plant (*Cassia angustifolia*) are used by Yemenite Jews to treat constipation, rheumatism and intestinal worms. The leaves are also a compound in preparations for darkening the hair and to prevent hair loss, and in a poultice to relieve headaches.[223] Indian senna (*Cassia acutifolia*) is imported by Iran from India where it is used as a purgative. In Iran and Iraq the seeds of the plant (*Cassia absus*) are used as a component in a bandage to cure wounds.[224]

In Iraq, the plant (*Cassia occidentalis*) which is called 'sana makki' is a medicinal plant used as a purgative, diuretic, a strengthener and to reduce fever. The leaves, roots and seeds are used as laxatives, while the leaves and seeds are used in medicinal preparations for curing skin diseases and to prevent menstruation.[225] Today, cassia leaves (senna) and its pods serve as a purgative because of their cynoside contents.[226]

Conclusions:
Cassia is a medicinal plant which is used until today among those supporting traditional medicine. According to researchers, the medical history of the plant began in the 9th century and its use became widespread by the Arabs who

[209] Maimonides, Regimen, 3:11; Maimonides, Aphorisms, 21:72; Maimonides, Sexual, Introduction, section 2.

[210] Feinbrun-Dothan, pp. 294-295; Morton, pp. 147-152.

[211] According to Maimonides, Glossaire, p. 77, No. 267; Issa, Dictionary, p. 42, Nos. 9-10; Dinsmore & Dalman, No. 649.

[212] Grieve, p. 168, 734-737; Collier, 734-737

[213] al-Kindi, p. 286.

[214] Hasselquist, p. 300.

[215] Malki, p. 63.

[216] Cohen, 18 Century, p. 325, No. 279.

[217] Assaph, 4, p. 401.

[218] al-Kindi, No. 211.

[219] For example: Maimonides, Regimen, 3:9; Maimonides, Aphorisms, 20:49; 21:69.

[220] Ibn al-Baytar, al-Jami, III, p. 32; Leclerc, No. 1236. Cf. al-Antaki, No. 201.

[221] Palevitz, p. 268. For the contents of active substances see: Plants & Animals, XII, p. 88; Hill, p. 257; Uphof, pp. 111-112; Grieve, pp. 734-737.

[222] Levey, Bedouins, p. 79; Osborn, p. 173.

[223] Reiani, p. 14, No. 21. For uses by the Jews of Iraq see: Ben-Yakov, p. 739.

[224] Hooper, p. 96.

[225] al-Rawi & Chaakravarty, p. 24, where the contents of active substances are given.

[226] Plants & Animals, XII, p. 88.

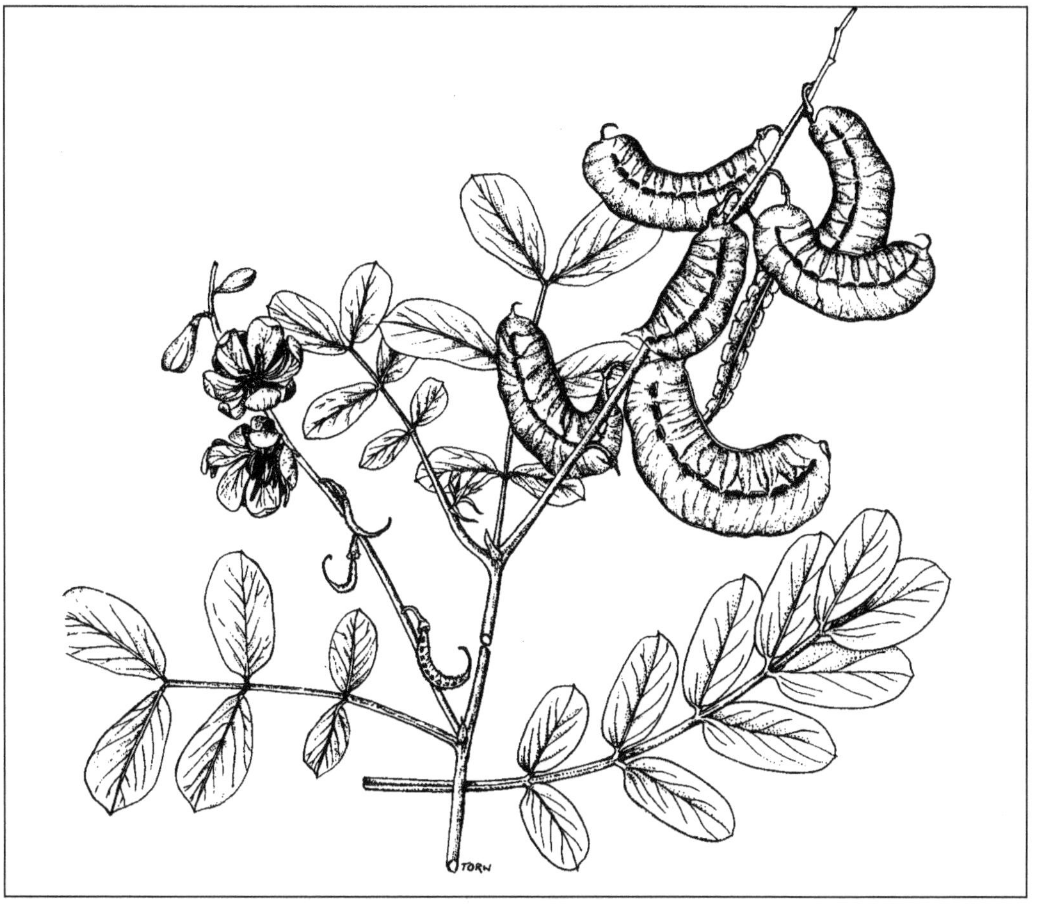

Figure 10 - Cassia (*Cassia italica*)

English	Scientific name	Synonym	Hebrew name
True Senna	*Cassia acutifolia*	*Senna alexandrina*	Kassia mehudedet
Senna	*Cassia obtusifolia*	*Senna obtusifolia*	Kassia kehah
Senna	*Cassia italica*	*Senna italica*	Kassia midbarit
Indian Senna	*Cassia angustifolia*	*Senna tinnevelly*	Kassia hodit

controlled its trade through the areas under Muslim rule, and later in Europe as well. From these sources we learn that the use of this plant for remedial purposes in Jerusalem during the 17th and 18th centuries was an accepted fact.

Celery

Scientific name: *Apium graveolens* (Umbelliferae)
Hebrew: Karpas Arabic: Karafs[227]

Description:
Annual or biennial plant that grows throughout the region in damp soil. Its wide leaves are trifoliate, its flowers white or reddish in colour, and its fruit pods are flattened and egg-shaped.[228]

History:
This plant has been cultivated for over 3000 years in China, Egypt, Greece and Rome. It is mentioned in the Bible only once, in the Book of Esther (1:6) but the term there is identified with cotton wool.[229] Dioscorides recommended using various kinds of *selinon* identified with celery, to treat the stomach, to ease breathing, for pains and coughs, and as a diuretic and emetic. He says that celery was an ingredient in theriac.[230] Celery is also mentioned by the Jewish Sages as an agricultural crop (Shevi'th 9,1).

Medicinal Uses in Jerusalem:
Refael Malki claims that the seed of the celery plant was a component in a general medicine (pill).[231] 'Karpas' was mentioned by David de Silva as a substance, that improves stomach function and also eliminates bad breath.[232]

Celery in the Levant:
Hayim Vital mentions 'sharab' (medicinal drink) made of bitter celery as a medication for a swollen stomach.[233]

[227] Maimonides, Glossaire, p. 62, No. 196. Cf. Dinsmore & Dalman, No. 746; Issa, Dictionary, p. 19, No. 5

[228] Plants & Animals, XII, p. 83; Feinbrun-Dothan, p. 480.

[229] Feliks, World, p. 288.

[230] Dioscorides, III.74, 75.

[231] Malki, p. 67.

[232] Amar, de Silva, p. 125.

[233] Benajahu, p. 98.

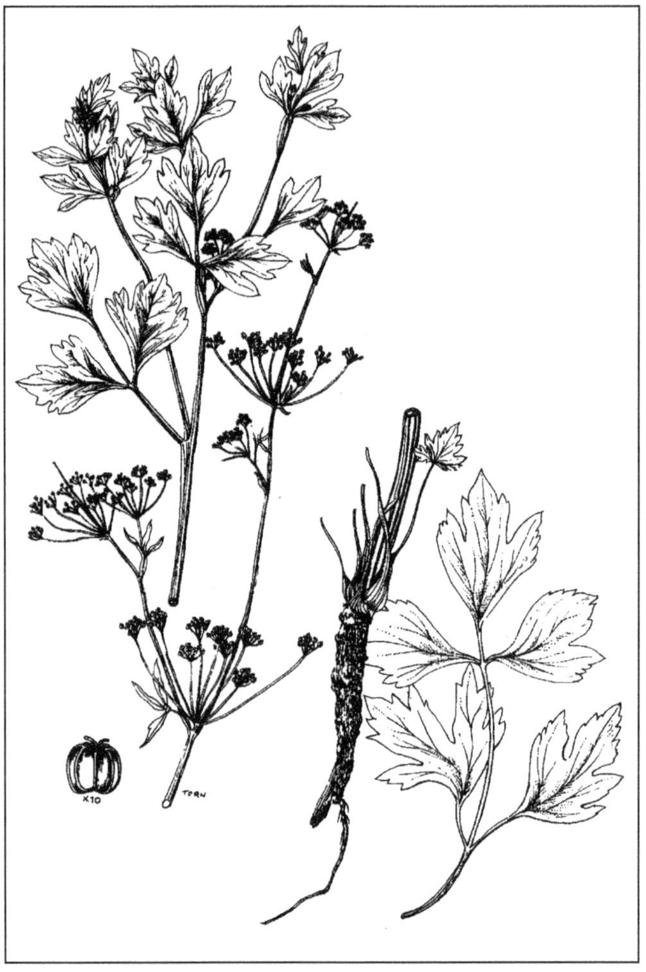

Figure 11 - Celery (*Apium graveolens*)

Medicinal Uses in the Medieval Period:
According to Assaph Harofe the plant which grew in streams was called 'karpasa damia' and was a hot drug used for curing kidneys, infected lesions, and skin diseases.[234] al-Kindi noted the use of celery seeds in treating stomach disorders and in the preparation of ointments to improve the memory.[235] Maimonides in his medical treatises mentions many uses of the plant. For instance: the oil in which celery seeds are fried was a component in a clyster and in theriac and also for urine flow, while the root of the plant was considered a general medication for strengthening.[236] Daud al-Antaki noted among other uses that it serves as a diuretic, a cure for jaundice, to promote appetite and memory, and to relieve respiratory problems.[237]

Traditional Medicine:
Arabs in Israel use marsh celery (*Apium nodiflorum*) to treat diseases of the spleen and it is also used as a stimulant.[238] Yemenite Jews use the aromatic celery to stimulate bowel movement, as a light purgative, to cure hemorrhoids, to dissolve kidney stones, to increase urine flow and to treat swellings. An extract from the seeds is used to treat toothache and gum inflammation.[239] In Iraq, the roots are used as a diuretic and the seeds as a stimulant, to dispel gases, arouse sexual desire, calm nerves and as component in a preparation against rheumatism.[240] In Egypt the seeds, which are sold in the bazaars, serve as a diuretic, emenagogue and to dispel gases.[241] Celery seeds are used in traditional medicine to dispel gases, as stimulants, emmenagogues, painkillers, nerve strengtheners and are effective against stomach pains.[242]

Cherry

Scientific name: *Prunus (Cerasus) sp.* (Rosaceae)

Description:
The cherry is a deciduous tree with fruit growing in bunches on spikes, or as individual berries on long thorns. The fruit ripens in summer and its colour is dark red (sweet cherry) or yellow, pink and black (sour cherry). The tree is cultivated in high, mountainous areas.[243] In our region there are two types of cherry which are used as food and for medicinal purposes:

Sweet Cherry (*Prunus avium*)	Hebrew: Gudgedan Arabic: Qrats mahlab
Sour Cherry (*Prunus vulgaris*)	Hebrew: Duvdevan hamutz Arabic: Qarasiya[244]

Identification:
In medieval literature the cherry was commonly called 'hab al-malukh' (king seed). The term 'kerasia' sometimes means *Prunus ursina* and sometimes *Prunus cerasia* because their morphological and linguistic similarity created confusion and caused an interchange of terminology.[245]

History:
The general name of cherry covers various types of fruit of the rose family. The Hebrew names 'gudgedaniot' (in the Mishna) and 'gadgedaniot' (in the Talmud) were wrongly identified by Jewish commentators with 'duvdevaniot.' It seems that the cherry was not known in the region during biblical, mishnaic and talmudic times, never held any place of importance in the economy and was not agriculturally cultivated.[246] From historical sources and archaeological-

234 Assaph, 4, p. 414.

235 al-Kindi, Nos. 1-2, 59, 113-114, 211, 225.

236 Maimonides, Poisons, p. 111; Maimonides, Aphorisms, 9:47; 18:32; 21:65, 70, 80.; Maimonides, Regimen, 2:10.

237 al-Antaki, p. 270. Cf. Ibn al-Baytar, al-Jami, IV, pp. 53-56; Leclerc, No. 1902.

238 Dafni, Edible, p. 69.

239 Reiani, p. 10, No. 11.

240 Hooper, p. 86; al-Rawi & Chaakravarty, p. 14 which gives detailed contents of substances.

241 Ducros, p. 31.

242 For details, including contents of substances, see: Uphof, p. 42. Cf. Grieve, p. 182.

243 Plants & Animals, XII, pp. 112-113.

244 Issa, Dictionary, p. 148, No. 18; Dinsmore & Dalman, No. 660; Maimonides, Glossaire, p. 103, No. 371.

245 Maimonides, Glossaire, p. 23, No. 330. Detailed discussion in Amar, Production, p. 107.

246 Feliks, Fruit Trees, pp. 265-267; Amar, Production, p. 107; Low, III, pp. 169-175.

botanical discoveries in Europe the cherry appears for the first time in the Roman period.[247] Dioscorides noted that the plant *kerasia* was used to treat the stomach and was known to cause constipation. The resin of the tree served as a remedy for cough, to improve appetite and the eyesight and to eliminate stones in the urinary tract.[248] It seems that the cherry tree arrived in the Land of Israel only during the Crusader period. The first evidence of its growth in the country is derived from the description by the Russian pilgrim, Daniel, who visited the Holy Land during the years 1106-1108 CE and noted their cultivation in the Hebron's mountains.[249]

Medicinal Uses in Jerusalem:
The use of the 'qarasiya' (cherry) leaves as part of the treatment for eye inflammation is referred to in a Muslim legal document of 1738. The treatment was applied by the Jerusalem physician and surgeon Hayim ha-Yehudi to his Christian patient Abraham Balata Ibn Alina.[250]

Cherry in the Levant:
During the Ayyubid period, al-Baghdadi noted that "cherries were not to be found in Egypt but could be found in al-Sham, in Asia Minor and in other countries."[251] In that same period (13th century) Ibn al-Baytar wrote that in Damascus there was a species known as 'qarasiya ba'albeki', which was also called 'hab al-malukh.'[252] al-Badri listed the names of seven species in al-Sham including this variety.[253] Maimonides describes the 'qarasiya' and claimed that its fruit resembled the plum though it was smaller, had a sour taste and could be found in Egypt and the Land of Israel.[254] According to al-Dimashqi, the 'qarasiya' was one of 90 species of plant growing in Mount Lebanon from which one could make a living by gathering its fruit.[255] During the Mamluk period the cherry was included among the rare fruits in the Land of Israel.[256] At the end of this period the cherry seems to have disappeared entirely from the plant life of the country as Rabbi Ovadia of Bartenura testifies: "One cannot find the 'gadganiot' which are the 'qarasiya' neither the sweet nor the sour kind."[257]

Medicinal Uses in the Medieval Period:
Maimonides claims that cherries are a light purgative.[258] Saladino d' Ascoli describes the 'grano rigon' - (royal seed) or 'hab al-malukh' - that had two types of fruit: small and large, and which was hot and dry and was used as a purgative and emetic. The seeds produced an oil resembling almond oil.[259] Daud al-Antaki claimed that the 'qarasiya' was a cold and dry medicine to treat depression, fainting fits, thirst, cough, loss of memory, internal wounds and for obstructions in the urinary tract.[260]

Traditional Medicine and General Uses:
The fruits are used for food and for the production of jams, compotes and alcoholic beverages. Oil produced from the seeds was used as food or in cosmetic preparations.[261] In Europe the fruit thorns of various types of cherry were used as an astringent a stimulant and a cure for respiration problems and anemia.[262]

Chicory

Scientific name: *Cichorium intybus* (Compositae)
Hebrew: 'Olash tarbuti Arabic: Hundaba

Other types: *Cichorium endivia, Cichorium pumilum*[263]

Description:
The chicory is an annual herbaceous plant, stiffly erect and branching with hairy stems and leaves. The leaves are split and the flowers are tongue-shaped, wide and blue-petalled with large cluster heads (3-4 cm.) This is one among nine different species in the world. The cultivated variety is similar to the wild one, but it is customary to break off the cluster heads in order to thicken the roots. Another cultivated variety is grown in India.[264]

History:
In the Mishna the 'olashim' are mentioned in connection with the laws for the sabbatical year and cross-fertilization. The reference is apparently to the common chicory which is one of the varieties which can be used as the bitter herbs required for the Passover meal.[265]

Dioscorides distinguished between the wild and the cultivated variety, which was called *endive* and was used as a remedy for the stomach, heart and eyes and for scorpion stings.[266] The Talmud also describes the two varieties of chicory. Some of the Jewish medieval commentators identified this plant by its Arabic name 'hundaba.'[267]

---

247 Zohary & Hopf, pp. 171-172.

248 Dioscorides, I.157.

249 Daniel in Raba, p. 51, n. 279, in the source cheresie.

250 Cohen, 18 Century, p. 327, No. 283.

251 al-Baghdadi, p. 76. A distinction should be made between 'kerasia' - cherry, and the rest of the section which refers to another fruit.

252 Ibn al-Baytar, al-Jami, IV, p. 8; Leclerc, No. 1749; Ibn al-Baytar, Tafsir, p. 148.

253 al-Badri, p. 116.

254 Maimonides, Glossaire, p. 23, No. 330. This description corresponds both to the sour cherry and also to (*Prunus cerasia*) which has two varieties: sweet and sour. Detailed discussion in: Amar, Ibn al-Baytar, p. 61, No. 34.

255 al-Dimashqi, p. 199.

256 al-Qalqashandi p. 87; Borchard, p. 87.

257 Rabbi Ovadia of Bartenura in: Ya'ari, Igrot, p. 132.

258 Maimonides, Regimen, 2:7.

259 Saladino, p. 98, No. 174.

260 al-Antaki, pp. 255-256.

261 Plants & Animals, XII, pp. 112-113.

262 Uphof, p. 430; Hill, p. 392.

263 Maimonides, Glossaire, p. 41, No. 114; p. 81, No. 285; Dinsmore & Dalman, No. 1032; Issa, Dictionary, p. 48, No. 12

264 Plants & Animals, XI, pp. 180-181. Description of cultivated varieties in: Loewenfeld & Back, p. 97; Hill, p. 377; Uphof, p. 130.

265 Feliks, Shevi'it, p. 168; Low, I, p. 287.

266 Dioscorides, II.132.

267 Discussion in: Feliks, Yerushalmi, p. 94, n. 394.

Medicinal Uses in Jerusalem:
Refael Malki was opposed to the medicinal use of 'iniaba' juice.[268] From an 18th century legal document in the Muslim court archives in Jerusalem, it appears that 'hundaba' juice was used as a remedy for the illness of pregnant women.[269] The details are described in the charge sheet brought by a Muslim Arab from the village of Silwan against the physician Salmon ben ha-Yehudi (who was acquitted by the judge). The physician had recommended using the water of chicory and the yellow pond lily to cure the illness of the pregnant wife, but her husband had given her cassia water which caused the woman to miscarry and to die. David de Silva asserted that chicory induces sleep and improve the conditions of the internal organs.[270]

Chicory in the Levant:
al-Ghafiqi quoted many physicians in connection with various types of 'hundaba.' Some of them attest that the plant was called 'antubiya' in Greater Syria.[271] Ibn al-Baytar in his entry 'antubiya' quotes Ibn Masawayh who claimed that this was the 'hundaba' to be found in al-Sham.[272] The plant 'hundaba' was listed among the crops grown in the al-Sham region during the Mamluk period.[273] Remains of cultivated chicory seeds were found in the Red Tower archaeological excavations (13th century) in the Sharon area.[274] According to Hayim Vital, the juice of the chicory called 'hindaba' was a component in a medication to relieve stomach swellings.[275]

Medicinal Uses in the Medieval Period:
According to al-Kindi, the chicory was used as an ointment for the nose and for treating skin rashes and the stings of scorpions and spiders.[276] al-Biruni described an unusual use of 'hundaba': as a component in a drugged drink which could cause death by an overdose.[277] Maimonides claimed that the seed of "the 'tarcascon' which is a bitter herb" was a component in a preparation for foul breath,[278] and recommended the 'hundaba' as the best medicine for curing diseases of the liver and to cure skin diseases.[279] al-Qazwini quotes Ibn Sina who described the use of the plant to treat rheumatism, eye inflammation, white spots in the eye, scorpion or wasp stings and malaria.[280] Daud al-Antaki in his entry 'hundaba' mentions uses such as: curing malaria, fever, headache, jaundice, and problems of the liver, spleen and kidneys. As a beverage, it strengthened the stomach, reduced swellings and prevented the inflammation of the eyes.[281]

Traditional Medicine:
The leaves of the common chicory are used as food and in sauces. The roots and cluster heads are a coffee substitute.[282] Arabs in Israel use chicory juice to clear the blood, to stimulate the urinary system, to treat constipation, arthritic pains, rash and light injuries, to eliminate intestinal worms and to cure internal diseases such as malaria and jaundice.[283] The roots of the cultivated chicory are considered as a strengthening substance and are used to cure diseases of the stomach and the gall bladder.[284] In Iraq, the plant is used as a diuretic, a purgative and a cure for stomach problems. The roots are used among other things as a cooling medicine to treat the gall bladder and also as a cathartic drug, a diuretic, a strengthener and to reduce fever.[285] The cultivated chicory is widely used as a remedy and a food in Europe as well.[286]

Cinnamon

Scientific name: *Cinnamomum zeylanicum* (Lauraceae)
Hebrew: Kinamon Arabic: Dar sini, Qirfah[287]

Description:
The cinnamon species comprises 275 varieties of large trees that grow in India and Eastern Asia. Some of these are of medicinal use, or used for spice, or grown as garden trees. The Ceylon cinnamon (from Sri Lanka) is a large, tall, tropical tree or shrub with a pungent scent. Its leaves are wide with prominent veins, its flowers are small and yellow and its fruit is a dark, grape-like berry. The spice, which is made from the bark of the tree is marketed till today, as it has been in the past, in the form of rolled pieces of bark or as a ground powder.[288]

History:
Cinnamon is one of the plants which have been used since early times as a condiment, for incense and for medication. It is mentioned in the Bible a few times and in various contexts such as: the brazen woman who perfumed her bed (Proverbs, 7:17) or as an ingredient in sacred anointing oil (Exodus, 30:23). The Talmud mentions the frankincense for the Temple in which cinnamon was one of the components.[289] Hippocrates wrote about it and listed its medicinal uses. Disocorides

268 Malki, p. 79.

269 Cohen, 18 Century, p. 325, No. 279.

270 Amar, de Silva, p. 119.

271 al-Ghafiqi, No. 263.

272 Ibn al-Baytar, al-Jami, p. 66; Leclerc, No. 181.

273 al-Badri, p. 175.

274 Pringle, p. 187.

275 Benajahu, pp. 97-98.

276 al-Kindi, Nos. 42, 52, 54, 173-174.

277 al-Biruni, II, p. 60.

278 Maimonides, Sexual, 7:1. Maimonides says that this is one of the names for chicory of the desert.

279 Maimonides, Aphorisms, 9:71, 106; 21:74.

280 al-Qazwini, p. 264. Cf. Ibn Sina, p. 298.

281 al-Antaki, p. 336. Cf. Ibn al-Baytar, al-Jami, IV, pp. 198-200; Leclerc, No. 2263; al-Biruni, I, p. 330

282 Dafni, Edible, p. 98; Chizik, p. 708.

283 Dafni, Edible, p. 98.

284 Uphof, p. 130.

285 Hooper, p. 99. Cf. Chizik, p. 731. Contents f substances in: al-Rawi & Chaakravarty, p. 26; Chizik, pp. 654-656.

286 Grieve, p. 197.

287 Maimonides, Glossaire, p. 37, No. 95; Issa, Dictionary, p. 49, No. 5; Ibn Rushd, No. 165.

288 Hill, p. 443; Zohary, p. 309.

289 For discussion about cinnamon in the Bible and Jewish sources see: Feliks, World, pp. 263-264.

described the *kinamomon* and stressed its use in regulating menstruation and in aborting the fetus. He also believed that the substance was effective in treating toxicity caused by poisonous creatures. Among the medicinal qualities he listed were: increasing urine flow, curing cough and kidney ailments.[290] The Talmud lists the 'zangbila and darzina' as the varieties of spices which a woman "puts into her mouth" on the Sabbath. The Gaonim and Rashi in their Talmudic commentaries, identify the 'darzina' with Chinese cinnamon. Another name that appears in the writings of the Jewish Sages and which is identified with cinnamon is the 'kilofa.' The research scholar, Feliks, identifies this with the cinnamon bark, which is called 'kirfa' in Arabic.[291]

Medicinal Uses in Jerusalem:
In the Genizah letters of the 11th century, cinnamon is mentioned as a merchandise traded in the Land of Israel including Jerusalem, Tyre and Ramlah.[292] According to Refael Malki cinnamon was a component in a general medicinal drink for the poor inhabitants of Jerusalem as well as an ingredient in other medicinal preparations.[293] Cinnamon was mentioned by David de Silva as a stomach strengthener, which also helps digestion and improves the sight.[294]

Cinnamon in the Levant:
In a 13th century register of customs duties, cinnamon was included in a list of imported merchandise traded in Acre.[295] The scholar, Ashtor, noted that these expensive products arrived overland by caravan route from Iran and Iraq because sea transportation would damage them.[296] Cinnamon also appears in a list of substances (1233 CE) imported by the Italians from Syria to Europe.[297] Cinnamon spice and other medicinal substances were purchased by Italian traders in Ramlah during the 15th century.[298]

Medicinal Uses in the Medieval Period:
Assaph Harofe described the "cinnamon which was called 'qirfah' in Arabic" and listed its uses: improving digestion, increasing urine flow, as an emmenagogue, for fetal abortions, as a cure for eyes, ears, cough, cold, skin disease and for removing obstructions in the urinary tract.[299] al-Kindi used the 'dar sini' as a medicine for general strengthening and cause a sense of well-being, to fortify the stomach and liver, and to treat the teeth and breathing problems.[300] The 'qirfah' is identified with the internal part of the cinnamon tree and served mostly as a substitute for the 'dar sini.' al-Kindi used it to cure deep depression, to improve hearing and to relieve neck pains.[301]

Maimonides listed many medicinal uses for cinnamon by all its different names: a component in cathartic drugs, in a medication against poisons, bites and stings by poisonous creatures, in a medicine against obstructions in the stomach and for hemorrhoids, as a strengthening medicine and as a spice.[302] Maimonides also noted its use as an effective preparation for coitus, to maintain erection during cohabitation, and in a medication called 'the great atriphal' which among other things strengthens the limbs and aids coitus.[303] al-Ghafiqi and Ibn al-Baytar in their entries 'dar sini' list the names, types and various medicinal uses of cinnamon.[304] In his entry 'dahan al-dar sini' Ibn al-Baytar described its use as medicinal oil, according to Dioscorides.[305]

Traditional Medicine:
Cinnamon is used by the Negev Bedouins as a medicinal drug against cough, throat pain and gases.[306] The use of cinnamon as a remedy is widespread among Yemenite Jews. The substance is considered as a medicinal drug that strengthens the body, lengthens life, induces good humour, relaxes the nerves, etc. Cinnamon is used as a medicine against insanity, to strengthen the eyesight, to relieve coughs and colds, to expel phlegm, to improve the voice, to relax the gullet, to cleanse the passages in the stomach, liver, kidneys and urinary tract. Cinnamon was a component in a medication to stop belching and hiccups, for fetal abortions, and to treat scorpion stings and drunkenness.[307] The Jews of Iraq used it in medications for many types of illness: kidney stones, scabies, to stop menstruation and for chills.[308] In Egypt, the 'dar sini' is a medicinal drug used for diarrhea, as a cure for stomach illnesses and as a stimulant[309] while in Iraq and Iran, the substance was used in making a tea, and to treat excessive secretion of saliva.[310] The use of the cinnamon tree for remedial purposes was also an accepted one in Europe.[311]

Medicinal Qualities and General Uses:
The bark of the cinnamon tree was used as a spice, mainly in baked goods and in confectionary. Cinnamon was also used in perfumes and in incense.[312] The bark of the tree contains

290 Dioscorides, I.13.

291 Feliks, World, p. 264.

292 For example: Gil, p. 142, No. 470; p. 272, No. 508.

293 Malki, pp. 62, 66-67.

294 Amar, de Silva, p. 136.

295 Assises, II, p. 173.

296 Ashtor, Levant, p. 33.

297 Venice Laws, p. 285. Translation and analysis in: Prawer, Colonial, p. 480.

298 Details and sources in: Ashtor, Trade, p. 290, n. 83.

299 Assaph, 4, p. 394.

300 al-Kindi, Nos. 3, 106, 213, 216. Cf. Ibn Sina, pp. 288-289; al-Biruni, II, pp. 92-93.

301 al-Kindi, Nos. 3, 68, 109. Cf. al-Biruni, I, pp. 265-266.

302 Maimonides, Aphorisms, 9:46; 13:6; 21:42, 80; 23:66; Maimonides, Poisons, pp. 103, 109.

303 Maimonides, Sexual, Introduction, 2; 13:1; Maimonides, Regimen, 3:11.

304 al-Ghafiqi, No. 232; Ibn al-Baytar, al-Jami, II, pp. 83-85; Leclerc, No. 841. Cf. al-Antaki, p. 149.

305 Ibn al-Baytar, al-Jami, II, p. 104; Leclerc, No. 902.

306 Abu-Rabia, p. 20.

307 Reiani, p. 16, No. 26.

308 Reference in: Ben-Yakov, p. 752.

309 Ducros, p. 181.

310 Hooper, p. 100.

311 Grieve, p. 202.

312 About the tree, its cultivation and marketing see: Uphof, p. 131; Hill, pp. 443-444; Loewenfeld & Back, p. 101.

essential oils and served as a stimulating drug, a light astringent and a disinfectant also intended for treating the stomach.[313]

Conclusion:
It appears that in ancient times as in our own day, products derived from Ceylonese cinnamon or related varieties are being marketed. Physicians and writers have tried to differentiate between them, but it appears that the uses for all of them are similar in principle, and in medieval times one variety could substitute for another in compound medications. In addition to its use as a spice, cinnamon has been used in traditional medicine and as a medicinal substance in various cultures from the early periods of history until present day. Evidence of such use in Jerusalem is given by Refael Malki. It seems that the medicinal use of the cinnamon tree was widespread in the Levant during the Middle Ages, since the international trade routes for cinnamon passed through the Land of Israel.

Clove

Scientific name: *Eugenia caryophyllata* (Myrtaceae)
Hebrew: Tziporen Arabic: Qaranful, Zir

Description:
The clove tree is an Asian evergreen tree which grows up to 10-13 meters. Its bark is hard and gray, its leaves are narrow and slightly pink when young, and then turn green. The flower buds contain a fragrant oil.[314]

History:
The clove tree was cultivated in the early periods of Asian history mainly for the flower buds which were plucked and dried.[315] Cloves as well as pepper, cinnamon and nutmeg were among the first spices mentioned in Indian and Chinese literature.[316] The etymological source for the name 'clove' comes from the French 'clou' which means nail (the Hebrew term 'tziporen' means fingernail). Historical evidence for the use of cloves can be found as early as the 3rd century BCE in China and as an imported substance in the 2nd century CE in Alexandria. By the 4th century the clove was a well-known spice in Europe and in the 8th century it became an important commodity in international trade between East and West. al-Qazwini provides us with interesting data, and reported that the clove is a tree that grows on certain Indian islands and its fruits are similar to the jasmine, though darker in colour. al-Qazwini adds that the islanders boiled the fruits before they exported them to prevent others from cultivating them elsewhere.[317]

Medicinal Uses in Jerusalem:
Benevenutus listed the clove among the substances in his 'Jerusalem Electuary' which he used to prescribe for curing cataracts. Other substances in this remedy were: honey, beaver testicle glands, saffron and coconut.[318] Refael Malki described some general remedies that were used to treat the poor members of the Jewish community in Jerusalem, and the clove was one of the important substances in these remedies.[319] In a letter dated 1045 CE found in the Cairo Genizah, a Jewish merchant from Cairo wrote to his partner in Jerusalem about a purchase of the expensive substance 'qirfah qaranful' identified as clove.[320] Clove was also mentioned as medicinal substances by David de Silva.[321]

Clove in the Levant:
The 'giroffle' (clove) was mentioned as a merchandise which was taxed in the Crusader Kingdom of Jerusalem during the 13th century,[322] and it was also listed among the substances exported to Europe.[323] This trade continued well after the Crusaders left the Levant. For example, cloves and other spices were mentioned as bought by a Venetian trader in the 15th century in Ramlah.[324] Clove was one of the delicate spices, light in weight and expensive, which were transported overland. The scholar, Ashtor, estimated that their price in the Levant was low and therefore European merchants found it worthwhile to buy and transport them to their countries.[325]

Medicinal Uses in the Medieval Period:
al-Kindi described the intensive use of the clove in medicinal preparations to freshen the breath, treat the gums and stomach disorders.[326] Maimonides reported on different medicinal applications of clove as a component in a general remedy which also included pomegranate seeds and sugar.[327] Elsewhere he quotes al-Tamimi who asserted that the clove was very useful as a cure for hysteria, epilepsy and as a component in a remedy used to treat heart palpitations.[328] Maimonides also claimed it was a component in an aphrodisiac pill used to stimulate erection and improve sexual pleasure.[329] al-Qazwini quotes Ibn Sina who asserted that the clove sweetened the breath, improved eyesight and prevented the loss of consciousness. al-Qazwini also wrote that the clove is effective against nausea, and that its scent strengthened the brain and heart and caused one to be cheerful.[330]

---

[313] Uphof, p. 131; Hill, p. 443; Reiani, p.16, No. 26; Contents of substances in Riaz.

[314] Singh, p. 227.

[315] Zohary, p. 455

[316] On the history of cloves and its various names see in detail: Singh; Maimonides, Regimen, p. 97.

[317] al-Qazwini, p. 299.

[318] Benevenutus, p. 37. On the source and its problematics see my introduction.

[319] Malki, pp. 62-63, 67.

[320] Gil, No. 485.

[321] Amar, de Silva, p.137.

[322] Assises, p. 174.

[323] Pegolotti, p. 63.

[324] Ashtor, Levant, p. 290. In detail: Ashtor, Spices.

[325] Ashtor, Levant, p. 33.

[326] al-Kindi, Nos. 3, 106, 108, 152, 213, 225-226; Cf. al-Biruni, I, p. 265; II, pp. 101-102.

[327] Maimonides, Answers, 21:6.

[328] Maimonides, Aphorisms, 21:96.

[329] Maimonides, Sexual, Introduction, 15.

[330] al-Qazwini, pp. 229-230. Cf. Ibn Sina, pp. 416-417.

Traditional Medicine and General Uses:
All parts of the clove tree contain oil which is used in the cosmetic industry as well as a component in soaps, toothpastes and mouth washes. Clove oil also serves as a digestive aid, a disinfectant and to relieve toothache.[331] Cloves are often used as a spice in certain beverages.[332] Yemenite Jews use cloves to prevent vomiting and nausea, to strengthen the stomach, liver, eyesight and heart, to disinfect the renal tracts, cure colds and relieve toothache. It is also used both as aphrodisiac and as a contraceptive.[333] In Middle Eastern countries the clove is still used as an expectorant, stimulant and for the treatment of throat irritations. Clove oil was also applied to relieve headache and toothache.[334]

Colocynth

Scientific name: *Citrillus colocynthis* (Cucurbitareae)
Hebrew: Avatiah ha-paku'a Arabic: Handhal[335]

Description:
The colocynth (also called bitter gourd or bitter apple) is a perennial herbaceous plant, which grows on sandy soil and in desert gorges. Its fruits are rounded, the size of oranges, and their taste is very bitter. This species grows mainly in the Arabian-Sahara region and scholars believe that it might be the original species for the domesticated watermelon.[336]

History:
The special characteristics of the colocynth were mentioned in the Bible (II Kings, 4:39-40). According to medieval Jewish commentators the plant was identified as 'handhal.' Colocynth oil is mentioned in the Mishna as one of the oils that may be used for lighting the Sabbath eve candles. The medicinal uses of the plant were known at that time as well. Dioscorides described the use of the *kolokunthis* pulp as a purgative, expectorant, abortive and to relieve toothache.[337]

Medicinal Uses in Jerusalem:
Refael Malki who worked in Jerusalem during the 16th century, wrote that "the 'colocontida' which is called 'handhal' in Arabic" was used as one of many substances in a general remedy for strengthening the heart and brain.[338]

Colocynth in the Levant:
Ibn al-Khair al-Ashbili informs us in his entry 'Handhal' that some people think this is the 'batih al-falastini' while other Andalusian contemporaries were of the opinion that the 'dala'a' is the 'batih al-falastini.'[339] We can learn about the use and trade of the plant from an unusual historical source - personal names. For example: Mahmad Ibn Mahmad Abu al-Tib al-Handhali (d. 948 CE), who was the 'kadi' (judge) of Ramlah, and the Jewish scholar, Rabbi Yehoshua Ben Yosef Handali (17th century) from Safed, who also worked in Jerusalem.[340] They were both named after the colocynth plant. In an Italian trade book of the 14th century, the 'coloquinta' was mentioned among other commodities that were traded in Mediterranean ports.[341]

Medicinal Uses in the Medieval Period:
Many medieval physicians inform us about the use of the colocynth as a medication, mainly as a strong cathartic. al-Kindi, for example, described an extensive use of the plant as part of certain remedies for the treatment of itching, arthritis, to cure insanity and as an expectorant.[342] Maimonides reports that its roots were part of a "very important" remedy for scorpion stings.[343] al-Qazwini wrote that its leaves cured hemorrhage, depression and epilepsy. He added that after boiling the fruit in milk it could be used as a purgative and that the roots are used to treat the bites of snakes and scorpions. It was also used as a remedy for leprosy, arthritis and other diseases. [344] Ibn al-Baytar mentions different ways of collecting the plant and the medical applications of its fruit: to treat constipation, headache, toothache, muscle pains and spasms, epilepsy, lung disease, depression, diseases of the kidney and of the urinary tract. The leaves were used to stop hemorrhages, reduce swellings, and treat skin diseases such as boils and leprosy. The roots were used to treat scorpion and snake bites, and to increase the quantity of milk for breastfeeding women.[345]

Oil pressed out of the colocynth seeds had medicinal qualities as well.[346] Saladino d'Ascoli, the Italian pharmacist of the 15th century, described similar uses of the plant and warned, as did Maimonides, of side effects such as causing harm to the liver, heart, stomach and internal hemorrhages.[347] Daud al-Antaki reported on the medicinal uses of colocynth fruit and oil such as: curing skin diseases, insanity, excessive phlegm, scorpion stings and to treat pains.[348] It should be mentioned that other wild varieties of the Cucurbitaceae family such as bryony (*Bryonia certica*) and squirting cucumber (*Ecballium elaterium*) and vegetable (*Luffa cylindrica*) were used as medicine in the Levant as well as the cultivated varieties: watermelon (*Citrillus vulgaris*) and apple cucumber (*Cucunis dudaim*).[349]

331 Uphof, p. 202.

332 Ibid.; Hill, pp. 445-446.

333 Reiani, p. 23, No. 45.

334 Hooper, p. 118.

335 Maimonides, Glossaire, p. 52, No. 158; Leclerc, Nos. 1317, 1741; Issa, Dictionary, p. 50, No. 9.

336 Plants & Animals, XII, 121-122; Feinbrun-Dothan, p. 655.

337 Dioscorides, IV.178.

338 Malki, p. 67.

339 al-Ashbili, p. 235.

340 Amar, Colocynthis.

341 Pegolotti; Heyd.

342 al-Kindi, No. 47, 138. Cf. Ibn Sina, pp. 316-317.

343 Maimonides, Poisons, p. 118.

344 al-Qazwini, p. 246.

345 Ibn al-Baytar, al-Jami, II, p. 36; Leclerc, No. 714. Cf. al-Biruni, I, pp. 131-132; II, pp. 89-90.

346 Leclerc, No. 952.

347 Saladino, p. 156.

348 al-Antaki, pp. 132-133.

349 See the corresponding entries in: Lev, Materials.

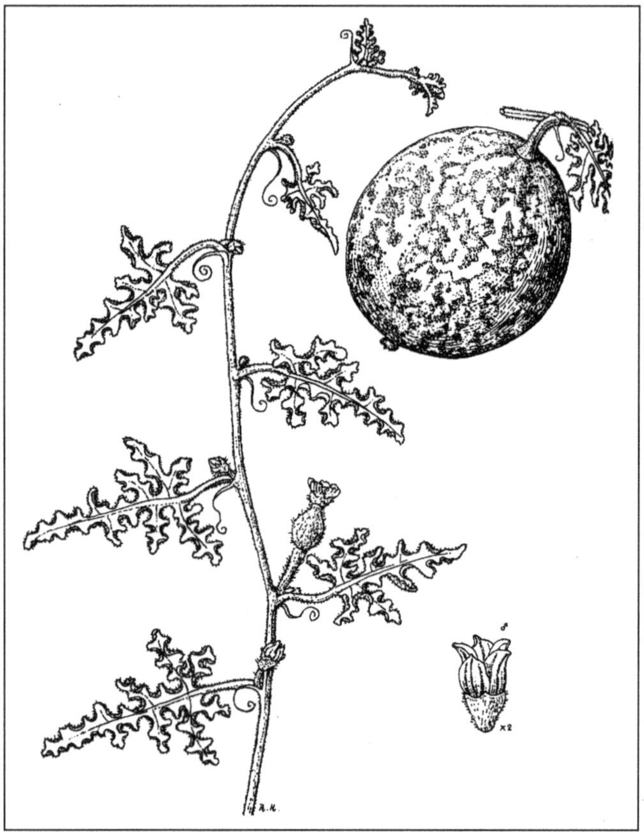

Figure 12 - Colocynth (*Citrillus colocynthis*)

Traditional Medicine:
Arab traditional medicines include the use of the fruit and seeds of the colocynth for treating diabetes, paralysis, face spasms, hemorrhoids, arthritis, and pains of the stomach and heart.[350] The Bedouins of the Sinai desert used the plant as a purgative and to treat muscle pain and toothaches.[351] Yemenite Jews used the fruits to treat stomach worms and jaundice.[352] The pulp of the colocynth was widely used in Europe, India, the Middle East and North Africa to treat various symptoms and diseases such as warts, and internal cancers (leukemia and breast cancer).[353]

In many countries it is also used as a cathartic drug in modern as well as traditional medicine,[354] because the pulp contains many glycosides, which irritate the stomach and intestines and cause vomiting and diarrhea. The seeds contain 17% oil, which is edible.[355] al-Qazwini reproted that the water in which colocynth fruits were soaked was used to kill fleas.[356] Ibn al-Baytar quotes Ibn Amran who wrote that oil which was boiled together with colocynth fruit's peel prevented graying hair and dyed it black.[357] In some regions of the Middle East, colocynth seeds are still eaten by people as well as animals.[358]

Conclusions:
The colocynth is a plant, which has medicinal uses known in the East for many centuries since earliest times. This plant is a good example of the ability of the ancients to locate medicinal plants. In this case, modern science has proved that this plant contained active substances, which were effective for the medicinal problems mentioned above.[359] The colocynth was an important medicinal plant in Jerusalem throughout the ages and was a valuable market commodity. We have evidence that Jewish citizens of Gaza in the 19th century bought quantities of colocynth fruits from the local Bedouins and distributed them throughout Europe for medicinal uses.[360] However, although this fruit is still sold in Jerusalem and in other Mediterranean markets for traditional uses, it is hardly used in modern medicine.

Deer Balls (Harts Truffles)

Scientific name: *Lycoperdon lividium* (Lycoperdaceae)
Hebrew: Avkit ma'afira Arabic: Ghushinah, Karshna, Kashnaj

Description:
Deer balls are species of fungi (mushroom) of the *Gasteromycetes* genus. The spore pods are globular (4-6 cm.) and are filled with spores that, when ripened, spread around like dust as soon as the pods are touched. Deer balls are common to Israel and the Levant. They grow in winter in forest groves, and the pods remain intact until the summer. The mushroom is edible before the spores are formed.[361]

Identification:
Issa identified the 'ghushna' as *Morchella esculenta*[362] which does not grow in Israel, while Leclerc says it is a species of Lycoperdon[363]. Another variety of this plant is the *Lycoperdon clavatum* which is called 'maskia' in Arabic and 'clubmoss' in English.[364]

In accordance with the medieval description of the mushroom plant and its habitat, we agree with Leclerc's identification and specify it more exactly as *Lycoperdon lividium.*

Medicinal Uses in Jerusalem:
Ibn al-Baytar claimed that the 'ghushinah' grows in Beit al-Maqdis (Jerusalem) and is also known as 'kashnaj.'[365] Daud al-Antaki wrote that the 'ghushinah' grows in the 'al-Haram'

[350] In detail: Palevitz et al, p. 17.

[351] Levey, Bedouins, p. 75.

[352] Reiani, p. 16, No. 28.

[353] Hartwell, p. 94; Grieve, pp. 49-50.

[354] Uphof, p. 133; Hill, p. 259.

[355] On the contents of the substances in the various parts of the plant and their medicinal uses see in detail: Darwish-Said et al; Hooper, p. 101.

[356] al-Qazwini, p. 246.

[357] Ibn al-Baytar, al-Jami, II, p. 116; Leclerc, No. 952; al-Antaki, p. 133.

[358] For example: Hooper, p. 101.

[359] Darwish-Said et al.

[360] Amar, Colocynthis.

[361] Plants & Animals, IX, p. 162.

[362] Zohary, pp. 118-119; Issa, Dictionary, p. 113, No. 3.

[363] Leclerc, Nos. 1644, 1938.

[364] Issa, Dictionary, p. 113.

[365] Ibn al-Baytar, al-Jami, III, p. 152.

(Temple Mount).[366] The medieval uses of the 'ghushinah'[367] and the 'kashnaj'[368] are described in the relevant entries by Ibn al-Baytar.

Traditional and Popular Uses:
Certain varieties of the Lycoperdon species are used for food in different countries of the world.[369] In early times and also in 19th to 20th century England, medicinal use of the spore pods was made.[370]

Dodder of Thyme (Lesser or Heath Dodder)

Scientific name: *Cuscuta epithymum* (Convolvulaceae)
Hebrew: Kashut ha-koranit Arabic: Aftimun[371]

Description:
There are 170 varieties of dodder and 11 of them grow in Israel. The dodder of thyme is a parasitic vine which entwines itself around plants of the Mediterranean region such as the headed thyme, prickly burnet and the local stachys in Israel. Its stems are threadlike and leafless, and do not contain any chlorophyll. It has small flowers and tiny seeds.[372]

History:
Dodder of thyme is known throughout the Near East and is mentioned in medical writings in Mesopotamia mainly as a remedy for stomach disorders.[373] Dioscorides notes the use of *Epithumon* especially for treating mucus and black bile.[374]

Medicinal Uses in Jerusalem:
al-Tamimi reported on the medicinal use of 'aftimun' in connection with Jerusalem.[375] Ishaq ibn Sulayman (Yitzhak ha-Israeli) noted that the 'aftimun' was call 'al-za'atira' by the people of Greater Syria, and that Jerusalem was one of the best sources for its supply.[376] In his entry "aftimun' Ibn al-Baytar describes the medicinal uses of the plant according to various physicians. One of them also claimed that Jerusalem was a good source for this medication.[377]

Medicinal Uses in the Medieval Period:
According to al-Kindi, the 'aftimun' was a component in a preparation for reducing fever.[378] Al-Biruni reported on its use for treating influenza, spasms, epilepsy and depression.[379] Ibn al-Baytar quoted the following medicinal uses of this plant according to classical and Arab physicians: treating various types of mucus (bile), nervous and mental disorders, muscular cramps, swellings and intestinal worms.[380] In a medical response to Sultan al-Afadhal, Maimonides notes that the dodder-'khasha' was a component of a medication for heart disease invented by Ibn Sina and that he recommends its use. In another letter, Maimonides does not recommend the use of dodder-'aftimun' jam because it causes the "purging of the intestines and their drying out." From other references it seems that the 'aftimun' served as a light purgative and was a hot and dry drug.[381] Saladino d'Ascoli mentioned the 'epitimu' as a medicine that should be found in every pharmacy and which retains its medicinal effectivity for the duration of a year.[382]

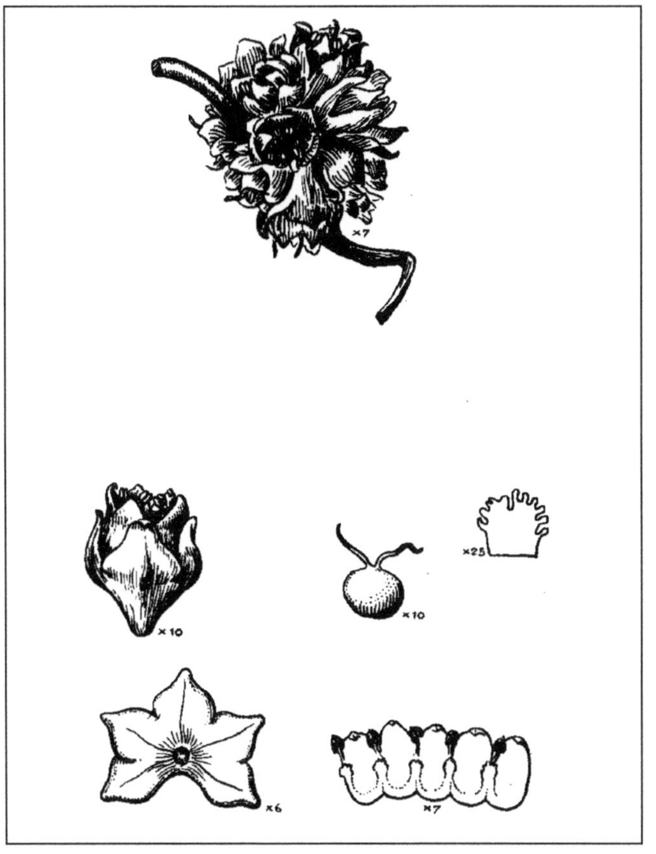

Figure 13 - Dodder of Thyme (*Cuscuta epithymum*)

Traditional Medicine:
The dodder plant is considered as a cathartic drug and a cure for liver complaints.[383] In Iran, Iraq and Europe it is used as an aid for digestion, to purify the blood and to reduce gases.[384]

[366] al-Antaki, p. 246.

[367] Ibn al-Baytar, al-Jami, III, p. 152; Leclerc, No. 1644; Ibn Sina, p. 469.

[368] Ibn al-Baytar, al-Jami, IV, p. 71; Leclerc, No. 1938.

[369] Uphof, p. 321; Grieve, p. 337.

[370] Grieve, pp. 337-338.

[371] Maimonides, Glossaire, p. 21, No.23; p. 60, No. 186; Serapion, No. 181; Issa, Dictionary, p. 63, No.6; Leclerc, No. 1161.

[372] Plants & Animals, XI, p. 41; Feinbrun-Dothan, p. 524.

[373] al-Kindi, p. 233, No.18.

[374] Dioscorides, IV.179.

[375] al-Tamimi, p. 19.

[376] Ishaq, p. 390.

[377] Ibn al-Baytar, al Jami, I, pp. 40-41; Leclerc, No. 112.

[378] al-Kindi, No. 113; al-Biruni, II, pp. 73-74.

[379] al-Biruni, I, pp. 35-36; Ibn Sina, pp. 201-202. Cf. al-Ghafiqi, No. 80.

[380] Ibn al-Baytar, al-Jami, I, pp. 40-41; Leclerc, No. 112.

[381] Maimonides, Answers, 3:13, 19; Maimonides, Aphorisms, 17:40; 21:80.

[382] Saladino, pp. 82, 112.

[383] Uphof, p. 165. Cf. Grieve, p.261.

[384] Hooper, p. 110. Cf. al-Rawi & Chaakravarty, p. 34 for the uses and qualities of substances of local varieties.

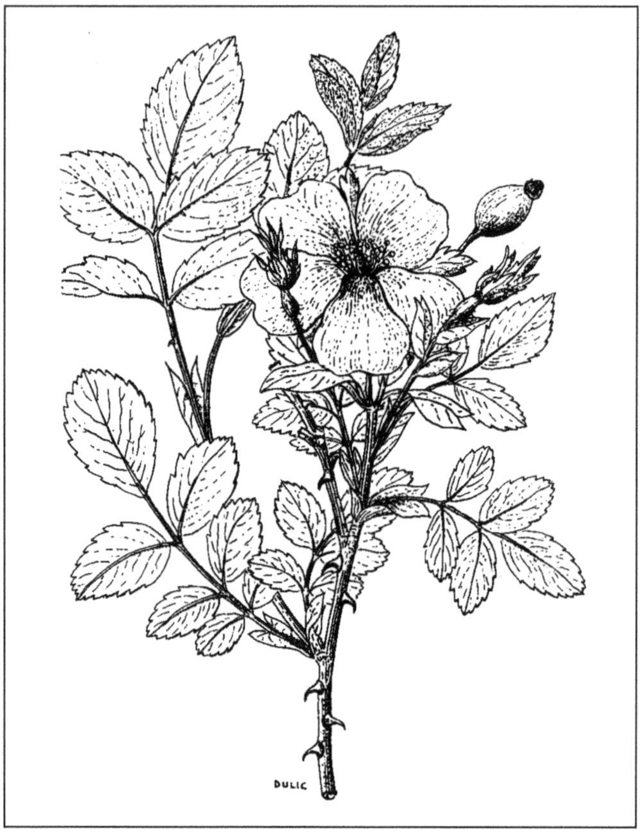

Figure 14 - Dog Rose (*Rosa canina*)

Dog Rose

Scientific name: *Rosa canina* (Rosaceae)
Hebrew: Vered ha-kelev Arabic: Nasrin, Ward[385]

Description:
The wild dog rose is a large shrub which grows in the mountains of Israel and in damp Mediterranean groves. Its leaves are pinnate and composite, and its flowers are pink with grape-like fruits or hips of a deep scarlet colour.[386] Another variety that is widespread in this region is the *Rosa phoenicia* - a large thorny shrub which blooms in the summer with abundant pink blossoms. The rose hips are shaped like tiny pears (1 cm. long) of a dark red colour.[387]

History:
The Latin name for the dog rose, from which the Hebrew name is derived, originates in story about a Roman soldier who cured himself of hydrophobia (rabies) by eating the root of the dog rose.[388] But the Hebrew name may also have been derived from the Persian 'lawarda'. The dog rose is not mentioned in the Bible, but many commentators have mistakenly identified it with the 'shoshan-shoshana' (lily).[389]

One of the first times that Rose was mentioned in literature was by Ben Sira (24:14) "as the rose seedlings in Jericho".

It seems that there was an increasing use of this plant during the Second Temple period. The Mishna mentions the rose as an ornamental plant and it was also used in the cosmetic industry, as a body lotion and for concocting medicines. The medicinal use of the dog rose is also described by physicians of the classical period. Dioscorides, for example, describes the medicinal use of *Kunosbaton*, which is identified with a variety of the dog rose, to treat stomach disorders, headaches, gynaecological problems, skin diseases, wounds, and for the eyes and gums.[390]

During medieval times the rose was cultivated as a highly prized agricultural crop in the Middle East because of the rose water produced from it - 'dahan al-jul' (rose oil) and 'julanjabin' (roses soaked in honey).[391] Several types of wild dog rose grow in the Land of Israel which became cultivated varieties.[392] According to the description of the plant, its habitat and uses during the Middle Ages,[393] it may be assumed that the variety, which was cultivated for agricultural and medicinal purposes in this region was the dog rose.

Medicinal Uses in Jerusalem:
Literary encomiums of Jerusalem mention rose water and perfumes distributed to those visiting the Dome of the Rock during the early Arab period.[394] al-Tamimi asserted that several species of roses had been used in remedies in Jerusalem including species named: 'Roman, Damascus, Ramleh and Jerusalem'.[395] Benevenutus reported that rose sugar was a component in a medication called the "Jerusalem pill" which was used to cure cataract, while 'dried rose leaves' were a component in a medication called 'Jerusalem colirium.'[396] Refael Malki noted that a rose concoction served as a light cathartic in Jerusalem. Rose water was part of a general medication called 'sharab' (medicinal syrup) and rose honey was a component in a pill to treat headaches and colds.[397] David de Silva mentioned two species of rose, of which medicinal use had been made: white and red. Both were used to produce rose water, rose oil, medicinal syrup and 'sukar rusano' - sweet rose water.[398]

Rose in the Levant:
During the Middle Ages rose growing was widespread and renowned mainly in the north of Israel and in the region of Damascus where they prepared "the best rose water in the

385 Maimonides, Glossaire, p. 74, No. 253; Issa, Dictionary, p. 157, No. 1; Plants & Animals, X, p. 133; Dinsmore & Dalman, No. 671.

386 Plants & Animals, X, p. 133.

387 Ibid, X, pp. 132-133.

388 Dafni, Edible, p. 36; Goor, Rose, p. 2.

389 Discussion in: Feliks, World, p. 283; Low, III, pp. 193-211.

390 Dioscorides, I.123.

391 Maimonides, Glossaire, p. 35, No. 85; p. 39, No. 106. Cf. Ibid, p. 44, No. 121.

392 In detail: Goor, Rose, pp. 1-52.

393 Amar, Production, pp. 115-117.

394 al-Wasti, p. 82 ; Ibn Katir, VII, p. 280.

395 Amar, Tamimi, p. 19; Ansari 77b, 28a.

396 Benevenutus, pp. 33, 44.

397 Malki, pp. 58, 62, 66.

398 Amar, de Silva, p. 119.

world."[399] The rose seems to have been grown in the Land of Israel since the 11th century.[400] Trading documents found in the Cairo Genizah contain information regarding the export of 'maraba' (rose jam)[401] from Tyre to Egypt. The jam was made from the meaty fruit and petals and stored in jars.[402] Elsewhere there is mention of exported "dried rose called azrar rose." [403] Levi ben Yefet the Karaite, who was active in the Land of Israel at the beginning of the 11th century, noted that it was permitted to take 'sharab al-ward al-maraba' (rose syrup) as a medication on the Sabbath.[404] Ibn al-Baytar mentions the rose fruit called 'dalik' which was used for medicinal purposes when ripened, and added that in al-Sham it was called 'zaram al-dik.'[405]

In a Jewish guide-book written at the beginning of the 14th century for travellers to the Land of Israel, some medical advices concerning the uses of the "expensive rose oil" are given.[406] During the Mamluk period the rose was listed as a perfume plant in the al-Sham region, and high quality rose water was exported to all countries.[407] Roses were also listed as Syrian products exported from Tripoli and Beirut.[408] The scholar al-Ghazzi praised the medicinal quality of the Damascus rose.[409] Hayim Vital described the use of rose water to treat obstructions in the urinary tract. Medicinal use was also made of rose oil which was a component in a medication to treat hemorrhoids and as an ingredient in rose honey.[410]

Medicinal Uses in the Medieval Period:
al-Kindi reported on the medicinal use of rose oil to treat hemorrhoids, stomach ulcers and swellings. It also served as a component in a preparation to treat liver diseases. The rose blossoms were used for treating disorders of the stomach, liver and spleen and for the preparation of medicines against pains of the throat and mouth, fever and mucus.[411] Maimonides says that the rose seed was a component in a medication to induce sleep, that rose oil and rose honey were a medication for snake bite, that rose water was a component in a poultice mixture to bandage bee stings, and that rose blossoms served as a light cathartic and a component in a strong purgative.

Roses were used also as a medication for general strengthening and as a component in 'the great atriphal' to fortify the heart, to delay old age and to increase sexual potency.[412] al-Qazwini quotes Ibn Sina who praised the plant and said that the scent "counteracted the smell of sweat." Other physicians recommended the plant for easing pain. Rose essence was also used to treat eye inflammation, hemorrhages and fainting fits.[413] In his entry 'nasrin' al-Qazwini quoted Ibn Sina who claimed that the rose was used to treat ear diseases, teeth pains and head pains and to stop hiccups.[414]

al-Biruni and al-Ghafiqi in their entry 'ward' described these and other uses.[415] Daud al-Antaki states in his entry 'nasrin' that this is a hot and dry drug used to strengthen the brain and sense organs, to dispel gases, cure colds, earaches, jaundice and hemorrhoids. The rose also served as an emmenagogue, to cleanse the skin, to improve scent, to act as a contraceptive and to dye the hair.[416]

Traditional Medicine:
The Arabs in Israel make a preparation from the fruit of the dog rose to strengthen the heart and brain, to regulate the menses and cure stomach disorders. The fruit (rose hips) are also used to cure chest diseases, to relieve coughs, to stop bleeding, to cure inflammation in the kidney and urinary tract.[417] Rose hips have been a food component for Europeans since Neolithic times.[418] Yemenite Jews use rose water externally to reduce swelling, to treat infections in the mouth, eyes, womb and anus, and internally to strengthen the heart and brain, to treat headache, breathing difficulties and to regulate lung functions. In addition, rose water was a component in a preparation for treating throat inflammation, coughs, digestive disorders, wounds and teeth.[419]

The people of Iraq use rose seeds to treat spasms and they are also considered as a diuretic and constricting drug. Rose hips serve as a source for Vitamin C. The fruits and seeds of closely related varieties such as *Rosa damascena* are also used as remedies.[420] The variety *Rosa gallica* is used in Egypt as a constricting substance and as a component in an eye medication[421] while the fruit serves as a diuretic as well as a cooling and constricting agent.[422]

General Uses and Medical Qualities:
The Damascene rose is the main source for producing ethereal oils for the cosmetic industry in the world. Dog rose petals

399 al-Dimashqi, pp. 195-198; Amar, Production, pp. 115-116.

400 Amar, Production, p. 115.

401 Low, III, p. 209.

402 Gil, III, Doc. 516, line 6. Cf. Doc. 514, in the margin of line 6.

403 Ibid., No. 275.

404 Levi Ben Yefet, p. 47a.

405 Ibn al-Baytar, al-Jami, p. 95; Leclerc, No. 877.

406 Kupper, p. 108.

407 al-Qalqashandi, p. 87.

408 Piloti, p. 136.

409 Hamarneh, Plants, p. 256.

410 Benajahu, pp. 91, 101, 110.

411 Collected references in: al-Kindi, pp. 345-346, No. 318.

412 Maimonides, Aphorisms, 21:67, 69; Maimonides, Sexual, p. 41; Maimonides, Poisons, pp. 111, 125.

413 al-Qazwini, p. 237. Cf. Ibn Sina, pp. 299-300.

414 al-Qazwini, p. 263. Cf. Ibn Sina, p. 374.

415 al-Biruni, I, p. 336; al-Ghafiqi, No. 273.

416 al-Antaki, p. 330.

417 Dafni, Edible, p. 36.

418 Loewenfeld & Back, pa. 211; Dafni, Edible, p. 36.

419 Reiani, p. 45, No. 105. Cf. Ben-Yakov, p. 728 for collected references to uses by the Jews of Iraq.

420 Hooper, pp. 165-166; al-Rawi & Chaakravarty, p. 83 for contents of active substances.

421 Ducros, p. 116.

422 Uphof, p. 454.

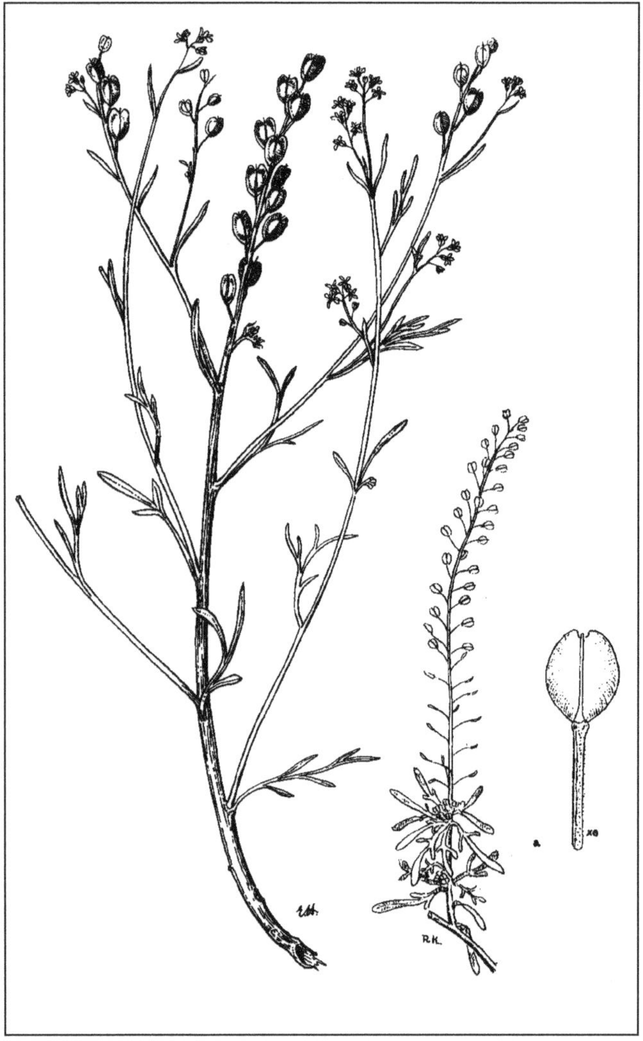

Figure 15 - Garden Cress (*Lepidum sativum*)

are a substitute for tea leaves, and the roasted seeds are used in Iraq as a coffee substitute.[423] Rose hips (especially of the dog rose) contains a high amount of Vitamin C as well as A, E, B, P and substances such as carotene and lemon acid.[424]

Garden Cress (Pepper Grass)

Scientific name: *Lepidium sativum* (Cruciferae)
Hebrew: Shahlayim tarbutiyim Arabic: Hurf, Hab al-rashad, Rashad al-bustani[425]

Description:
The garden cress is an annual plant, short (up to 40 cm.) with branching stem in the upper section. Its leaves are split at the base, the stem leaves are small, the flowers are white and the fruit is flattened and double-seeded.[426]

[423] Hill, p. 179; Uphof, p. 454; al-Rawi & Chaakravarty, p. 83.

[424] Loewenfeld & Back, p. 211. For detailed list of contents including seed substances see: al-Rawi & Chaakravarty, p. 83.

[425] Maimonides, Glossaire, p. 53, No. 163; al-Biruni, II, p. 88; Issa, Dictionary, p. 108, No.1; Dinsmore & Dalman, No. 136; Crowfoot & Baldensperger, p. 101.

[426] Plants & Animals, X, p. 112.

History:
Assyrian medicine used the garden cress for curing the eyes, mouth, ears, head, breathing and stomach as well as coughs.[427] Dioscorides reported on the use of *kardamon*, which is identified with garden cress, as an emmenagogue, for causing abortion, to let blood, and to cure skin diseases and internal wounds.[428] Garden cress is mentioned in the Mishna, Tosefta and Talmud.[429]

Medicinal Uses in Jerusalem:
In his medical treatise, al-Tamimi listed the 'shitraj al-shami' among the types of medicines.[430] Ibn al-Baytar claimed in his entry 'hamsha' that this is the name for 'shitraj' which is given by the residents of Jerusalem and its environs in the al-Sham region.[431]

Agriculture and Medicinal Uses in the Levant:
According to Ibn al-Baytar, the 'lividiyun' is a herb which is known in Egypt as the 'Sultan's herb' and that the "chroniclers say it is a herb widely found in Damascus and that it is pungent."[432] In his entry 'hurf al-stuh' Ibn al-Baytar writes that "this type is the one known in al-Sham as 'harpak' while the people of Egypt and Alexandria call it 'harfuf' and as 'hashishat al-sultan.' Among its uses, Ibn al-Baytar lists the curing of skin diseases, as an emmenagogue, and to cure intestinal disorders.[433] 'Hurf al-stuh' has been identified by certain researchers with garden cress,[434] but others claim it refers to the type *Lepidium campestris*.[435] The Jewish physician, Kohen al-Attar known as al-Israili, wrote that "'Ares' is 'al-shitraj,' and the people of al-Sham call it 'al-hamsha' ..."[436]

In his entry 'zanb al-hurf' Ibn al-Baytar notes that this is the basis for producing 'razda lividiyun' known in Spain. It is similar to the 'hurf' but slightly bigger than it. In Africa and al-Sham (Greater Syria) this name is given to another plant.[437]

Medicinal Uses in the Medieval Period:
According to al-Kindi, various types of cress were used to treat black spots on the skin, stomach ulcers, weakness, and the gums, and were a component in a medication for mumps

[427] Thompson, Art, p. 59.

[428] Dioscorides, II.156.

[429] For remarks on its identification see: Amar, Production, p. 286; Low, I, pp. 505-506; Feliks, Yerushalmi, II, p. 147; Feliks, World, p. 107.

[430] al-Tamimi, p. 46b.

[431] Ibn al-Baytar, al-Jami, II, p. 46; Leclerc, No. 751.

[432] Ibn al-Baytar, Tafsir, pp. 202-203.

[433] Ibn al-Baytar, al-Jami, II, p. 17; Leclerc, No. 654. Cf. Maimonides, Glossaire, p. 109, No. 399; al-Antaki, p. 122; Dietrich, pp. 41-44.

[434] See editor's remarks in Ibn al-Baytar, Tafsir, pp. 202-203.

[435] Issa, Dictionary, p. 107, No.9. Discussion in Amar, Ibn al-Baytar, p. 75, n.75.

[436] al-Israili, p. 209. According to Issa, Dictionary, p. 108 this relates to garden cress, but in Amar's opinion this is a local term for tall cress.

[437] Ibn al-Baytar, al-Jami, II, p. 126; Leclerc, No. 1004. According to Issa, Dictionary, p. 154, No. 19 this concerns a variety of mignonette, but Leclerc identifies it as one of the cress varieties.

(parotitis)[438]. al-Qazwini relates in his entry 'hurf' that eating this plant adds to intelligence and wisdom and it increases sexual potency. He quotes Ibn Sina who claimed that the plant in effective against skin diseases (scurvy), wounds, bites and stings. A high dosage is liable to cause abortion.[439] Ibn al-Baytar in his entry 'hurf' lists medicinal uses such as: curing pains of the side and head, elimination of intestinal worms, softening the stomach, reducing swelling of the spleen, increasing sexual desire and curing bites, stings and skin diseases.[440]

Traditional Medicine:
The seeds of the 'rashad' are listed among the components of the 'arba'in' medication, which is widely used among the Arabs of Israel.[441] In Iran and Iraq the plant is used as a strengthening drug, stimulating the appetite and sexual desire, as a diuretic and for the prevention of scurvy.[442] In Egypt the seeds are used as a drug stimulant, a diuretic and as a component in a medication for mumps.[443] The Jews of Iraq called various plants 'rashad' including prickly cress, watercress, cakile, etc. and used them for medicinal purposes.[444]

Modern Medicine and General Uses:
Various kinds of cress, mainly garden cress, are used around the world in the making of salads. The roots are used for sauces and edible oil is derived from the seeds.[445] Natural and popular medicine makes use of the plant to purify the blood, to cleanse the liver, to cure mumps and to dissolve kidney stones.[446] According to Chizik, the use of cress as a medicinal plant in early times as well as today is due to its high vitamin content, mainly Vitamin C and also A, B, and E.[447]

Garlic

Scientific name: *Allium sativum* (Liliaceae)[448]
Hebrew: Shum Arabic: Thum[449]

Description:
Garlic is a perennial herb which has a bulbous root composed of small cloves. It has spear-shape leaves and its flowers are pink or white. The cultivated specie is the *Allium cepa,* a well known ancient agricultural crop.

History:
Garden garlic was widely cultivated in Egypt and Rome. It is mentioned in the Bible (Numbers 11:5) and by the Jewish Sages[450] who described its medicinal uses in treating toothache and wounds. The Talmud says that it "satisfies, anoints and brightens the face, increases sperm and kills intestinal worms, and some say it even generates love and expels jealousy." Dioscorides notes that the *skorodon* (a species of garlic) kills intestinal worms and is a most effective medicine against snakebite and the bite of a rabid dog. It eliminates lice, cures baldness and also acts as an emmenagogue.[451] Garlic is a medicinal plant even in the Muslim holy scriptures and in the treatises of many Arab physicians.[452]

Medicinal Uses in Jerusalem:
al-Tamimi mentioned the 'thum bari' (wild garlic) as one of the substances he used to make the theriac. He praised its medicinal actions and asserted that the plant itself can replace the composite theriac.[453] David de Silva described other medicinal uses of garlic such as diuretic, emmenagogue, to improve the eyesight and the voice. As he did in other cases, de Silva brought quotations from the Talmud to support his remarks.[454]

Garlic in the Levant:
At the end of the 12th century the 'thum' was listed among the vegetables sold in Acre.[455] Hayim Vital described the use of garlic to treat thigh pains by means of a clyster made of "a boy's urine and olive oil in which two bulbs of garlic are fried in their skins."[456] He also mentions its use in treating arthritis and colds by "inhaling the smoke from the roots of burnt garlic bulbs" as well as poultices of crushed garlic with frankincense in a bandage over the forehead.[457]

Medicinal Uses in the Medieval Period:
Assaph Harofe described the uses of wild garlic which grows on the mountains as: 'a strong antidote to fatal drugs and snakebite and for all poisonous plants, from which one may drink and be healed." Elsewhere he recommends 'garlic water' to cure eye inflammation.[458] al-Kindi reported on the use of garlic to reduce pains of lung inflammation.[459] Maimonides stated that the 'shum' was an easily digested food and called it the 'village theriac' because of its medicinal properties. He also recommended that garlic be eaten by those who were bitten.[460] Ibn al-Baytar described the plant in his entry 'thum'

438 al-Kindi, Nos. 9, 31, 38, 81.

439 al-Qazwini, p. 224. Cf. Ibn Sina, p. 314.

440 Ibn al-Baytar, al-Jami, II, pp. 15-16; Leclerc, No. 654. Cf. al-Antaki, p. 122.

441 Crowfoot & Baldensperger, p. 101.

442 Hooper, p. 136. Cf. for contents of substances in: al-Rawi & Chaakravarty, p. 59.

443 Ducros, p. 72.

444 In detail: Ben-Yakov, pp. 606-607.

445 Plants & Animals, X, p. 112; Uphof, p. 308.

446 Ibid.

447 Chizik, p. 635.

448 Plants & Animals, XII, p. 81

449 Issa, Dictionary, p. 9, No. 15.

450 Summary of sources in: Feliks, Plants, p. 156; Feliks, World, p. 172; Low, II, pp. 138-148.

451 Dioscorides, II.182; Historical summary in: El Gammal, Garlic.

452 Ibn Qayyim, p. 193.

453 Amar, Tamimi, p. 18; Anzari, p. 70b, 78a.

454 Amar, de Silva, p. 140.

455 Ibn Jubayr, p. 314.

456 Benajahu, p. 104.

457 Ibid. p. 109.

458 Assaph, 4, p. 418.

459 al-Kindi, No. 123.

460 Maimonides, Aphorisms, 20:49; 21:39, 80; Maimonides, Poisons, p. 133; al-Biruni, I, p. 102.

and listed its names and uses among the physicians of his time and of the classical period.

Garlic is considered by the medieval Arabic physicians a hot and dry drug used to eliminate intestinal worms, to cleanse the throat, to relieve chronic coughs and toothache, to treat diseases of the skin, eyes, teeth and as an emmenagogue, as well as to cure the stomach, to treat bites and stings and to increase urine flow.[461]

Traditional Medicine:
In the local traditional medicine in Israel, garlic is usually used to expel intestinal worms.[462] The Arabs also use it to treat earache, eye inflammation, vomiting and hemorrhoids, as a poultice to bind wounds and to purify water.[463] The Jews of Yemen and Iraq use the garlic bulb and leaves for the external treatment of teeth and gum inflammation, for styes, for backache, snakebite, scorpion stings and for insanity. Internal uses include treatment of inflammation in the digestive tract, thirst, increase in sexual potency, elimination of worms and as an immunization agent against diseases. Garlic is an expectorant, a carminative and a diuretic.[464] In Iran and Iraq it is used as a digestive aid and a stomach stimulant.[465]

Medical Qualities:
The plant has anti-bacterial properties, it disinfects, causes sweat, and is an expectorant. It is also used to treat coughs, colds, high blood pressure and nerves. Popular medicine uses it to treat toothache and earache and to expel worms,[466] and credits the plant with the power to reduce the level of sugar and cholesterol in the blood and to strengthen the heart.[467]

General Uses:
Garlic is used in cooking and in sauces, in the industrial production of garlic salts and sausages.[468]

Conclusions:
Garlic is a food plant, condiment and medicinal herb well known in popular medicine today. Its medicinal uses are of ancient origin and are mainly for elimination of intestinal worms and the treatment of bites and stings. Many sources refer to its uses during medieval times and others describe its cultivation and trade in the Land of Israel. al-Tamimi and David de Silva mentioned its medicinal uses in Jerusalem and Hayim Vital described its uses in the Levant.

461 Ibn al-Baytar, al-Jami, I, pp. 151-153; Leclerc, Nos. 453-453. Cf. al-Antaki, p. 101; Ibn Sina, pp. 449-450.

462 Chizik, p. 733. The Negev Bedouins do so as well. See Abu-Rabia, p. 21.

463 Krispil, p. 1461.

464 Reiani, No. 5. References in Ben-Yakov, p. 757.

465 Hooper, p. 82; See al-Rawi & Chaakravarty, p. 10 for contents of active substances. Cf. Ducros, p. 60.

466 Uphof, p. 25; Hill, p. 372; Contents of substances in: El Gammal, Garlic, pp. 86-67.

467 Plants & Animals, XII, p. 81. for example, also in Singer, Garlic.

468 Uphof, p. 25a; Hill, p. 372; Plants & Animals, XII, p. 81.

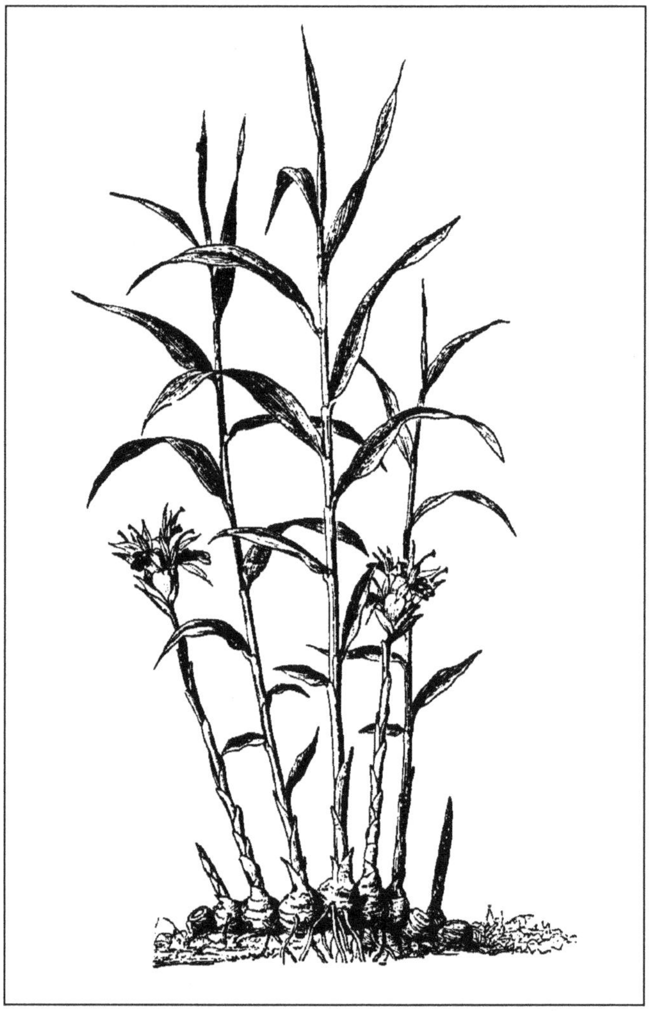

Figure 16 - Ginger (*Zingiber officinale*)

Ginger

Scientific name: *Zingiber officinale* (Zingiberaceae)
Hebrew: Zangbil refu'i Arabic: Zanjabil, Zangabir[469]

Description:
Ginger is one variety of a tropical species that includes 1300 plant types with bulbous roots, many of which contain essential oils, and it serves as spice and a medicinal herb. The stalks grow to a height of up to one meter.[470]

History:
It appears that the plant was cultivated in China and introduced to Europe by the Greeks and Romans. Dioscorides notes in his entry *Zingiberi* - identified with ginger - that the bulbous stalk has heating qualities and is used to treat stomach disorders and to counteract poisons.[471] According to the Jewish Sages, the 'zingbila' was generally chewed, probably to sweeten the breath, or as a remedy. Ginger drink is mentioned in the Koran in the description of Paradise (Koran 76: 15-17).

469 Maimonides, Glossaire, p. 49, No. 145; p. 98, No. 353; Issa, Dictionary, p. 191, No. 11.

470 Zohary, p. 651; Hill, p. 439.

471 Dioscorides, II.190.

Medicinal Uses in Jerusalem:
Refael Malki claimed that the 'zingbil' was a component in a general medication for the Jerusalem poor.[472] According to Moshe Poriat, one could obtain in the Jerusalem markets, during the first half of the 17th century, various perfumes and spices including ginger.[473] David de Silva mentioned ginger in his medical book and wrote that it softens the stomach, makes food hot and spicy, and treats eye diseases.[474]

Ginger in the Levant:
Evidence of the ginger trade in the Land of Israel during the Crusader period can be found in the 13th century taxation lists of Acre where the 'gingimbre' is mentioned.[475]

Sources from that period show that the quality of the ginger traded in Syrian markets was superior because it arrived overland and was not damaged by a sea voyage. The merchandise was brought by traders who exported it to Europe.[476] From trade records of 1414 CE it appears that the ginger was bought in Ramlah by a Venetian trading company with the purpose of export to Europe. The spice was marketed in packages, and large quantities of it were brought by caravans from Mecca. The sources mention two varieties: 'zanjabil baladi' and zanjabil mecca.'[477]

Medicinal Uses in the Medieval Period:
According to al-Kindi, ginger was a component in various medications such as in a preparation for improving the eyesight and for treating pains in the throat, ears and stomach.[478] Shabtai Donolo brings ginger as an example for a thick root and explained how to prepare medicine from it.[479]

Maimonides reported that ginger was a component in a medication called 'the great atriphal' which "strengthens the heart and limbs, delays ageing, fortifies the senses and even aids coitus." The plant is also used for the 'great theriac' and the 'walnut theriac', and it is listed among the hot and moist drugs.[480] Ibn al-Baytar quotes important physicians of his time and described the medicinal uses of the 'zanjabil': improvement of sexual potency, expulsion of stomach gases, treatment of stomach and liver disorders, draining of mucus, heating the body and curing eye diseases.[481]

Daud al-Antaki notes that the 'zanjabil' opens blockages, eliminates mucus, expels gases, cures the intestines and jaundice, stimulates the memory and improves the appetite.[482]

Traditional Medicine:
Bedouins of the Negev use ginger to cure throat infection, colds, hoarseness, and liver diseases, to treat gases and to strengthen sexual potency.[483]Among Yemenite Jews, ginger was a component in a medication to strengthen the eyes, to treat cough and excessive mucus. Ginger by itself was used for treating stomach and throat pain and to increase sexual potency.[484] The Jews of Iraq also used ginger for medicinal purposes such as: to treat dysentery, gases and bronchial infections, to improve the memory and increase sperm.[485] In Europe, the root stem which contains ethereal oils is used as a carminative and a digestive stimulant.[486]

General Uses:
Ginger serves as a spice and it is also used as an ingredient in the confectionery industry, in cake baking, in wine and in brandy, as well as in the perfume industry.[487]

Grape Vine

Scientific name: *Vitis vinifera* (Vitaceae)
Hebrew: Gefen ha-yayin Arabic: Karam, Zebib (raisins), Hazram (sour grapes)

Description:
The grape vine is a climbing plant with woody vines and leaves which fall in the winter. In spring, after the leaves sprout, small green flowers blossom. The juicy fruit is in cluster formation and ripens in the summer.[488]

History:
The grape vine is an ancient cultivated crop and was widely grown throughout the world. The cultivated vine is derived from a species originating in Asia Minor.[489]

Grape seeds from the Mousterian period have been found in the Kebara caves on Mount Carmel.[490] Grape juice was used as a basis for many remedies in ancient Babylonia, and other products such as vinegar, wine and raisins have also been used as medicinal cures.[491]

Grape vine is one of the seven species with which the Land of Israel has been blessed (Deuteronomy, 8:8). The cultivation of grapes, which was very widely grown in this region, is mentioned in many Jewish sources such as the Bible, Mishna, Tosefta and Talmud, as well as in pagan and Christian sources. It was also evident in archaeological finds such as an apparatus for grape products.

---

472 Malki, p. 62.

473 Ya'ari, Travels, p. 278.

474 Amar, de Silva, p. 120.

475 Assises, p. 176.

476 Ashtor, Levant, p.33.

477 Ibid., pp. 285, 297, 299.

478 al-Kindi, Nos. 72, 109, 154, 216, 225-226.

479 Donolo, p. 17, n.114.

480 Maimonides, Aphorisms, 21:81; Maimonides, Regimen, 3:11; Maimonides, Poisons, p. 109, 115.

481 Ibn al-Baytar, al-Jami, II, pp. 167-168; Leclerc, No. 1125.

482 al-Antaki, p. 18. Cf. al-Biruni, I, p. 169; Ibn Sina, p. 302.

483 Abu-Rabia, pp. 16-17.

484 Reiani, p. 53, No. 126.

485 Ben-Yakov, pp. 97, 105, 118, 147, 150.

486 Zohary, p. 651; Uphof, p. 562; Hill, p. 440.

487 Uphof, p. 562 for detailed content of substances; Hill, pp. 431-439.

488 Plants & Animals, XII, p. 115.

489 Zohary, p. 476.

490 Lev, Kebara, p. 57.

491 al-Kindi, p. 306, No. 207.

The grape and its products were used mainly as food and drink, for industries and for ritual ceremonies. Medicinal uses of the grape and its products are also mentioned in various sources.[492] Dioscorides, for example, noted the medicinal use of grapes to improve the appetite, to relieve stomach pains, to treat dysentery and he also recommended wine to reduce fever.[493]

Medicinal Uses in Jerusalem:
Benevenutus claimed that white wine was a component in a medication for cataract,[494] and in another medication for the eyes called 'Jerusalem colorium'.[495]

Refael Malki described the many uses of the grape and its products such as the use of old sweet wine boiled with sugar as a medication for the eyes. Another medical treatise mentions the use of raisin wine and of Hebron raisins.[496] Many pilgrims described the cultivation of the grape vine and the careful nurturing of its products in the Land of Israel in general and in Jerusalem in particular. For example, Moshe Poriat describes grape honey which was offered for sale in Jerusalem markets.[497]

Grape Vines in the Levant:
Grapes were an important agricultural crop in the Land of Israel in ancient times, and continued to hold a central place in agricultural cultivation during the medieval period as well. Evidence of grape cultivation and the use of its various products, mainly wine, vinegar, grape honey and raisins, can be found in Christian, Muslim and Jewish sources.[498] In a 12th century document from the Genizah, there is mention of the 'hazram' (vinegar grapes) which were sent from Ashkelon to Egypt[499] and its medicinal use was mentioned by Maimonides who practiced medicine in Egypt during that period as well as by the physician Ibn al-Baytar.[500] Hayim Vital reported on the use of wine which was an important component in many medications, including various preparations to treat obstructions in the urinary tract, kidney stones[501] and hemorrhoids.[502] Vinegar was used as a component in a preparation for gargling and in a medication against mouth disease.[503]

Medicinal Uses in the Medieval Period:
Assaph Harofe claimed that "Lebanon wine, Carmel wine, the wine from the mountains of Jerusalem and of Samaria, Cretan wine and Egyptian wine, are the seven kinds of wine superior to all other varieties in the world. The other types of wine are worthless compared to these because they differ in quality, taste and smell and for medicinal purposes by virtue of their strength."[504] Ibn al-Baytar in his entry ''anab' mentions the medicinal uses of grapes.[505]

The following is a survey of the medicinal uses of the different grape products without reference to period or physician. Because of the numerous sources for this subject, only some of them are mentioned and only a few of their uses:

Wine: Used as a major component in many medications (more than ten references are made by Maimonides) against fatal drugs, snakebite, stings of poisonous creatures, and in medications for curing various diseases.[506] Shabtai Donolo in his medical treatise also notes the many uses of wine mainly as a basis for liquid medications (syrups).[507]

Vinegar: Used as an important component in medications as in a preparation for treating attacks by poisonous creatures, in cathartic medicines and for hemorrhoids. A medication combining vinegar and honey called 'sikanjbin' (also known as 'aksumili') was frequently used by Maimonides and physicians of his time.[508]

Vine leaves: Used as a medication for the stomach and especially as a poultice to bandage wounds.[509]

Raisins: Mentioned as effective for liver complaints and used as a component in cathartic medications and in various medicines.[510] Ibn al-Baytar in his entry 'Zebib' mentions various contemporary medicinal uses.[511]

Vine roots: According to al-Kindi the roots of the grape vine were used as a component in a preparation for treating swellings and carbuncles.[512]

Vinegar grapes: These are called 'hazram' in Arabic and are also mentioned in connection with medicinal uses.[513]

[492] Comprehensive survey in: Goor, Fruits, pp. 27-53; Feliks, World, pp. 17-24; Goor, Wines; Shapira, Wine. On the cultivation of the grape vine in the Land of Israel and Syria during the Middle Ages, see: Amar, Production, pp. 72-105.

[493] Dioscorides, V.3.

[494] Benevenutus, p. 19.

[495] Ibid, p. 41.

[496] Malki, pp. 60-62, 66.

[497] Ya'ari, Travels, p. 280. In this connection see additional sources is Amar, Dibs.

[498] In detail: Amar, Production, pp. 72-105.

[499] Goiten, Jewry, p. 225.

[500] Maimonides, Regimen, 4:14; Ibn al-Baytar, al-Jami, II, pp. 22-23; Leclerc, No. 679.

[501] Benajahu, pp. 91-92.

[502] Ibid., p. 99.

[503] Ibid, pp. 106, 110.

[504] Assaph, 4, p. 175.

[505] Ibn al-Baytar, al-Jami, III, p. 141; Leclerc, No. 1595. Cf. al-Antaki, p. 240.

[506] Maimonides, Regimen,; Maimonides, Aphorisms; Maimonides, Poisons, pp. 105, 107.

[507] Donolo, pp. 14-15, 17, 19, 23; Assaph, 4, pp. 400-401.

[508] Maimonides, Poisons, pp. 102, 105, 1107; Maimonides, Regimen, 3:5, 6; Maimonides, Aphorisms, 9:77; 21:19-27.

[509] Maimonides, Aphorisms, 9:105; 21:31.

[510] Maimonides, Regimen, 1:13; 3: 5, 6. Raisins are mentioned 14 times in Maimonides, Aphorisms, mainly 23: 19, 20.

[511] Ibn al-Baytar, al-Jami, II, pp. 153-155; Leclerc, No. 1084.

[512] al-Kindi, No. 121

[513] Maimonides, Regimen, 4:14; Ibn al-Baytar, al-Jami, II, pp. 22-23; Leclerc, No. 679.

Grape honey: Daud al-Antaki described the method of producing 'dibs' (grape honey) and listed it medicinal uses. The 'dibs' was a hot and moist drug and was used as a component in many medicinal preparations to treat obesity, to purify the blood, to open obstructions in the body and to cure jaundice, heart disease, depression and epilepsy.[514]

Grape juice: According to al-Kindi, grape juice was a component in a preparation to treat neck pains.[515]

Vine resin: Used for treating skin diseases.[516]

Traditional Medicine:
Yemenite Jews made extensive use of the grape vine and its products for remedies. Grapes were used as a component in a medication against insanity and to calm the nerves. Raisins were used to increase sexual potency and to strengthen the memory. Vine leaves were used to treat open wounds, and the gum resin from pruned vines were used to treat the eyes. Wine was a component in medications for treating stomach pains, fever, colds and rheumatism. ''ark' (grape resin) served to treat colds, toothache, gum infection and growths in the nose. Vinegar was used to eliminate intestinal worms, to treat colds, skin diseases, fever, headaches, chills and toothaches.[517] In Iraq, the gum resin from the pruned vines served to treat skin diseases, the vine leaves to cure diarrhea, the juice of sour grapes to treat throat infection, and raisins to induce diarrhea, as a cooling agent, for stomach pains, coughs, hoarseness, high fever and so on.[518]

General Uses:
The grape vine and its products are used worldwide for food, drink, industry and for ritual ceremonies.[519]

Gum Arabic (Babul Acacia)

Scientific name: *Acacia arabica* (Leguminosae)
Hebrew: (tree) Shitah Aravit (gum) Gumy Aravi
Arabic: (tree) Zant, Sant, Akakia; (gum) Samgh[520]

Description:
The acacia species includes 750 varieties of trees and shrubs widespread throughout tropical and sub-tropical regions. Most of them grow in desert areas, and some of the trees and shrubs are thorny. The leaves are composite and pinnate, the flowers are small and bloom abundantly in round blossom clusters. The fruits are cylindrical or flattened seed capsules, elongated or curled and contain a few seeds. The main varieties that flourish in this region are: *Acacia albida, Acacia raddiana, Acacia tortilis* and *Acacia gerrardii*.[521]

History:
The use of acacia gum was widespread in Egypt since the second millennium BCE, and in Sudan during the first century CE.[522] The Bible describes the use of acacia wood for building the Sanctuary in the desert and for making ritual objects such as the Holy Ark, the altar, the table and the pillars (Exodus, 25-27). Acacia is also mentioned in the prophetic books (Isaiah 41:19). The Talmud mentions the use of 'akakia' (acacia gum) for remedial purposes and as a contraception. Because of its low cost and its appearance, acacia gum was sometimes used as a deceptive substitute for the more expensive myrrh and frankincense. Dioscorides mentions *akakia* identified as *Acacia vera*, claiming that it grew in Egypt and noting especially the use of its gum to cure diseases of the eyes and intestines, as well as mouth sores, and to dye the hair black.[523]

Medicinal Uses in Jerusalem:
According to Refael Malki, the 'samaj 'arabi' soaked in wine was a component in a general medication or pill.[524]

Acacia Products Traded in the Levant:
A letter dated 1110 CE found in the Genizah and sent by Natan ha-Kohen of Ashkelon to Ola ha-Levi in Fustat, describes a consignment of 'rab al-zant' (acacia concentrate) sent from Ashkelon to Egypt.[525]

Medicinal Uses in the Medieval Period:
According to al-Kindi, 'akakia' was a preparation for the teeth and for wounds, and 'gumi arabicum' was a component in medications against cough and to treat eye diseases.[526] Shabtai Donolo claimed that the 'komos' was a variety of gum resin used as a remedy and was melted by fire.[527] Maimonides quotes al-Tamimi and notes that the 'akakia' was a component in a medication for fracture. Elsewhere he describes the use of 'gumi arabica' to cleanse the body and head from liquids and mucus. The "juice of acacia seed pods" was used as a component in a preparation to constrict the glans and strengthen the penis, as well as in a preparation to restore virginity. The 'akakia' (juices of the fruit and seed pod) and 'gumi arabica' were considered a hot and dry drug.[528]

Ibn al-Baytar in his entry 'samgh' described gum arabic and listed its medicinal uses such as: to dilute bitter medication, to cure diseases of the eyes and intestines, to relieve coughs,

[514] al-Antaki, pp. 150-151. On the identification of 'dibs' its production, trade and uses during the Middle Ages, see: Amar, Dibs.

[515] al-Kindi, No. 106.

[516] Assaph, 4, p. 400.

[517] Reiani, p. 52, No. 124. Similar uses were made by the Jews of Iraq. Cf. Ben-Yakov, pp. 714, 710, 743, 749.

[518] al-Rawi & Chaakravarty, p. 98 for content of substances.

[519] Uphof, pp. 547-548; Hill, pp. 397-399.

[520] Maimonides, Glossaire, p. 19, No.12; p. 80, No. 278.

[521] Plants & Animals, X, pp. 141-145; Morton, p. 137. For synonyms see: Dinsmore & Dalman, Nos. 654-657; Issa, Dictionary, pp. 1-3.

[522] Hill, p. 151.

[523] Dioscorides, I.133.

[524] Malki, p. 67.

[525] Gil, I, p. 484, Nos. 501, 588.

[526] al-Kindi, Nos. 57, 103-104, 111, 150, 159, 172-173, 175, 177; al-Biruni, I, pp. 37-38.

[527] Donolo, p. 18, n. 151.

[528] Maimonides, Aphorisms, 9:123; 13:13; 21:73, 78; Maimonides, Sexual, 8:11; 17:2.

to splint fractures and as a component in a cathartic medication. Gum arabic was so frequently used that the word 'samgh' alone came to mean 'samgh arabi.'[529] In the entry 'karat' identified with the acacia of the Nile, Ibn al-Baytar described the tree that few in Egypt, listed its medicinal uses and noted that this was the 'zanat' (gum arabic).[530]

Traditonal Medicine:
The Sinai Bedouins used *Acacia raddiana* to treat pus in the eyes, inflammation of the eyes, heart pains and pains in the ribs. The bitter gum was used to wean breastfeeding infants.[531] Yemenite Jews used the gum internally to treat coughs and hemorrhages in the lungs, as well as to strengthen the lungs and stomach, and they used it externally to strengthen the teeth, to treat hemorrhoids, burns and bleeding gums, as well as to relieve pains in the womb, spine and back. The gum also served to bathe the eyes, to strengthen eyesight and to treat wounds.[532] In Iraq and Iran the *Acacia senegal* was the main source for 'gumi arabi' used as a remedy, and it was traded throughout the Levant.[533] In Egypt the seeds are used today as a component in a medication against diarrhea and also for the tanning industry, and the gum was used as a cathartic, a softening drug, and to treat stomach ulcers, blood expectoration and eye diseases.[534]

General Uses:
Gum arabic is a softening drug, stabilizes liquid solutions and was a component of the preparation of writing ink. It is also used in the textile industry, for painting and for confectionery. The bark of the Nile acacia is used as a tanning substance.[535]

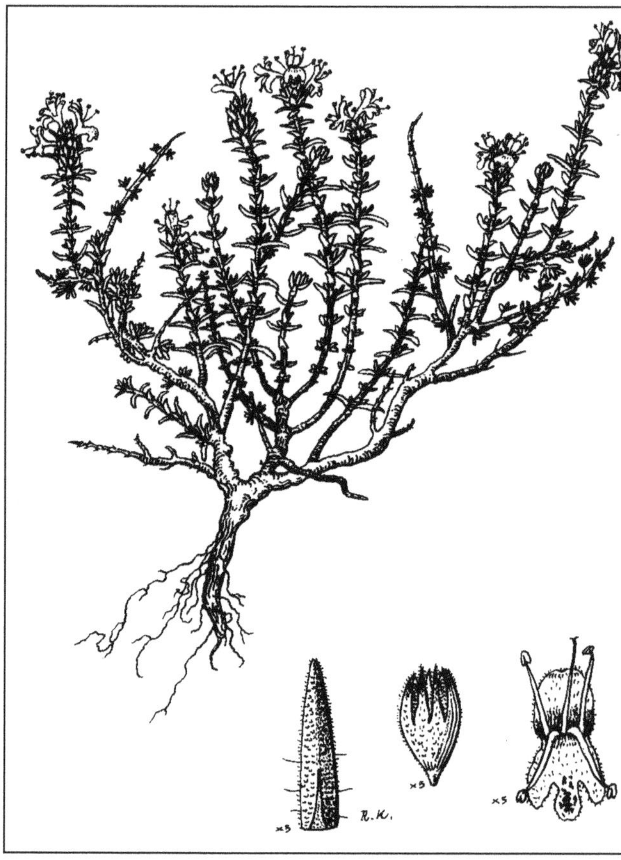

Figure 17 - Headed Thyme (*Coridothymus capitatus*)

Headed Thyme

Scientific name:
***Coridothymus {Thymus} capitatus* (Labiatae)**
Hebrew: Koranit mekurkefet
Arabic: Sa'tar parsi, Sa'tar al-hamir, Hasha[536]

Description:
Headed thyme is a dense bush branching out from the base, blossoming abundantly with small, purplish pink flowers. It has a very strong scent.[537]

History:
In Ancient Egypt the plant was used for embalming the dead. Dioscorides noted the *Erpullos* and listed its medicinal uses such as: an emmenagogue, to open obstructions in the urinary tract, to relieve the pain of bone fractures, sprains and bruises, to cure inflammations of the liver, to neutralize snake poison, to aid in the treatment of asthma and intestinal worms.[538] According to the Jewish Sages, the 'koranit' was a plant used for seasoning and for firewood, and it was also a food plant for man and beast.[539]

Identification:
The identification of the varieties of thyme is not a simple matter because, in different areas of this region, general names were give to plants that had similar features and qualities. Maimonides, for example, in his entry 'sa'tar' gave details about several varieties and tried to identify them.[540] Different condiment plants called 'za'tar parsi' and 'hasha' were mainly of the Labiatae family. However, according to the Arabic and Spanish names, the descriptions of the plants and the frequency of their use, they are one of the two varieties: Savory of Crete or Headed Thyme.[541]

Since there is some confusion among medieval writers as to the names and varieties of the Labiatae species - even among modern researchers - it seems impossible or perhaps mistaken

529 Ibn al-Baytar, al-Jami, p. 85; Leclerc, No. 1407.

530 Ibn al-Baytar, al-Jami, IV, pp. 14-15; Leclerc, No. 1758.

531 Levey, Bedouins, p. 84. Additonal medicinal uses and folklore in: Krispil, pp. 1503-1514.

532 Reiani, p. 7, No. 1. Cf. Ben-Yakov, p. 749.

533 Hooper, p. 79. For uses and methods of production see: Morton, pp. 137-141. For the uses of gum arabic in Eastern regions, see in detail: Howe et al.

534 Ducros, pp. 29, 143. Cf. Grieve, pp. 4-6 for uses in Europe.

535 Reiani, p. 7, No.1; Hill, p. 121. For production of the gum and additional uses see: Ibid, p. 151 and also Howes, pp. 17-38.

536 Maimonides, Glossaire, No. 319; Issa, Dictionary, p. 163, No. 10.

537 Description: Plants & Animals, XI, pp. 81-82.

538 Disocorides, III.46.

539 Feliks, Yerushalmi, II, pp. 146, 159.

540 Maimonides, Glossaire, pp. 90-91, No. 319.

541 Issa, Dictionary, p. 163, No. 10; p. 180, No. 223; Dinsmore & Dalman, Nos. 1348, 1350; Maimonides, Glossaire, p. 52, No. 157; Witztum & Gruber; Amar, al-Baytar, p. 72, n. 65.

to identify and distinguish between varieties that are closely related in form, habitat and usages. The two varieties mentioned above are therefore presented with their distinctive characteristics.

Medicinal Uses in Jerusalem:
Ibn al-Baytar described the 'hasha' which the inhabitants of Spain and herbalists knew as 'sa'tar al-hamir.' According to him, the plant grew widely in the 'lands of Bayt al-Maqdis" (Land of Jerusalem) and its suburbs.[542] Refael Malki says that 'the waters of sa'tar parsi' was a component in a syrup as a general medication for the Jerusalem poor. In his view, hyssop water was an effective substitute for the water of 'sa'tar parsi.'[543]

Varieties of Thyme in the Levant:
Ibn al-Baytar mentions elsewhere that the 'thymbra' is the 'za'tar al-farsi' - a well known plant among the Spaniards which they call 'shteria' and he goes on to say that "this type of thin-leaved za'tar is found in the cultivated areas of Egypt and in their orchards, as well as in al-Sham."[544]

Medicinal Uses in the Medieval Period:
According to Assaph Harofe, the plant is a "slender tree" called in Greek 'oregani,' in Aramaic 'zifa raba,' and in Latin 'shturiya - sturaya'. It is effective in treating pains in the kidneys and in dissolving kidney stones, for urine flow, for opening blockages in the ears, treating the intestines and eye diseases.[545] al-Kindi brings examples for various kinds of thyme: 'sa'tar parsi' served as a component in a medication for external treatment of growths on the neck;[546] 'hasha' was a component in a medication for the liver, stomach and swollen spleen;[547] while the drug 'hashi' was a component in an expectorant drink to cleanse the lungs as a result of asthma.[548] Ibn al-Baytar in his entry 'hasha' listed uses such as: an emmenagogue, diuretic, opening blockages, curing disorders in the breathing system, elimination of intestinal worms, improving the eyesight, cleansing the liver and stomach and inducing diarrhea.[549] In the entry 'thuma' Ibn al-Baytar notes that this is a synonym for 'hasha.'[550] al-Qazwini described the plant in his entry 'hasha' and quotes Ibn Sina who described its use in straightening curly hair and improving the eyesight.[551]

Traditional Medicine:
The Arabs of Israel use the plant internally to cure heart diseases, to eliminate excess water in the stomach, to relieve pains of the joints, stomach and nerves, to reduce the effect of poisons and drugs, to treat diabetes and cure palsy and blindness.[552] The Bedouins of the Negev use 'Sa'tar hamir' which is also called 'Sa'tar parsi' to cure colds, throat pains and cough.[553] Among the Yemenite Jews the plant served in the treatment of coughs and colds, to regulate breathing and intestinal functions, as a diuretic, a general relaxant, to relieve toothache, to coagulate the blood, strengthen eyesight, eliminate worms, douche the womb, and to treat burns and scorpion stings with a powder made from the plant.[554] Among the Jews of Iraq, the plant was a component in a medication to treat bone fractures, colds and diarrhea.[555]

Medical Qualities:
One of the main ingredients of its essential oils is the thymol.[556] Alternative medicine today uses the ethereal oil derived from the plant as a disinfectant, to prevent spasms, for strengthening, to dispel gases, to relieve coughs and colds, to clean the gullet and as an expectorant.[557]

Hedge Mustard (London Rocket)

Scientific name: *Sisymbrium sp.* (Cruciferae)
Hebrew: Todra   Arabic: Tudari[558]

Description:
Hedge mustard is an annual, biennial or perennial plant, either bald or hairy, with erect stems. The leaves are dissected and pinnate and the flowers, which bloom in clusters are generally yellow in colour, but are sometimes white or pink. The fruit is a narrow, elongated capsule, either flat or curled. Seven varieties of hedge mustard grow in Israel. Two of the more prominent ones used for remedies are the *Sisymbrium officinale* and the *Sisymbrium irio*.[559]

History:
Dioscorides described the *sisumrium eteron*, which is identified with *Sisymbrium nasturtium* mainly used for food and to treat sunburn.[560]

Medicinal Uses in Jerusalem:
In his entry 'Tudari' Ibn al-Baytar notes that it is also called 'tudrij' and he quotes Hunian ibn Ishaq who claimed that this plant was the Greek remedy *orosiman*. According to him, the plant was well known in Jerusalem and its environs by the name of 'ashjara' and among its medicinal uses he listed:

---

542 Ibn al-Baytar, al-Jami, II, pp. 2-3; Leclerc, No. 548.

543 Malki, p. 63.

544 Ibn al-Baytar, Tafsir, p. 224.

545 Assaph, 4, pp. 411-412.

546 al-Kindi, No. 70. Cf. al-Biruni, I, pp. 205-206.

547 al-Kindi, Nos. 6, 8.

548 Maimonides, Asthma, 12:1,3.

549 Ibn al-Baytar, al-Jami, II, pp. 2-3; Leclerc, No. 548. Cf. al-Antaki, p. 113.

550 Ibn al-Baytar, al-Jami, I, p. 153; Leclerc, No. 456; al-Antaki, p. 113.

551 al-Qazwini, p. 244. Cf. Ibn Sina, pp. 314-315.

552 Palevitz et al, p. 143.

553 Abu-Rabia, p. 20.

554 Reiani, p. 49, No. 116.

555 Ben-Yakov, p. 289; Krispil, p. 1218. Cf. Hooper, p. 178.

556 Uphof, p. 519; Plants & Animals, XI, p. 82.

557 Grieve, p. 811; Reiani, p. 49, No. 116; Palevitz et al, p. 144.

558 Maimonides, Glossaire, p. 106, No. 384; Issa, Dictionary, p. 170, No. 6. Cf. Ghaleb, p. 229, No. 4840; Dinsmore & Dalman, No. 95; Chizik, p. 727.

559 Feinbrun-Dothan, p. 226.

560 Disocorides, II.156.

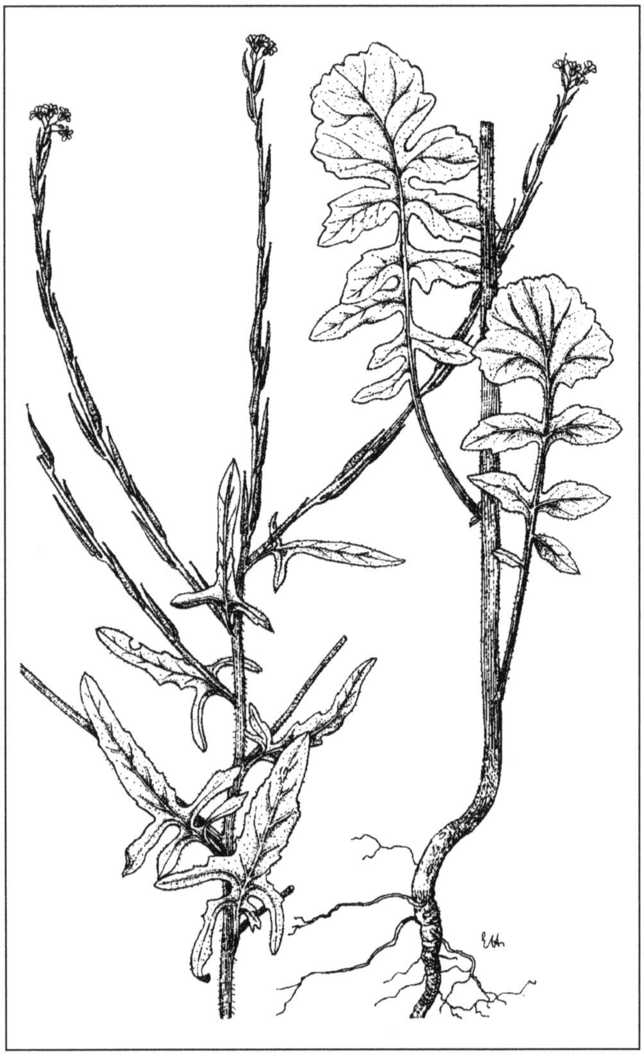

Figure 18 - Hedge Mustard (*Sisymbrium officinale*)

diseases of the breathing tract, reducing swellings and treating cancer.[561] Elsewhere, Ibn al-Baytar brings additional synonyms for the 'tudari' including 'ashjara' 'irsion' and 'shandla.'[562]

In his entry 'ashjara', Ibn al-Baytar quotes al-Tamimi who related that in al-Sham the leaves were eaten after being boiled in 'anfak' oil and salt and served as a sauce. This dish warmed the stomach, dispelled gases, and drained mucus, and it was used as an emmenagogue and to relieve constipation.[563]

Medicinal Uses in the Medieval Period:
Assaph Harofe described the 'tidra' and listed its uses: to treat wounds and contusions, to improve eyesight and cure diseases of the lung and liver.[564] According to al-Biruni, the plant was used to treat skin diseases.[565] Maimonides says that 'white todra' was a compound in a medication which was "very effective for coitus, increased the sperm, strengthened the kidneys and was fattening,' while 'red and white todari' was used as a compound in a concoction for aiding coitus.[566] Daud al-Antaki in his entry 'Tudari' also described the plant and listed its uses: to reduce swellings, to cure coughs and diseases of the chest, liver and spleen, to relieve rheumatism, cleanse wounds, dispel body odours and to cause fattening.[567]

Traditional Medicine:
Negev Bedouins use the leaves of the *Sisymbrium irio* for eating with yoghurt made from goats' milk which served as a remedy for throat inflammation and colds.[568] The seeds of other varieties, which are called 'tudari' in Iran and Iraq, are considered as stimulants for sexual desire, for fattening, for purifying the blood and to relieve stomach pains.[569] *Sisymbrium officinale*, which is called 'samara' in Iraq, is used as an expectorant, to cure chest diseases, to reduce fever, to constrict, to stimulate and as a diuretic.[570] Chizik described the use of 'asis matmarot' identified with *Sisymbrium officinale* to cure hoarseness.[571]

Modern Medicine:
The variety *Sisymbrium sophia* was used as an external remedy for canker sores because it contains various glycosides. The seeds are bitter and serve as an expectorant, as a strengthener, to reduce fever, to eliminate worms, to treat diseases of the breathing tract, dysentery and problems of the urinary tract.[572]

General Uses:
Sisymbrium irio is used by Negev Bedouins as a substitute for tobacco. At the beginning of the 20th century the plant was used in Jerusalem as a butter sauce and as food.[573] Various types of hedge mustard are used in Europe and Asia for sauces and in Mexico for the production of a drink. *Sisymbrium officinale* serves as a stimulant, an irritant, diuretic and is effective in treating scurvy.[574]

Hyssop

Scientific name: *Hyssopus officinalis* (Labiatae)
Hebrew: Ben-ezov refui Arabic: Zufa yabis[575]

Description:
The hyssop is a lowly shrub which grows on walls and rocks. It is square-stemmed with dark green leaves, and it flowers in

561 Ibn al-Baytar, al-Jami, I, p. 143; Leclerc, No. 436.

562 Ibn al-Baytar, al-Jami, III, p. 71; Leclerc, No. 1348.

563 Ibn al-Baytar, al-Jami, I, p. 34; Leclerc, No. 82. The editor identified it with 'arismin' but this is not plausible.

564 Assaph, 4, p. 405.

565 al-Biruni, II, p. 83.

566 Maimonides, Sexual, Introd. pp. 7, 11.

567 al-Antaki, p. 98. Cf. Ibn Sina, p. 443.

568 Abu-Rabia, p. 22.

569 Hooper, pp. 171-172. Cf. also al-Rawi & Chaakravarty, p. 89.

570 Ibid., p. 88. Cf. Grieve, pp. 570-571 for uses of hedge mustard varieties in Europe.

571 Chizik, p. 727.

572 Chopra et al, p. 31.

573 Plants & Animals, X, p. 102; Crowfoot & Baldensperger, p. 38.

574 Uphof, p. 486.

575 Issa, Dictionary, p. 97, No. 10. Additional names in al-Biruni, I, pp. 170-171.

the summer with feathery blossoms of blue, purple or white. The plant grows in Asia, Southern Europe and in the Middle East.[576]

Identification:
In Arabic medieval literature the plant was known as 'zufa yabis' and according to its name and description it has been identified with the *Hyssopus officinalis* to differentiate it from 'zufa ratab' which according to Maimonides means 'oil on wool.'[577] Although the plant does not grow wild in the Levant, it may have been cultivated in Jerusalem and its environs in rock gardens and on walls.

History:
The plant appears to have been well known in ancient Mesopotamia where it was used for remedial purposes and was called 'zufa' in Chaldean.[578] Classical medicine also recognized it as *Ussopus* and, according to Dioscorides, it was used to treat asthma, coughs and colds, to eliminate worms and drain mucus.[579]

Hyssop in Jerusalem and the Levant:
According to Ibn al-Khair al-Ashbili the 'zufa yabis' was a type of 'za'atar' (savory) which was frequently found in 'Jabal Bayt al-Maqdis' (the Jerusalem hills).[580] Ishaq Ibn Amran described the 'zufa yabis' and was quoted by Ibn al-Baytar: "It is a plant which grows in the hills of Jerusalem 'Bayt al-Maqdis,' its branches spread out at the height of one cubit, and some say it has leaves and stalks that resemble the form of the 'marzanjush' (cultivated hyssop) which has a good smell and a bitter taste, and is gathered in the spring."[581] According to Ibn Rushd, "the two varieties 'al-zufi' and 'al-zufa' are one and the same. It is a plant with a slender, square stem and leaves like the thin 'za'atar' leaves, which is called 'al-yabis' (the dry) of the mountain and garden variety. It contains strong properties that are beneficial to the chest and lungs, for chronic coughs and for the stomach. It is used in some villages in Syria and the Lebanon."[582]

It seems that the former description corresponds more closely to the type of thyme, which is called by a similar name even today.[583] Among its medicinal uses Ibn al-Baytar listed the heating ability of the plant and the fact that it was a component in a medication to eliminate chronic coughs, swelling in the lungs, asthma, colds, excess mucus and breathing difficulties. The plant also served to soften the stomach, to treat jaundice, to dissolve blood clots in the eyes, to cure diphtheria and to relieve toothache and earache. From the words of other physician Ibn Suleiman it seems that the plant was also used to treat dropsy, insect bites and excess tears.[584] From another sources, Abu al-Kassam al-Ghassani it appears that 'zufa yabis' was gathered in the Jerusalem hills and exported to North Africa.[585] Daud al-Antaki notes that the plant grew in the Jerusalem hills, and the medicinal uses he mentions are similar to those given by Ibn al-Baytar.[586]

Medicinal Uses in the Medieval Period:
According to al-Kindi, the 'zufa' was a component in a medication to reduce fever and to treat malaria.[587] Maimonides says that the hyssop was a hot and dry remedy.[588]

Traditional Medicine and General Uses:
A special kind of honey is made by bees from the nectar of the hyssop. The plant is also used in sauces, salads and soups, in meat dishes and in liqueurs.[589] In Europe the hyssop is used as a component in medications against cough, to reduce swellings, to stabilize blood pressure, to relieve colds and to treat throat pains, lung diseases, and the nerves. The plant is also utilized to produce ointment for treating and curing infections of the eyes, ears and throat, as well as bites and stings.[590]

In Iraq and Iran, the plant serves as a stimulant, an expectorant and to cause sweating.[591] Among the Jews of Iraq, the 'zufa' was a component in various medications to cure eye diseases, coughs and colds.[592] The plant is also known for its ability to cure heart problems.[593]

Conclusions:
Hyssop is a cultivated plant that was grown in the Land of Israel during the Middle Ages. From certain sources it appears that the plants grown in Jerusalem were so effective as cures that they were exported to North Africa. The plant had already served as a remedy in ancient Mesopotamia and was also mentioned in classical medicine. Its medicinal use has been quite consistent throughout history and included treating fever, colds, coughs, diseases of the eyes, lungs and the respiratory tract.

Jericho Balsam (Egyptian Balsam)

Scientific name: *Balanites aegyptiaca* (Zygophyllaceae)
Hebrew: Zakum mizri **Arabic: Zakum**[594]

Description:
Jericho balsam is a tree or prickly shrub that grows up to a height of six meters. It is a rare Sudanese plant, and is prevalent

[576] Loewenfeld & Back, pp. 149-152; Hooper, p. 128; Uphof, p. 278.

[577] Maimonides, Glossaire, p. 47, No. 136; Assaph, 4, pp. 38, 411.

[578] al-Kindi, p. 277, No. 131.

[579] Dioscorides, II.25. The editor has identified it with savory.

[580] al-Ashbili, p. 365.

[581] Ibn al-Baytar, al-Jami, II, pp. 172-173; Leclerc, No. 1136.

[582] Ibn Rushd, No. 102. Cf. Tuhfat, p. 16, No. 141.

[583] Dinsmore & Dalman, No. 1346.

[584] Ibn al-Baytar, al-Jami, II, pp. 172-173; Leclerc, No. 1136.

[585] al-Ghassani, p. 105.

[586] al-Antaki, p. 272.

[587] al-Kindi, No. 113. Cf. Ibn Sina, pp. 302-303.

[588] Maimonides, Aphorisms, 9:88. Cf. 'Zufa ratab' in Ibid., 23:49.

[589] Loewenfeld & Back, pp. 149-152; Uphof, p. 278.

[590] Loewenfeld & Back, pp. 149-152; Grieve, p. 426.

[591] Hooper, p. 128.

[592] Ben-Yakov, pp. 92, 165, 295, 317.

[593] In detail, including content of substances in: Uphof, p. 278.

[594] Ibn al-Baytar, al-Jami, II, p. 166; Leclerc, No. 1118.

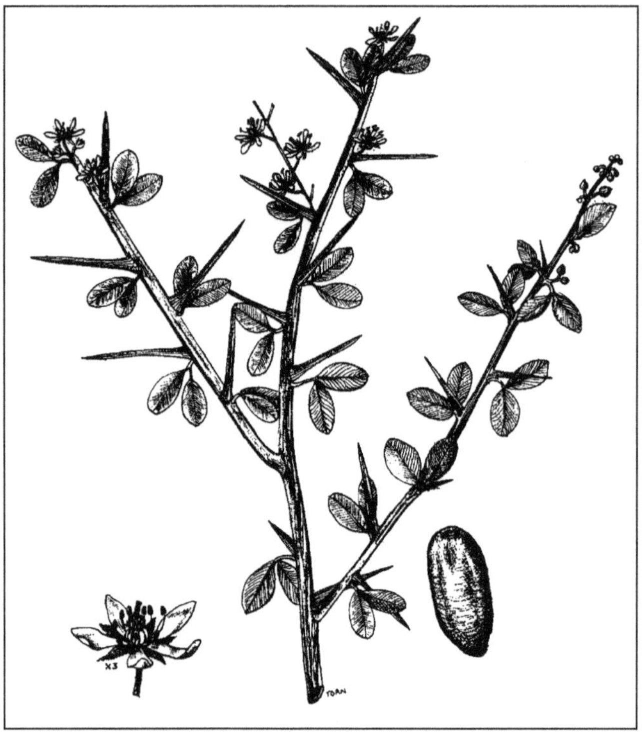

Figure 19 - Jericho Balzam (*Balanites aegyptiaca*)

in the Land of Israel, in desert oases and in hot, desert ravines mainly in the Dead Sea valley. Its leaves are leathery and fall in the winter, and its flowers are small and green. The fruit has a large kernel (up to 3 cm.), the pulp is juicy, and the kernel contains oil.[595]

History:
The fruits of this tree were among the gift offerings, which the ancient Egyptians presented to their gods. The tree was therefore sacred and its fruit was used for ritual purposes.[596] The researcher, Chizik, identified the tree with the biblical 'mesukan' (Isaiah 40:20). Other scholars tried to identify the gum resin of the Jericho balsam with the biblical 'tzori.'[597] Monks in the Judean desert used to extract oil from the kernels and sell it to pilgrims as 'tzori Gilead' (the balm of Gilead).[598]

Medicinal Uses in Jerusalem:
In his entry 'Dahan al-Zakum al-Shami' (Syrian balsam oil), Ibn al-Baytar quotes al-Tamimi who noted that Jericho balsam oil was produced in Jericho valley in 'Bilad al-Quds' (the district of Jerusalem). According to his description, the kernel oil served as a cathartic substance and a medication for rheumatism, women's sweat and paralysis. The pulp of the fruit was used as food for the poor, although it sometimes caused nausea and vomiting.[599]

In his entry 'Zakum ahar' Ibn al-Baytar described the tree: Thorny, with fruit the size of almonds, small leaves and yellow flowers. He also noted that Jericho balsam oil was fire-resistant more than any other oil, that it was pungent and was used as a medication against paralysis.[600] Daud al-Antaki noted in his entry 'Zaku' that the plant was known in 'al-Quds' (Jerusalem) and was used to reduce swellings, to suture wounds, to cure skin diseases, joint and muscle pains, to reduce gases and to open internal obstruction. The plant was considered a hot and dry drug.[601]

The wood of the Jericho balsam tree is used for building and woodcraft manufacturing, and its seeds contain oil which is used in Africa for food, and also as a remedy, or for anointing, and it is recommended in the production of soap. The leaves and fruit are edible, and in the Congo they are used in a preparing an alcoholic drink.[602] The Arabs of Israel use the oil derived from the seeds to treat joint pains and to relax the nerves and muscles. The juice or smoke of the roasted seeds serves to treat dizziness, fainting and amnesia.[603] In Egypt, the fruit of the Jericho balsam is used to treat illnesses such as: syphilis, diarrhea, vomiting, chills, worms and diabetes.[604] The bark of the tree and its roots are considered as cathartic substances and as effective in eliminating worms.[605] In India, the seeds, fruit, tree bark and leaves are all considered as cathartic substances.[606]

Medical Qualities:
The ripe fruit of the Jericho balsam contains steroids which are hemolytic substances that are poisonous mainly for cold-blooded creatures.[607] The fruit contains 30%-60% oil and 7% saponins. The saponins are liable to cause deterioration of the blood and this led to the use of the fruit pulp to poison fish. The effect of this substance on humans is negligible.[608]

Job's Tears

Scientific name: *Coix lachryma-jobi* (Gramineae)
Hebrew: Dema'ot iyov Arabic: Amdharian, Damu'a iyob[609]

Description:
This plant is a tall annual cereal grain (up to 80 cm.) with ribbon-like leaves and grayish white berries shaped like pears, which are hard and shiny. The fruits have an egg-shaped capsule (tears).[610]

595 Plants & Animals, X, p. 200; Feinbrun-Dothan, p. 396.

596 Gal, p. 149; Krispil, p. 196; Dafni, Dudaim, p. 29.

597 Feliks, World, p. 248.

598 Dafni, Dudaim, p. 29; Krispil, p. 196.

599 Ibn al-Baytar, al-Jami, II, p. 114; Leclerc, No. 944. Cf. al-Antaki, p. 179

600 Ibn al-Baytar, al-Jami, II, p. 166; Leclerc, No. 1118; al-Biruni, I, p. 168.

601 al-Antaki, p. 179.

602 Zohary, p. 491; Uphof, p. 63. In detail: Chopra et al, p. 24.

603 Palevitz et al, p. 68; Crowfoot & Baldensperger, p. 86.

604 Kamel, Zakom; Gal, p. 149. Popular medical uses in: Dafni, Dudaim, p. 29; Palevitz et al, p. 69.

605 Uphof, p. 63.

606 Chopra et al, p. 23.

607 Ibid, p. 24.

608 Dafni, Edible, p. 39.

609 Issa, Dictionary, p. 53, No.20; Ghaleb, p. 97, No. 1989.

610 Zohary, p. 639.

History:
The medicinal use of the plant is first mentioned in China (3rd cent. CE) since when it has been widely utilized in Chinese medicinal prescriptions.[611] Today it is a cultivated plant in many tropical countries.[612]

Medicinal Uses in Jerusalem:
According to Ibn al-Baytar, the 'amdharian' is a plant found in abundance in 'Bayt al-Maqdis' (Jerusalem) and on the Temple Mount itself within the Haram al-Sharif.

He claimed further that it also grew in the cemeteries near the gates of Damascus and in Alexandria. The plant resembles a tree with large leaves and is strongly scented.[613]

Medicinal Uses in the Medieval Period:
Among the medicinal uses of 'amdharian' that were noted by Ibn al-Baytar were: the opening of obstructions, strengthening of the liver, reducing swellings both internal and external, treating of wounds, skin diseases and the cooling of wounds and swellings. It also served to cure the bites of dogs and snakes, and scorpion stings.[614] Daud al-Antaki stated in his entry "amdharian' that its Arabic name was 'damu'a iyob' (Job's tears) and that its seeds were used to make prayer beads. The plant was grown mainly in cemeteries and was used to open blockages, to relieve stomach pains, to neutralise scorpion stings and to leach pus. The plant was a hot and dry drug.[615]

Traditional Medicine and General Uses:
This ornamental plant is commonly grown in lawn gardens. It berries are used to make bead necklaces, rugs and prayer beads, and they are also used as food for man and beast, for the beer and tea industry, and in certain countries for remedies as well.[616] The plant was used to treat infections, to relieve pain, to reduce fever, to stimulate spleen activity, to lower the amount of sugar in the blood, and to cause diarrhea. It was also used to treat rheumatism, problems of the urinary tract and oedema (dropsy) of the lungs.[617]

Conclusions:
Ibn al-Baytar is the only known source that mentions Job's tears in connection with the Land of Israel and with Jerusalem in particular. So far no further evidence has been discovered for the presence of this plant in Israel in early times. It is not part of the natural flora of the country and there is no proof that it was an agricultural crop.

Lentisk

Scientific name: *Pistacia lentiscus* (Anacardiaceae)
Hebrew: Elat ha-mastik Arabic: Mastaki, Luban, Saris[618]

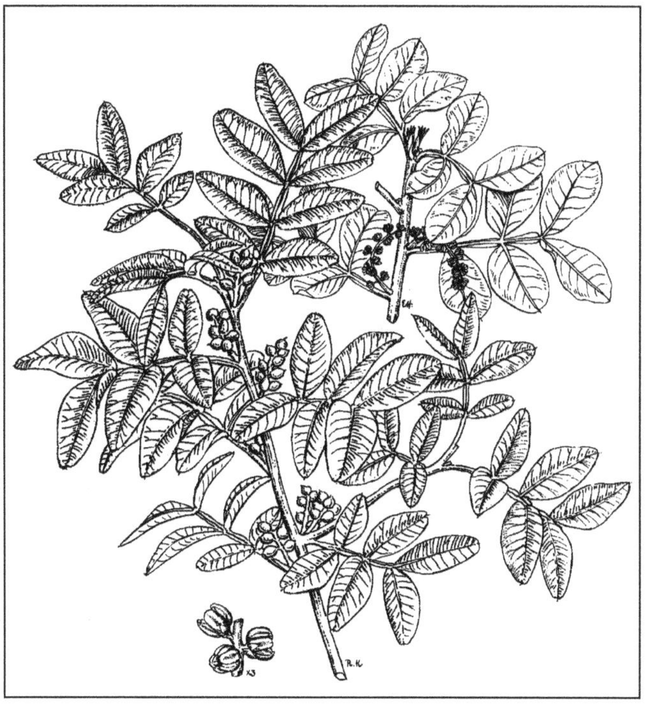

Figure 20 - Lentisk (*Pistacia lentiscus*)

Description:
The lentisk is a small tree or evergreen shrub (up to 2 m.). It is one of the most common plants in the forests, maquis and garigues of the Mediterranean phytogeographic zone. The green leaves are pinnate and the red fruits ripen in the summer. The leaves and other parts of the plant contain fragrant resin that drips when the plant is slashed.[619]

History:
Since early times, a pungent gum was derived from the lentisk resin and this gave it the Hebrew name 'mastik'. The plant was identified with the 'bekhaim' (mulberry trees) mentioned in the story about King David and the Philistines (II Samuel, 5:23).[620] Dioscorides recommended the use of *schinos* (lentisk resin) to brighten the facial skin, cure wounds, treat dysentery, stop bleedings, constrict the gums and prevent bad breath. The resin was also used in a remedy to treat snake bites, the fruits were used to treat scabies among people and dogs, and the oil derived from the plant served as a purgative.[621] The Jewish Sages described the use of lentisk resin 'mustiky' for medicinal applications and for bad breath. Lentisk resin production, uses and trade still exist today in the Greek Islands.[622]

Medicinal Uses in Jerusalem:
A list of goods belonging to a deceased person in Jerusalem (1391 CE) included several 'saris' branches which might have been used for basketwork, or subsequently for medical purposes.[623] 'Saris' is the Arabic term for lentisk.[624] The Arab

[611] Bown, p. 264.

[612] Hill, p. 332.

[613] Ibn al-Baytar, al-Jami, I, p. 56; Leclerc, No. 148.

[614] Ibid.

[615] al-Antaki, p. 57.

[616] Uphof, p. 143; Hill, p. 333; Chizik, p. 740.

[617] Bown, p. 264.

[618] Assaph. 4. p. 416; Maimonides, Glossaire, p. 70, No. 232.

[619] Plants & Animals, X, p. 212.

[620] Feliks, World, p. 102.

[621] Dioscorides, I.89.

[622] Howe, pp. 307-308.

[623] al-Asali, Wata'iq, II/1 p. 33.

[624] Dinsmore & Dalman, No. 405; Issa, Dictionary, p. 141, No. 12.

village of Saris near Jerusalem was named for the lentisk shrubs growing in that area.[625] Refael Malki asserted that the 'al-mastika' (lentisk resin) was a component in a pill applied to strengthen the brain and the heart.[626] David de Silva describe the use of 'mastiga' as a diuretic drug and for the treatment of internal diseases.[627]

Lentisk in the Levant:
Hayim Vital reported that the 'levona mastik' was a component in a remedy to cure abscess in the throat.[628] The resin was mentioned indirectly by al-Zahari with regard to the 'mastikey al-Shamiya' (Syrian lentisk resin) which he saw in Crete.[629] al-Israeli also gives a description of this plant.[630] The 'mastico' was one of the substances sold in the markets of Acre in the 13th century.[631] The traveler Rauwolf who visited the Land of Israel in 1573, says he saw lentisk growing on the route from Jaffa to Ramlah and that resin gum was produced from it.[632]

Medicinal Uses in the Medieval Period:
Ibn al-Baytar wrote about several medicinal applications of the plant and its parts: the leaves were used to induce urination, cure wounds, treat cancerous wounds, mend broken bones, stop womb secretions and strengthen and brighten the teeth. Oil derived from the lentisk fruit induced constipation. The resin was used as an expectorant, an analgesic for toothache and stomach pains, to improve the taste of food and increase the appetite, to brighten the skin and strengthen the stomach.[633]

Daud al-Antaki mentions these uses and added others such as: to treat leprosy, eye diseases, dysentery and constipation.[634] According to Maimonides, lentisk resin was a component in a remedy to strengthen the heart[635] and in a syrup to improve the digestion.[636] The resin was also used as a component in a remedy for eye diseases, and water boiled with lentisk resin was used to strengthen the stomach and liver.[637]

Traditional Medicine:
Arabs in Israel have several uses for the different parts of the lentisk plant. The fruits are used to treat paralysis, for bad breath, and to clean the teeth. The leaves and young branches are used to treat high temperature, cure internal inflammations, relieve throat and stomach pains, jaundice, kidney stones, fungi and diarrhea.[638] Yemenite Jews use the resin to congeal wounds, cure liver and lung ailments, ease breathing and back pains, strengthen the function of the intestines, treat tuberculosis, inflammations and swelling of the intestines, and to stop bleedings.[639]

Modern Medicine:
Lentisk resin is used as an expectorant, stimulant and as a component in dental plaster.[640] It is also used as an incense, to coat paints and metals and also as a glue, a spice and a preservative (mainly for wine).[641] In Greece and Syria, a traditional liqueur is made out of the resin and the Arabs in Israel often place the fruits on the oven to enjoy the fragrance.[642]

Madonna Lily (White Lily)

Scientific name: *Lilium candidum* (Liliaceae)
Hebrew: Shoshan zahor Arabic: Sawsan[643]

Description:
The Madonna lily is a rare perennial herbaceous plant, with a bulb root and tall, erect stem (1.5 m.) without branches. Its tapering leaves are dense and its flowers, which rise up in clusters of five to ten blossoms on each stalk, are large (up to 10 cm.) and white. The flowers contain nectar of a sweet fragrance and open mainly at night. The fruit is a large capsule with many flat seeds inside.[644]

History:
The Hebrew name is derived from the number of petals in its corolla, and is often mentioned in the Bible as a symbol of beauty (Song of Songs, 6:2), as a symbol for the flourishing nation of Israel (Hosea, 14:6) and for its pleasant fragrance.[645] It is also mentioned in the Mishna, Talmud, Ben Sira and in Greek and Roman writings where it is a symbol of beauty and a source for remedies. Dioscorides praised the fragrant oil produced in Phoenicia and Egypt from a thousand lily blossoms *susinon* steeped in oil with the addition of myrrh and sweet calamus. This oil was the basis for medication against the bites of venomous creatures and for bandaging wounds. The bulb root was used for cosmetic purposes and to calm the nerves, while the seeds were used against snakebite.[646] The researcher, Feliks, identified the biblical 'shoshan' with the Madonna lily, according to the description of the plant by the Jewish Sages and other sources.[647]

---

625 Vilnai, p. 458.

626 Malki, p. 67.

627 Amar, de Silva, p. 127.

628 Benajahu, p. 106.

629 al-Zahari, p. 176.

630 al-Israeli, p. 235. Cf. Maimonides, Glossaire, p. 31, No. 66.

631 Pegolotti, p. 64. On the trade in the plant and resin gum in the Middle Ages see: Heyd, II, pp. 633-635.

632 Rauowlf, p. 460.

633 Ibn al-Baytar, al-Jami, IV, pp. 158-159; Leclerc, No. 2139. Cf. Ibn Sina, p. 360.

634 al-Antaki, pp. 299-300. Cf. al-Biruni, I, p. 306.

635 Maimonides, Answers, 3:19; 4:15, 20.

636 Maimonides, Regimen, p. 76.

637 Maimonides, Aphorisms, 9:46; 13:44; 22:39.

638 Palevitz et al, p. 35.

639 Reiani, p. 42, No. 94.

640 Uphof, p. 413. Additional uses in: Palevitz et al, p. 37.

641 Chizik, pp. 580, 729; Uphof, p. 413; Hill, p. 161; Howe, pp. 307-309.

642 Dafni, Dudaim, p. 16.

643 Maimonides, Glossaire, p. 73, No. 247; p. 78, No. 272; Issa, Dictionary, p. 109, No. 2.

644 Plants & Animals, XI, pp.209-210.

645 Additional references and discussion of identity in: Feliks, World, pp. 234-240.

646 Dioscorides, I.62.

647 Feliks, World, p. 238.

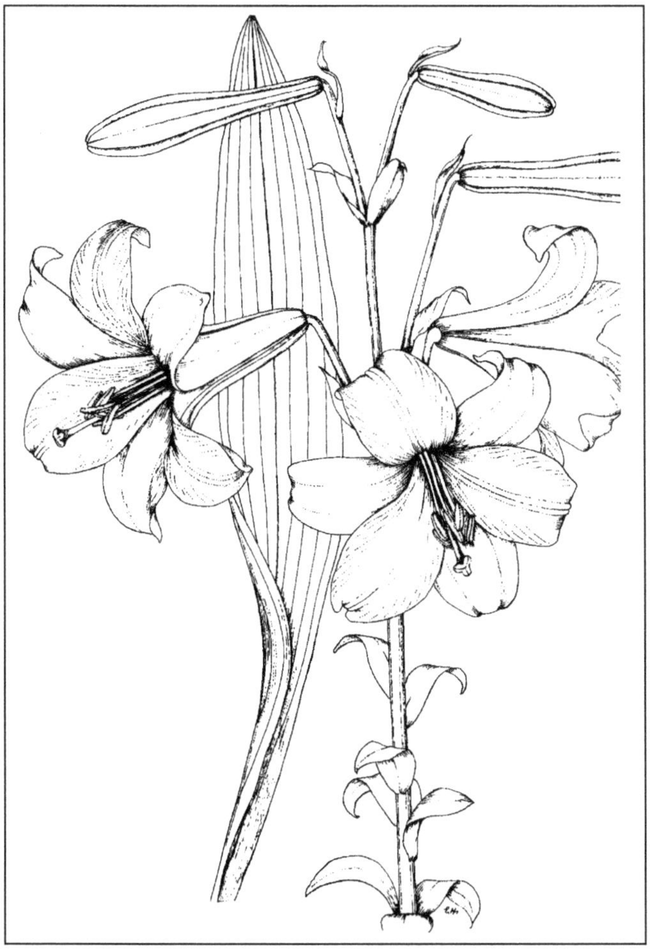

Figure 21 - Madonna Lily (*Lilium candidum*)

During the Middle Ages the plant was identified with the biblical 'shoshan' and since Christians saw it as a symbol of purity it was dedicated to Mary, mother of Jesus (the Madonna). It is assumed that this is the reason for it having been continually plucked by the Crusaders and nearly becoming extinct in the Land of Israel. In modern times, during the 1920's, it was newly discovered in the north of Israel.[648] The researcher, Levey, claimed that during the Middle Ages the Arabic name 'sawsan' was the term for various kinds of iris, nuphar and other types of lily.[649]

Medicinal Uses in Jerusalem:
According to Refael Malki, the oil of the Madonna lily was a light cathartic drug.[650]

Madonna Lily in the Levant:
Hayim Vital reported on the use of Madonna lily oil and the root of 'lidio morado' (Spanish purple lily) in preparing a medication to treat hemorrhoids.[651]

Medicinal Uses in the Medieval Period:
al-Kindi reported on the use of Madonna lily oil to treat swellings in the ears, hemorrhoids, and pus-infected wounds in the mouth.[652] Shabtai Donolo tells of the medicinal use of lily water which was a basis for various medications.[653] Maimonides quotes Galen and describes the use of the lily roots to prepare a medication for treating asthma and to clear the lungs.[654] Ibn al-Baytar in his entry 'dahan al-sawsan al-abiz' describes the lily oil and quotes a section from al-Tamimi's treatise *al-Marshad*.[655] According to al-Qazwini, the 'sawsan' was a plant with a soporific fragrance and the ability in external application to remove freckles and to relieve headache. It was also effective in treating snakebite. The powder of the plant was used to treat skin diseases and to improve facial skin.[656]

Traditional Medicine and General Uses:
The flowers were used as a source for essential oils in the cosmetic and perfume industries.[657] Natural medicine makes use of the flowers soaked in wine as a disinfectant, and the bulb of the lily soaked in milk to prepare poultices, while lily water was used for cosmetic purposes.[658] In Iraq, the Madonna lily is called 'sawsan abiad' and its flowers are used as a drug against spasms, the bulb root is used as a drug for strengthening and softening, as a diuretic, an expectorant, and more recently also as a cure for dropsy and an effective treatment for vomiting.[659]

Marjoram

Scientific name: *Origanum sp.* (Labiatae)

There are two species of marjoram which were extensively used in Jerusalem and the Levant: Wild Marjoram and Sweet or Cultivated Marjoram.

Identification:
The identification of the different species of marjoram mentioned in medieval literature was a complicated matter and has been discussed by the Jewish Sages.[660] Babylonian Jewish scholars identify the 'ezov' (wild marjoram) with the plant 'shomshok' and Assaph Harofe specifies different varieties of the 'ezov.'[661] In a letter found in the Genizah, the writer made a clear distinction between the two species - the wild 'sa'tar' and the cultivated 'mardakosh.'[662] Maimonides also distinguishes between these two species and provides

648 Plants & Animals, XI, p. 209.

649 al-Kindi, p. 289, No. 160.

650 Malki, p. 79.

651 Benajahu, p. 101.

652 al-Kindi, Nos. 52, 75, 125, 146.

653 Donolo, pp. 14-15.

654 Maimonides, Asthma, 14:3, 5; Maimonides, Aphorisms, 16:55; 21:76.

655 Ibn al-Baytar, al-Jami, II, pp. 100-101; Leclerc, No. 895.

656 al-Qazwini, p. 252. Cf. Ibn al-Baytar, al-Jami, III, pp. 43-45; Leclerc, No. 1253; al-Antaki, p. 165; Ibn Sina, pp. 382-383.

657 Uphof, p. 312.

658 Dafni, Dudaim, p. 84.

659 al-Rawi & Chaakravarty, p. 59. Cf. Grieve, pp. 484-484 for uses in Europe.

660 For example in Mishna, Parah 11:7.

661 Assaph, 4, p. 408.

662 Goitein, Jewry, p. 204.

many synonyms for the cultivated species[663] and in his entry 'sa'tar' he described several other species.[664] Since the key differences between the species dealt with in this study are listed below, further identification of other species will be left for future research.[665]

Wild Marjoram (Hyssop)

Scientific name: *Origanum syriacum* (*Majorana syriaca*)
Hebrew: Ezov Arabic: Sa'tar, Za'tar,

Description:
Wild marjoram is a perennial, Mediterranean dwarf shrub (up to 60 cm.) with green-gray hairy leaves and small, white flowers. There are six varieties of wild marjoram, but only the *Origanum syriacum* grows in the Land of Israel.[666]

Sweet Marjoram

Scientific name: *Majorana hortensis*
Hebrew: Ezov tarbuti Arabic: Marzangosh, Mardakosh, Habat al-cana[667]

Description:
This is a small, perennial plant, with narrow, gray leaves and whitish-pink flowers which bloom from April to September. It originates in Europe and has been cultivated in the Levant for centuries.[668]

History:
This plant is mentioned in the Bible in various contexts: in relation to the Passover in Egypt (Exodus, 12:22), purification of the leper (Leviticus, 14:4), the ashes of the red heifer (Numbers 19:6 and 18),[669] and for its purgative qualities (Psalms, 51:9).[670]

Dioscorides claimed that the plant was used as a cure for dropsy, oedema, inflammations, excess urination and to regulate menstruation.[671] He also praised 'marjoram oil' which was brought from Egypt.[672] From the Jewish Sages we learn that the plant was used as food as well as for ritual purposes. It seems that the name 'ezov' was a common term for certain plants which shared similar qualities and were all used as foods, sauces and medicinal substances. The plant also appears in the folklore of other cultures in the region.[673]

Medicinal Uses in Jerusalem:
In a merchant's letter found in the Genizah (1065 CE) the name of a Jewish trader called Ibn 'Alush al-Jazar was mentioned as coming from Tyre to Jerusalem and bringing different substances including 'henna,' 'sa'tar' and 'markadosh.' This last name was a misspelling of 'mardakosh' i.e. marjoram.[674] Here we have clear evidence of the existence of the two different species of marjoram. According to Refael Malki, marjoram was one of the many substances used in a syrup made by the synagogue 'gabbaim' in Jerusalem as a remedy for the poor members of the community.[675]

David de Silva mentioned the medicinal uses of the 'ezov', mainly as a treatment for the stomach, and as a digestive and an appetizer.[676]

Marjoram in the Levant:
During the Mamluk period, cultivated marjoram was one of the perfume and medicinal plants grown in the Holy Land.[677] Hayim Vital of Safed reported that one of the main substances in a special syrup to cure asthma was 'zufa' (wild marjoram).[678]

Among the remedies for hemorrhoids, Vital mentions boiled marjoram, cumin and the powder of peach seeds as well as another remedy consisting of marjoram and frogs fried in oil.[679]

Medicinal Uses in the Medieval Period:
Assaph Harofe asserted that marjoram was used to cure many illnesses, mainly gynecological, kidney and urinary tract disorders.[680] Maimonides stated that marjoram was an easily digested food[681] and he quotes al-Tamimi who claimed that it was used to treat anemia.[682] al-Qazwini says in his entry 'sa'tar' (wild marjoram) that it was as remedy for toothache, intestinal worms and snakebites.[683] In his entry 'marzangosh' (sweet marjoram) al-Qazwini testifies to its good scent and says that it was used as a cure for migraines, headaches, constipation and paralysis.[684] Similar medicinal uses were described by Daud al-Antaki as well.[685]

---

663 Maimonides, Glossaire, p. 71, No. 236.

664 Ibid., pp. 90-91, No. 319.

665 See discussion of marjoram and its names in Amar, Production, p. 40.

666 Plants & Animals, XI, p. 79.

667 For additional names see the discussion in 'Identification' above. In the English Bible the name for this plant is translated as 'hyssop.'

668 Plants & Animals, XII, pp. 90-91; Amar, Production, p. 40.

669 The Samaritans still use bunches of marjoram leaves to prevent blood clots and claim that 'za'atar for the blood is like water for sugar." Experiments conducted by the Hebrew University have not confirmed this theory. On this subject in detail, see: Crowfoot & Baldensperger, p. 78.

670 For detailed identification of the biblical hyssop (sweet marjoram) see: Feliks, World, pp. 177-178; Fleisher, pp. 232-233.

671 Dioscorides, III.30.

672 Ibid., I.58.

673 Palevitz et al, p. 22; Dafni, Dudaim, p. 12.

674 Goitein, Jewry, p. 204.

675 Malki, p. 63.

676 Amar, de Silva, p. 111.

677 Suriano, p. 221; al-Amari, p.26.

678 Benajahu, p. 96. Cf. Ibn Sina, p. 302.

679 Ibid., pp. 98, 100.

680 Assaph, 4, p. 408.

681 Maimonides, Aphorisms, 20:49.

682 Ibid., No. 20:84.

683 al-Qazwini, p. 254.

684 Ibid., p.262. Cf. Ibn Sina, p. 367.

685 al-Antaki, p. 292.

Traditional Medicine:
Marjoram is used by the Arabs of Israel to relieve headache, cure gum inflammations and for whitening and strengthening the teeth. It is also used to ease cough, strengthen the heart, cure dizziness, expel worms, and to treat internal inflammations of the stomach, lungs, and liver.[686] Yemenite and Babylonian Jews used to make a medicinal tea from marjoram leaves to ease labour pains, as a general sedative, to cure heart pains, and reduce body swellings, mainly in the legs. Marjoram was also used as a component in remedies to ease headaches, earache and stomach pains, and to disinfect the female sex organs.[687]

General Uses:
Marjoram was used in the past for heating, and the wild species is a main substance in the famous eastern spice called 'za'atar.' Ibn Masawayh suggested using 'marzangosh' oil while staying in the hot bathhouse (hamam)[688] Arab villagers ('fellahin') used to pad their shoes with wild marjoram leaves in the winter for warmth and disinfection of the feet.[689] The seeds of the plant consists of essential oils used in the food and cosmetic industries.[690]

Conclusions:
Sweet marjoram is one of the typical plants of the Land of Israel. Its use as a traditional spice is very common among all the local inhabitants until the present day. Large quantities of the plant and its products are exported to neighboring Arab countries and for this reason it has been declared a protected species in Israel.

The history of the medicinal uses of this plant is a long one and historical evidence can be found in sources from different historical periods. Modern pharmacological researches have revealed that some of the ancient medicinal uses proved to be true, and it is therefore no wonder that traditional medicine in Israel and in the Levant still makes use of this plant.[691] Cultivated sweet marjoram and its medicinal uses were rooted in the Levant and both species of marjoram are mentioned in medieval sources. Three different sources, from the 11th, 17th, and 18th centuries, describe the medicinal uses and trade of both species of marjoram in space Jerusalem.

Mignonette (Dyer's Weed)

Scientific name: *Reseda alba* (Resedaceae)
Hebrew: Richpa levana Arabic: Jalbhang[692]

Description:
The genus has 60 species that flourish in various phytogeographic zones in the region. In Israel there are 12 species, half of them in the desert areas and the rest in the Mediterranean area. The mignonette is an annual plant, upright and growing to a height of 30-100 cm. It can be found close to human habitation such as walls and refuse dumps. Its flowers are clustered spikes of white blossoms, its leaves are lance-shaped, and its seeds are encapsulated.[693]

History:
The Latin meaning of the scientific name, *Reseda*, is restful - which is the medicinal quality attributed to the plant. Pliny was the one who gave it that name and recommended it for pain relief. Dioscorides described the *Sesamoeides mikron* identified with *Reseda canescens* and listed its medicinal uses: removing mucus, causing diarrhea, and curing swellings.[694]

Medicinal Uses in Jerusalem and the Levant:
Ibn al-Baytar in his entry 'Dhanb al-haruf' (sheep's tail) quotes Abu al-Abas al-Nabati who described various kinds of mignonette growing in the regions under Muslim rule and noted that the inhabitants of North Africa and Greater Syria used this name for a different variety which was used to cure eye diseases. He added that: "I saw it in Bayt al-Maqdis (Jerusalem)… and its effectivity against dog bites."[695]

Medicinal Uses in the Medieval Period:
Ibn al-Baytar in his entry 'jalbhang' Describes the plant and lists medicinal uses such as: curing wounds, removing mucus, and causing vomiting and diarrhea. In his view the plant was toxic.[696]

Modern Medicine and General Uses:
Another species, *Reseda luteola*, has been used since pre-historic times as a colouring substance[697] and was frequently mentioned by the Jewish Sages.[698] *Reseda odorata* served as a source for essential oils used for cosmetic purposes.[699]

Myrobalan (Cherry Plum)

Scientific name: *Terminalia sp.* (Rosaceae)
Hebrew: Amlag Arabic: Halilaj

Description:
The *Terminalia* genus includes 200 species. The trees are tall and their fruit contains 30% tannin which is used for remedial and industrial purposes. Indian myrobalan (*Terminalia arjuana*) is a tall tree with leaves that cluster close to the ends of the branches, and its globular fruit is a large, tasty drupe containing 50% oil, which is used for food.

686 Palevitz et al, p. 21; Crowfoot & Baldensperger, p. 78.

687 Reiani, p. 30, No. 64; Ben-Yakov, pp. 77, 103, 116, 129 ff.

688 Ibn Masawayh, p. 250.

689 Plants & Animals, XI, p. 80.

690 Ibid, XII, p. 91.

691 Fleisher; Fleisher et al.

692 Issa, Dictionary, p. 154, No. 15. Cf. Dinsmore & Dalman, No. 187; Ben-Yakov, p. 599.

693 Plants & Animals, X, p. 122; Feinbrun-Dothan, p. 271.

694 Dioscorides, IV.153.

695 Ibn al-Baytar, al-Jami, II, p. 126; Leclerc, No. 1004.

696 Ibn al-Baytar, al-Jami, I, p. 165; Leclerc, No. 496. Cf. Ibid, Nos. 67, 345, 1231, for synonyms and additional species such as 'samsam bari'

697 Zohary, p.402; Hill, p. 130; Uphof, p. 446.

698 For example: Feliks, Shevi'it, II, pp. 122-124.

699 al-Rawi & Chaakravarty, p. 81 including content of active substances; Uphof, p. 446.

Most of the varieties listed below[700] grow in India and Madagascar.[701]

Other known species are: *Terminalia citrina, Terminalia chebula, Terminalia bellerica, Terminalia emblica.*

History:
The use of the myrobalan fruit for remedy is well known in India and China since early times. In Greek and Roman medical treatises, neither the tree nor its fruit is mentioned.[702] In the Middle East the plant is mentioned from the early Islamic period in connection with the medicinal use of its fruit. In the West, there is no information about this plant until the Middle Ages when trade in its fruit began.

Medicinal Uses in Jerusalem:
In a Genizah letter dated 1053 CE, Abraham ben Shmuel of Ramlah requests Shlomo ben Yehuda of Jerusalem to send him a little 'halilaj' besides the 'khol' "to remove the white spot from the eye of my little daughter."[703] In another letter dated 1040 CE, Moshe ben Ya'akov of Jerusalem, writing in the name of his sister, requests Naharai ben Nissim of Fustat to buy some 'cabli' - probably referring to 'halilaj caboli' - and to bring it to Jerusalem.[704]

Myrobalan in the Levant:
In a Genizah letter dated 1060 CE from Ya'akov ben Yosef of Ashkelon to Naharai ben Nissim of Fustat, the writer requests that a consignment of yellow 'amlag' be sent to him. Another letter of that same year describes the sale of 'amlag' in Tyre on behalf of a trader in Fustat.[705] 'Amlag' (Helileth) is mentioned in a list of substances that the Crusaders in Acre traded in during the 13th century.[706]

Medicinal Uses in the Medieval Period:
al-Kindi reported on the use of black 'halilaj' which was a cathartic drug intended also for the cure of ear diseases and throat pains, while the yellow 'halilaj' was used to counteract swellings in the mouth and was also used as a component in an abortive medication.[707] Maimonides mentions several uses for different varieties of myrobalan such as a decoction of 'myrobalanash' that was defined as a medication which could also be used by healthy persons. Elsewhere he indicates that the 'myrobalani caboli' 'andi' and 'balilaj' were all components of 'the great atriphal.' These varieties were also components in a cathartic syrup.[708] 'Balilaj' and 'amlag' served as components in a decoction to strengthen breathing, to "revive the spirit, stimulate coitus, harden the penis and increase sperm." All the species of myrobalan are cold and dry drugs.[709]

Ibn al-Baytar described the different varieties of the 'halilaj' and quotes many physicians in reference to it. Most of the information deals with the various uses of the 'amlag' fruit for causing or preventing diarrhea by means of the varieties which have pungent and astrigent qualities. These qualities also aid in treating hemorrhoids. Ibn al-Baytar quotes al-Ghafiqi who praised this medication for preventing diarrhea, and for strengthening the gums, teeth and brain, and he called it "one of the most important and useful medications."[710]

Frederick Hasselquist testifies that when he visited Egypt they used 'myrobalan' there. According to the information he gathered, he described each of the different terms - 'caboli' 'asfar' 'balili' 'ambalili' 'hindi' and cabjiri' - their various qualities and the ripening stage when the fruit was picked. Hasselquist assumed that the references were to a specific tree which grew in India and Malabar, and that its fruit was brought by caravan to Egypt. The main use of the fruit was to cause diarrhea.[711]

Traditional Medicine:
Yemenite Jews called the dried, sour fruit of the *Terminalia chebula* by the name 'halilaj' and used it to cure eye inflammation and excess tears, to strengthen the lungs and to treat jaundice, an excess of stomach juices and respiratory difficulties. The substance also served as a component in a medication to increase sexual potency and to treat hemorrhoids, backache and stomach ache.[712] The Jews of Iraq had similar uses for the different varieties of the 'halilaj.'[713] The fruits of the *Terminalia bellerica* called 'balila' in Persia, are brought to Iran from India and serve as an astrigent, to improve digestion, as eye ointments and as strengtheners. Other varieties, mainly the 'caboli' (*Terminalia chebula*) are found in the markets of Iran, Iraq and Israel, and are used mainly as cathartic substances and as medication for stomach pains.[714] In Egypt, the 'caboli' variety is used till today as a cathartic substance.[715]

General Uses:
The fruits of most varieties are used in the leather industry because of their astrigent properties. The wood of the Indian 'amlag' is used in industry and for building.[716]

700 According to Korner, p. 651; Issa, Dictionary, pp. 178-179; Maimonides, Glossaire, p. 41, No. 112; p. 103, No. 374; Maimonides, Hemorrhoids, 4:1, 19.

701 Zohary, p. 459; Hill, pp. 123-124.

702 According to Levey, see: al-Kindi, p. 342.

703 Gil, p. 421, No. 230.

704 Ibid., p. 106, No. 460.

705 Ibid., p. 187, No. 487; p. 210, No. 494; p. 215, No. 496.

706 Assises, p. 176.

707 al-Kindi, Nos. 68, 71-71, 75, 211. Cf. Ibn Sina, pp. 271-271; al-Biruni, I, p. 76; II, pp. 80, 104.

708 Maimonides, Regimen, 2:9; 3:9, 11.

709 Maimonides, Sexual, 1:5. Cf. al-Ghafiqi, No. 124; Maimonides, Aphorisms, 21:73.

710 Ibn al-Baytar, al-Jami, IV, p. 190; Leclerc, No. 2261. For similar uses see also: al-Antaki, p. 62.

711 Hasselquist, p. 300.

712 Reiani, p. 48, No. 114.

713 Collected references in: Ben-Yakov, p. 708.

714 Hooper, p. 177.

715 Ducros, p. 14.

716 Reiani, p. 48, No. 114; Hill, pp. 123-124; Uphof, p. 415.

Myrrh

Scientific name: *Commiphora myrrha* (Burseraceae)
Hebrew: Mor Arabic: Murr[717]

Description:
This species has 50 varieties that grow in the deserts of Africa and Arabia. Myrrh is a small, deciduous tree or thorny shrub exuding an aromatic resin that emerges from ducts found in the stem and branches. The crystallized resin is reddish-yellow in colour and is produced by slashing the stem and gathering the resin after it dries.[718]

History:
Myrrh resin is one of the most ancient medicinal substances. It is mentioned in the Ebers papyrus as a component in various medications and an ingredient in incense in other cultures.[719] The Bible mentions it twelve times in connection with its use as a perfume and incense (e.g. Song of Songs 4:14), and in the Talmud, Jewish Sages have also noted its uses. Dioscorides in his entry *Smurna* describes the production of the resin and claimed that the pure variety causes heat, induces sleep, dries and constricts, serves as an external and internal medication and as incense.[720] In the Mishna, myrrh ointment is mentioned as softening the skin and depilating it. Myrrh is listed among the valuable merchandise traded in the East and in the Arabian peninsula in particular throughout the course of history.[721]

Medicinal Uses in Jerusalem:
Refael Malki relates about the use of choice myrrh which was contributed by wealthy people for the general medicine recommended for the poor to strengthen the heart and brain.[722]

Myrrh in the Levant:
Myrrh is mentioned in the will of Kalaf ben Yeshua' (d. 1043), the agent representative of the lepers in Tiberias. It may be that it was a component in a medication to treat leprosy.[723] Ibn al-Khair al-Ashbili claimed that the name of myrrh resin in Tripoli in the al-Sham region was 'samgh al-murr'.[724] Myrrh is mentioned in a document dated 1233 as one of the substances exported from that region to Europe (Venice).[725]

Medicinal Uses in the Medieval Period:
According to al-Kindi, myrrh was a component in many medications (28) to treat stomach ulcers, pus-infected sores, toothache, contaminated wounds, eye diseases and hemorrhages.[726] Ibn Wahshiya described the production process of myrrh resin and noted its uses: a hot drug for remedial purposes, for cultic rituals and as incense.[727]

According to Maimonides, the myrrh was the main component in the 'great theriac' and in a medication against snakebite, as described by Galen. It was also an ingredient in a theriac intended for bites by stray dogs.[728] Elsewhere, Maimonides warns against the use of myrrh in a cathartic medication or drinking it with wine.[729] Ibn al-Baytar quotes many physicians in connection with the medicinal uses of myrrh, including: congealing of wounds, treating intestinal worms, curing chronic cough and stomach ulcers, draining pus, preventing miscarriage, speeding up the birth process, aborting the fetus, improving the voice, sweetening the breath, and strengthening the teeth and gums.[730]

Traditional Medicine and General Uses:
Myrrh resin in a superb ingredient used in the perfume industry and also serves as incense in various Eastern cultures.[731] In Iraq, myrrh is a component in a medication for backache and to cure intestinal diseases.[732] Among the Jews of Iraq, myrrh is called 'masakh' and is a component in a medication for infertility and to strengthen the heart.[733] Yemenite Jews used myrrh extensively for treating intestinal worms, coughs, weakness of the lungs, pains of the throat, stomach and back, and to strengthen the teeth and gums.[734]

Modern Medicine:
Myrrh is used as a disinfecting drug in preparations for mouth rinses. It is used as a tonic for the womb, and as an emmenagogue, a stimulant and a component in various medicines for children.[735] Pharmacological studies conducted for myrrh resin have revealed its active medicinal properties.[736]

Nutmeg

Scientific name: *Myristica fragrans* (Myristicaceae)
Hebrew: Muskatit reihanit Arabic: Jauz buwwa, Jauz al-tib[737]

Description:
The Nutmeg is an evergreen tree with small flowers, growing in tropical Asia, mainly in the islands of the eastern Indian

[717] Issa, Dictionary, p. 55, Nos. 1, 6; Maimonides, Poisons, p. 112, n.151.

[718] Zohary, p. 482; Hill, p. 173.

[719] Amarna, No. 269.

[720] Dioscorides, I.77.

[721] In detail: Groom.

[722] Malki, p. 67.

[723] Gil, No. 253.

[724] al-Ashbili, pp. 531-532.

[725] Venice Laws, translation in: Prawer, Colonial, p. 480.

[726] Collected references in: al-Kindi, pp. 333-334, No. 283. Cf. Ibn Sina, p. 368.

[727] Ibn Wahshiya, II, p. 1256.

[728] Maimonides, Poisons, p. 112, 116, 130.

[729] Maimonides, Aphorisms, 14:49.

[730] Ibn al-Baytar, al-Jami, IV, pp. 145-147; Leclerc, No. 2102; Ibn al-Baytar, al-Tafsir, I, No. 55.

[731] Hill, pp. 173-174; Uphof, p. 146; Chopra et al, p. 70.

[732] Hooper, p. 103.

[733] Ben-Yakov, pp. 261, 361.

[734] Reiani, p. 19, No. 33.

[735] In detail: Michie & Cooper.

[736] In detail: Houh et al; Jones & Nunn.

[737] Maimonides, Glossaire, p. 32, No. 71; Leclerc, Nos. 464, 846, 1443; Issa, Dictionary, p. 122, No. 6.

Ocean. The fruit is fleshy and peach-shaped with a single, large seed or kernel. The seed or nut is encased in a red, net-like aril or mace which is also used as a spice and for medicinal purposes.[738]

History:
The use of the fragrant nutmeg as a remedy was known to physicians of the classical period. Nutmeg is mentioned by Dioscorides[739] who stated that it was a constricting drug used for treating blood in the sputum, dysentery, and diarrhea. In the Mishna, the expression 'rashei besamim' (chief of the spices) is mentioned and scholars interpret it to mean 'jauz buwwa.'[740] Maimonides also included the 'basbasa' (mace) among the main spices.[741] The Arabs began to trade in it in the 6th century CE and by the 12th century it was already well known in Europe.[742]

Medicinal Uses in Jerusalem:
According to Benevenutus, the nutmeg was one of the components in a famous medication call the 'Jerusalem Electuary' used mainly to treat cataract.[743] Refael Malki reported on the medicinal use of the seeds - ' egoz mushkada' - which were a component in a medicinal syrup for the Jerusalem poor during his period, as well as and in a pill to strengthen the heart and brain.[744] Moshe Poriat described the purchase of the seeds and their shells in the Jerusalem market and noted that they were not as commonly found in Jerusalem as compared with other spices found in abundance and at low cost.[745] David de Silva asserted that one of the uses for nutmeg was to treat eye diseases.[746]

Nutmeg in the Levant:
Ibn al-Baytar relates that the nutmeg aril (mace), which is called in Arabic 'makr' or 'basbasa' was used as a remedy and was named 'darkisa' in the al-Sham region.[747] Nutmeg was a delicate and expensive merchandise in the major markets of the Land of Israel, as it appears from the tax lists of Acre during the first half of the 13th century.[748] This merchandise was transported overland from India via Mecca to the ports of the Levant and from there to Europe.[749] The export of nutmeg in large quantities to Europe was also conducted from Egypt during this same period.[750]

[738] Zohary, p. 306.

[739] Dioscorides, I.110.

[740] Epstein, p. 145.

[741] Maimonides, Mishna, p. 452.

[742] Watson, Innovation, p. 195.

[743] Benevenutus, p. 33.

[744] Malki, pp. 63, 67.

[745] Ya'ari, Travels, p. 279.

[746] Amar, de Silva, p. 110.

[747] Ibn al-Baytar, Tafsir, p. 132. Discussion in Amar, al-Baytar, p. 52, n.52.

[748] Assises, p. 174, par. 8; Ashtor, Levant, p. 53.

[749] Ashtor, Trade, p. 297.

[750] Ashtor, Levant, p. 33.

Additional evidence for its high value and overland transport is given in a letter dated 1411 written by an Italian trader who describes the caravans from Mecca to Damascus and from there to Ramlah which brought the nutmeg seeds and flowers. Half of the merchandise remained in Ramlah and the rest was taken by Italian ships to Europe.[751]

Hayim Vital reported that he used nutmeg in a poultice for abscess of the throat,[752] and he also recommended putting nutmeg under the tongue during the entire night to counteract 'toxicity of the throat.'[753]

Medicinal Uses in the Medieval Period:
According to al-Kindi, nutmeg was a component in a medication to strengthen breathing.[754] Maimonides quotes the Jerusalem physician al-Tamimi who described the 'royal beverage' containing nutmeg which served as a medication for the elderly, for colds and for rheumatic pains. It was also prescribed to strengthen the stomach, improve the appetite and sexual desire.[755] According to Maimonides, nutmeg was a hot and dry drug.[756]

Daud al-Antaki described the various uses of 'jauz al-buwwa' and noted that it was paramount among the spices. He compared the shape of the nutmeg seed to the 'shami' nut and among the main medicinal uses he listed were: treatment of various skin diseases, paralytic symptoms, vomiting, fainting fits, obstructions in the urinary tract, gases, jaundice, rheumatic pains, the prevention of dropsy, relief for headache and earache and to sweeten the breath.[757]

Traditional Medicine:
The Jews of Iraq used nutmeg extensively to treat various illnesses such as colds, lung problems, infertility, heartburn, as well as to strengthen pregnant women and increase sexual potency.[758] Yemenite Jews used it to regulate the activity of the liver, spleen and intestines, to treat vomiting, fever, colds, tuberculosis, intestinal worms and skin diseases.[759] In Europe, it was used in a preparation for digestion, a medication against vomiting and as an expectorant.[760] The nutmeg tree grows today in Iraq and Iran and nutmeg is used to make sauces and for remedial purposes.[761] In Egypt, it serves as a strengthening drug, as a stomach relaxant and as a component in ointment.[762]

[751] Ashtor, Trade, p. 297.

[752] Benajahu, p. 106.

[753] Ibid., p. 108.

[754] al-Kindi, p. 213.

[755] Maimonides, Aphorisms, 21:96

[756] Ibid., 21:75; Maimonides, Regimen, p. 109.

[757] al-Antaki, pp. 110-111; al-Biruni, I, p. 114; Ibn al-Baytar, al-Jami, II, p. 93; Leclerc, No. 281. Cr. Ibn Sina, p. 27.

[758] Ben-Yakov, p. 702.

[759] Reiani, p. 32, No. 70.

[760] Watson, Innovation, p. 195; Uphof, p. 355; Hill, p. 461.

[761] Hooper, p. 142.

[762] Ducros, p. 37.

General Uses and Medical Qualities:
Nutmeg is used as a spice in cooking and baking and also in the food, perfume and cigarette industries.[763] The seed contains the alkaloid 'Myristicin' which has narcotic properties, and extensive use is liable to have negative effects.[764]

Plum

Scientific name: *Prunus domestica* (Rosaceae)
Hebrew: Shezif Arabic: Ijjas, Anjas[765]

Description:
The plum tree is a deciduous fruit tree, relatively large, with a hardwood trunk and white flowers. Its dark coloured fruit is round and in some species it is elongated. When ripe, the skin softens and the fruit becomes sweet, juicy and fragrant.[766]

Identification:
The identification of the plum in medieval sources is a complicated matter because of the large number of species and the alternate names given for similar varieties such as: peach, pear, apricot, and bear's plum.[767] According to these and other sources, it appears that the plum was called 'ijjas' or 'anjas'.[768]

History:
Growing in this region is a wild variety called *Prunus ursina* (bear plum). In the course of time, certain wild varieties were cultivated and some were brought into the region by the Greeks and Romans.[769] The Jewish Sages mention the plum by various names: 'dormaskana' 'ahon', 'ahonia', 'paga'in'.[770] According to Jewish sources, the plum also served as a remedy. In Greece and Rome the plum - *Kokkumelia,* was used for medicinal purposes, and physicians such as Dioscorides praised it for its efficiency in the digestive system, for restraining intestinal activity and preventing diarrhea.[771]

Medicinal Uses in Jerusalem:
Refael Malki reported on the use of "dried plums" as a "superb" general medication for the Jerusalem poor.[772] David de Silva asserted that boiled plums soften the stomach, its bark was useful for rinsing the mouth and the resin gum was praised for curing kidney diseases.[773]

Plums in the Levant:
al-Muqadassi listed the 'anjas al-kapori' among the special crops in the region of 'Falastin' (Palestine).[774] In a trading document of 1065 CE the 'anjas' is mentioned among the products purchased in Tyre.[775] Ibn Wahshiya relates that the plum tree was widespread in the al-Sham region and also in the area between al-Sham and the desert of Paran.[776] Bear's plum, which is a wild variety of plum, is mentioned by al-Baghdadi during the Ayyubid period. According to him, the plum was a fruit widely grown in Syria for use as food.[777]

During the Mamluk period, the 'Ijas' was included among the agricultural products of Greater Syria and was traded as merchandise.[778] Ibn al-Baytar, in his entry 'ijas' described the Syrian variety 'al-shami' especially "what is found of it in Damascus."[779]

Medicinal Uses in the Medieval Period:
al-Kindi reported on the use of 'ijas' as a general medicine[780] while Maimonides noted that plums were constricting fruits and a mild form of medication.[781] In his entry 'ijas' Ibn al-Baytar noted its medicinal uses: as a cold and moist drug, a cathartic substance and a regulator of bowel activity.[782] The resin gum of the plum tree was used to suture wounds and abscesses, to dissolve kidney stones, cure skin diseases, improve the lungs and treat cough, small pox and skin diseases.[783] al-Qazwini listed different medicinal uses including: to prevent gum bleeding, to relieve thirst and to stabilize the temperature of the heart.[784] Daud al-Antaki also listed the medicinal uses of the plum such as: relieving thirst, headache, throat pains, nausea and vomiting, opening blockages and drying wounds. The leaves were used to eliminate worms.[785]

Traditional Medicine:
The fruits are eaten raw, dried or as preserves. In Iraq and Iran, the dried fruit (prune) is used in cooking and to clean metal.[786] The Jews of Iraq used the plum extensively, especially for medicinal purposes to treat the kidneys, various kinds of skin diseases, pneumonia, sexual diseases and also to reduce fever.[787] In Europe, the plum fruit serves as a

763 Uphof, p. 355; Hill, pp. 460-461.

764 Watson, Innovation, p. 195.

765 Maimonides, Glossaire, p. 19, No. 13; al-Antaki, p. 38; al-Biruni, I, p.24; al-Ghafiqi, No. 10; Issa, Dictionary, p. 149, No.1; Dinsmore & Dalman, No. 660.

766 Plants & Animals, XII, p. 111.

767 Discussion in: Amar, Production, pp. 282-285.

768 Ibid, p. 284; Leclerc, Nos. 1269, 1615; Amar, al-Baytar, p. 75, n.74.

769 Goor, Fruits, p. 259.

770 Feliks, Fruit Trees, pp. 234-238; Goor, Fruits, pp. 264-265; Low, III, pp. 163-169.

771 For example: Disocorides, I.174.

772 Malki, p. 45.

773 Amar, de Silva, p. 141.

774 al-Muqadassi, p. 181.

775 Gil, III, p. 253, Doc. No. 503.

776 Ibn Wahshiya, I, p. 644.

777 al-Baghdadi, p. 76.

778 For example: al-Qalqashandi, p. 87. In detail: Amar, Production, p. 285.

779 Ibn al-Baytar, al-Jami, I, pp. 13-14; Leclerc, No. 21; Amar, al-Baytar, p. 75, n.74.

780 al-Kindi, Nos. 211, 214.

781 Maimonides, Regimen, 1:13; 2:7.

782 Ibn al-Baytar, al-Jami, I, pp. 13-14; Leclerc, No. 21; al-Ghafiqi, No. 10.

783 Ibn al-Baytar, al-Jami, III, p. 86; Leclerc, No. 1409.

784 al-Qazwini, p. 217.

785 al-Antaki, pp. 38-39. On medicinal uses cf. Ibn al-Baytar, al-Jami, I, pp. 13-14; Leclerc, No. 21.

786 Uphof, p. 430; Hooper, p. 158.

787 Collected references in: Ben-Yakov, p. 758.

cathartic substance and the oil produced from the flower buds is used in traditional medicine, especially in Hungary.[788]

Modern Medicine:
The seeds of the plum, similar to those of the almond, apricot and peach, contain the substance amygdaline which is commercially known as laetrile and is used in Mexico as an anti-cancerous substance. In the 1970's arguments broke out as to the efficiency of this substance.[789]

Prickly Burnet

Scientific name: *Sarcopoterium spinosum* (Rosaceae)
Hebrew: Sira kotsanit Arabic: Bilan[790]

Description:
The prickly burnet is a small, round, entangled bush, short (30-40 cm.) with paired sets of leaves. It is wide-leaved in winter and prickly-leaved in summer. Its flowers are greenish with small, rounded berries (up to 5 mm.), which are dispersed by water currents.[791]

History:
The Bible mentions the prickly burnet a few times mainly in connection with the wasteland of "nettles and brambles" (Isaiah, 34:13), thorny hedges (Hosea, 2:6) or as stubble for lighting a fire (Nahum, 1:10). The Jewish Sages considered the 'sirim' as the kind of prickly bush which lay in the path of the Israelites in the desert, and especially noted the thorns which had various uses such as fastening of the slave's ear to the doorpost and to cure boils. (Tosefta, Sota 4:2; Mishna, Keritot 3:7).[792]

Medicinal Uses in Jerusalem:
al-Biruni described the 'bilan' and noted that in 'Falastin' (Palestine) it was used as a broom, while its seeds had constricting qualities used in treating hemorrhoids.[793] Ibn al-Baytar quotes Abu al-Abas al-Nabati who described the 'bilan' which grew in al-Sham and mainly in Jerusalem, as well as its uses which according to him were: a medication against skin diseases such as scabies, and to treat hemorrhoids.[794]

Traditional Medicine:
Minority communities in Israel use the prickly burnet among other things for heating their homes and for industrial purposes (e.g. to produce lime), as well as to erect hedges and make brooms.[795] The Arabs in Israel use the root of the prickly burnet to relieve toothache and stomach ache, to regulate digestive problems, treat diabetes and temporary paralysis, to cure external inflammation and to relieve pain. The seeds are used to regulate blood circulation and the berries to release obstructions in the urinary tract.[796]

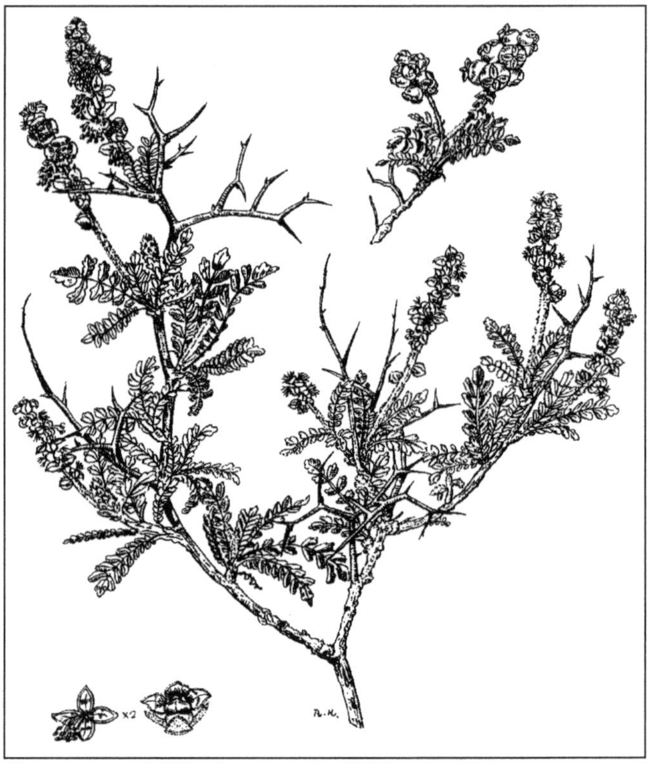

Figure 22 - Prickly Burnet (*Sarcopoterium spinosum*)

Modern Medicine:
The skin of the burnet root contains a substance effective against diabetes. Another crystallised substance derived from the plant was discovered as an active anti-cancerous agent.[797]

Purslane

Scientific name: *Portulaca oleracea* (Portulacacea)
Hebrew: Raglat ha-gina Arabic: Baqlah hamka[798]

Description:
Common or garden purslane is an annual herbaceous plant listed among the most commonly found plants in the world. Its leaves are fleshy and juicy, its flowers are small and yellow, and the fruit is in the form of small capsules (1 cm.) with a lid and contain tiny seeds.[799]

History:
Dioscorides described the use of the plant *Andrachne* to treat stomach problems.[800] Other classical physicians such as

788 Grieve, p. 659.

789 Palevitz, p. 269.

790 Dinsmore & Dalman, No. 669; Issa, Dictionary, p. 148, No. 1.

791 Feinbrun-Dothan, p. 285; Plants & Animals, X, pp. 133-134.

792 In detail: Feliks, World, p. 218.

793 al-Biruni, II, p. 79.

794 Ibn al-Baytar, al-Jami, I, pp. 113-114; Leclerc, No. 348.

795 Dafni, Dudaim, p. 58; Crowfoot & Baldensperger, p. 49; Krispil, pp. 796-812.

796 Palevitz et al, p. 116; Dafni, Dudaim, pp. 55-56; Abu-Rabia, p. 19. For other uses see: Krispil, pp. 801-804.

797 Shani et al, p. 117.

798 Maimonides, Glossaire, p. 29, No. 59; Issa, Dictionary, p. 147, No. 10; Amar, Production, p. 272; Dinsmore & Dalman, No. 306.

799 Plants & Animals, X, pp. 47-48.

800 Dioscorides, II.151.

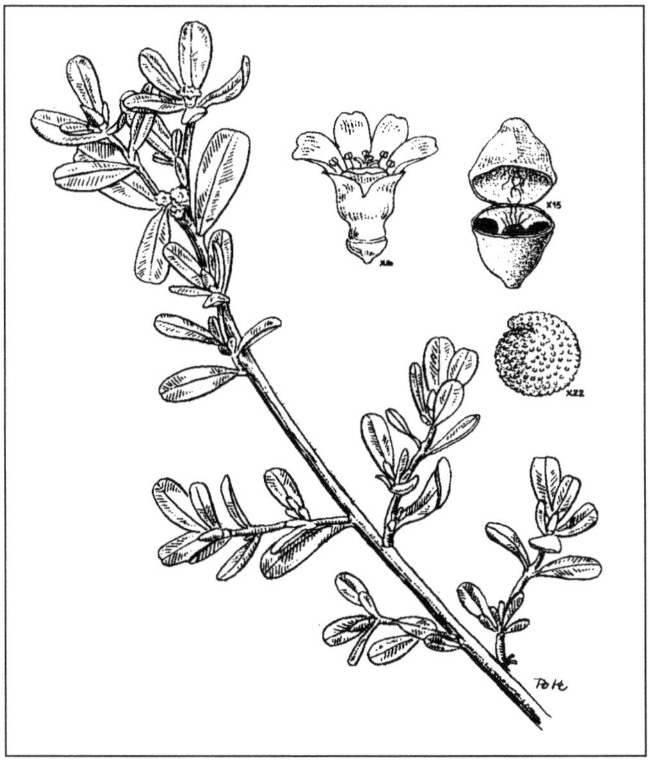

Figure 23 - Purslane (*Portulaca oleracea*)

Hippocrates, Theophrastus, Pliny and Galen reported on its use to treat diseases of the digestive tract as well as external wounds and burns. The plant was apparently cultivated in Europe and used for food.[801] The source for the Hebrew name is the Mishna where it is also called 'halaglogot' and in the Talmud it is termed 'farfahina.' These names, which appear in Jewish rabbinical writings, are identified with 'raglat ha-gina' (purslane).[802] The Arabic name retains the one used by the Jewish Sages. Medieval commentators identify the plant correctly and called it 'regel ha-orev' (raven's foot) and 'bazar ragla.'[803]

Medicinal Uses in Jerusalem:
According to Refael Malki, the 'mai ha-virdolagas' was an ineffective medication used in Jerusalem.[804]

Purslane in the Levant:
According to Maimonides, the 'baqlah yamina' was called 'al-farfahin' in Syria.[805] The purslane plant was listed among the typical agricultural crops in Greater Syria during the Mamluk period.[806] al-Badri listed the 'baqlah al-hamka' among the green produce growing in Syria.[807]

Medicinal Uses in the Medieval Period:
According to al-Kindi, the plant was a component in a medication to treat pustules on the lips, the spitting of blood, throat pains and inflammation of the teeth and gums. The seeds were used for rinsing the mouth.[808] According to Maimonides, the 'halaglogot' were a mild and safe medication.[809] He also reported that the 'laglogot' were an external medication for erysipelas. He quotes al-Tamimi in saying that the 'laglogot' stop the emission of blood from the intestines.[810] Purslane also serves as a component in an internal medication to treat the stings of bees and wasps, and as a medication against poisons.[811] In his entry 'baqlah al-hamka' Ibn al-Baytar describes the purslane plant and lists the medicinal uses such as: treatment of stomach problems, stones in the kidney and urinary tract, and causing diarrhea.[812]

Traditional Medicine:
In India and Pakistan the plant serves as a mild diuretic, as a cure for sores, as a cold drug to treat the diseases of the skin, liver, kidneys, wounds and burns as well as for scurvy. In China the plant is used as a softening drug and its leaves for treating growths, stomach ulcers, severe wounds and gonorrhoea (venereal disease). In Iraq the leaves and stalks serve as a diuretic and the seeds as a medication to expel worms. In Europe purslane is recommended as a treatment for scurvy, and the plant juice is recommended to treat damaged teeth and gums.[813] It is used as a strengthener and as a medication for irregularities in the blood system.[814] Large concentrations of potassium from the soil are found in the purslane plant and it is therefore used in Africa as a source for special medications.[815] It also increases the ability to coagulate the blood and serves as a cathartic drug.[816]

General Uses:
The plant is edible and can be used as a salad or in salads as an acidic additive. In Israel it was once used as chicken feed. It can be made into a soup or preserved for winter use.[817]

Quinine (Peruvian bark)

Scientific name: *Cinchona sp.* (Rubiaceae)
Hebrew: Kinin Arabic: Kina, Kina kina

Description:
Various types (15) of the Cinchona species are grown in South America on the slopes of the Andes. A few of these trees supply the well known Peruvian bark. The bark and the root

[801] Plants & Animals, X, p. 48.

[802] Low, III, pp. 70-75; Feliks, Shevi'it, I, p. 383; II, p. 215.

[803] In detail: Amar, Production, No. 272.

[804] Malki, p. 77. The editor identifies it with purslane and this may be accepted as a probable identification.

[805] Maimonides, Glossaire, p. 29, No. 59.

[806] al-'Umari, p. 26; al-Qalqashandi, p. 87.

[807] al-Badri, p. 174.

[808] al-Kindi, Nos. 88-90, 116, 179, 214.

[809] Maimonides, Regimen, 2:10; Maimonides, Aphorisms, 20:47; Maimonides, Answers, No. 6; 19(3).

[810] Maimonides, Aphorisms, 9:106; 20:84; 21:84.

[811] Maimonides, Poisons, pp. 124, 150.

[812] Ibn al-Baytar, al-Jami, pp. 102-103; Leclerc, Nos. 313, 1035, 1680. Cf. Ibn Sina, p. 275.

[813] Uphof, p. 426; al-Rawi and Chaakravarty, p. 77; Grieve, p. 660; Dafni, Edible, p. 112.

[814] Loewenfeld & Back, p. 209.

[815] Plants & Animals, X, p. 48; Loewenfeld & Back, p. 207.

[816] Chizik, p. 732.

[817] Plants & Animals, X, p. 48; Uphof, p. 426.

contain 30 kinds of alkaloids including quinine and quinidine. Quinine is marked as a white powder which has a bitter taste and is used to cure malaria.[818]

History:
The South American Indians used the bark to treat relapses of malarial fever. In the 17th century after the discovery of America, the bark was brought to Europe. Quinine was mentioned in medicinal treatises in England (1667) and was later exported to India. Since that time, quinine has become known for its effectiveness in curing malaria. The great demand for Peruvian bark led to the destruction of most of the trees in their original habitat, and the English and Dutch began to grow them in India and Java. These plantations supplied 90% of the world's needs, but in modern times the demand decreased because of the synthetic production of medicines for malaria.[819]

Medicinal Uses in Jerusalem:
The Franciscan monk, Elazar Horn, described the use of large quantities of quinine to reduce fever among the elderly, the lame and the blind in Jerusalem.[820] David de Silva mentions the quinine as a tree that can be found in Africa. Its main medicinal uses were treating high fever and other "cold diseases".[821]

Traditional Medicine:
The bark of the Cinchona tree is sold in the markets of the East from Iran to China.[822] In Europe, quinine was a drug to reduce fever and to stimulate, constrict and strengthen as well as to treat malaria, influenza and nervous illnesses.[823]

Summary and Conclusions:
Quinine is a unique example for the introduction of Western medicine in this region. Cinchona is a tree from the New World which was introduced into Europe and its use quickly spread throughout the world, mainly by the colonial settlements established by Britain and Holland. Quinine was apparently brought to the Land of Israel by Franciscan monks who used it to treat patients with high fever. The evidence of the use of quinine at the beginning of the 18th century in Jerusalem is particularly important as a landmark in the research for that period.

Rhubarb

Scientific name: *Rheum sp.* (Polygonaceae)
Hebrew: Ribas Arabic: Ribas, Rawand[824]

Description:
The rhubarb species has 50 varieties which were widespread in the temperate, sub-tropical regions of Asia and Central Europe. Rhubarb is a perennial herbaceous plant with thick roots and large leaves that lie spread out over the ground. It has an impressively tall, flowering stem with many blossoms. In the Land of Israel two varieties are grown: *Rheum palaestinum* - an endemic type which grows in the Negev, and *Rheum ribes* - which grows in the region of Mount Hermon.[825]

History:
Rhubarb has served as a medicinal substance in ancient China since the 27th century BCE and written evidence from the 1st century BCE describes its use as inducing vomiting which makes it effective against poisons. It also served to reduce fever, to cause constipation, as an emmenagogue, as well as for treating skin diseases, for hemorrhages and to lower the level of cholesterol in the blood.[826] Dioscorides called the plant *Rha* and described its use in strengthening the stomach, to reduce gases, to treat spasms and cure hemorrhoids, the liver, kidneys, chest, asthma, dysentery, malaria and chronic pneumonia.[827]

Medicinal Uses in Jerusalem:
Refael Malki mentions the use of 'raont' in a general remedial syrup for the Jerusalem poor. According to him, the plant was also a cathartic substance and a component in pills.[828]

Rhubarb in the Levant:
Ibn al-Baytar says that the 'ribas' was not to be found in Spain or the Maghreb (North Africa), but that it was "prevalent in al-Sham" and in northern countries.[829] Elsewhere he notes that the 'rawand al-shami' which was brought from the "district of Ammon in the al-Sham region" was not used to a great extent for remedial purposes, meaning that it was of poor quality.[830] Al-Dimashqi mentions both the 'ribas' and the 'rawandan' and listed them among the 90 varieties of useful herbs in Mount Lebanon which could provide a living by their harvesting.[831] From various medieval sources it appears that rhubarb was an important seasoning spice which was imported overland by the Crusader kingdom from eastern countries such as India or China.[832] According to Hayim Vital, the rhubarb was a component in a medication against stomach swelling and in an ointment to treat hemorrhoids.[833]

Identification:
The research scholar, Amar, suggested identifying the rhubarb mentioned in the sources of the medieval period, especially that of Ibn al-Baytar, with the desert rhubarb. The 'rawand' was presumably *Rheum officinale* and the 'rawand al-shami'

[818] Zohary, p. 548; Tal, p. 140.

[819] Zohary, p. 548; Uphof, p. 130; Hill, pp. 248-251.

[820] Horn, p. 181.

[821] Amar, de Silva, p. 138.

[822] Hooper, p. 99.

[823] Grieve, p. 630.

[824] Maimonides, Glossaire, p. 98, No. 350; Dinsmore & Dalman, No. 1507; Issa, Dictionary, p. 155, Nos. 19-22.

[825] Feinbrun-Dothan, p. 112; Plants & Animals, X, p.42.

[826] For the history of the plant, its medicinal uses and trade see:Foust.

[827] Dioscorides, III.2

[828] Malki, pp. 62-65.

[829] Ibn al-Baytar, al-Jami, II, p. 147; Leclerc, No. 1072.

[830] Ibn al-Baytar, al-Jami, II, p. 131; Leclerc, No. 1018.

[831] al-Dimashqi, p. 199.

[832] Prawer, History, pp. 125-127. Further details on its trade in: Heyd, pp. 665-667.

[833] Benajahu, pp. 97, 103.

was garden rhubarb which was a plant cultivated in the region.[834]

Medicinal Uses in the Medieval Period:
Maimonides noted that varieties of the 'rabiobrabari; were used as a cathartic substance and were effective for the liver.[835] Ibn al-Baytar in his entry 'ribas' described the plant and listed its medicinal uses such as: strengthening the stomach, improving its smell, softening the faeces, cessation of thirst and vomiting, relieving jaundice, regulating the heart beat and improving the appetite. His quotations from other physicians indicate that the plant was also used to treat hemorrhoids, small pox and pustules as well as to cool the blood.[836] In his entry 'rawand' he listed medicinal uses such as: relieving various pains, curing internal ailments and strengthening internal organs.[837] al-Qazwini added that the rhubarb was effective against the plague, sharpened the eyesight, cured jaundice, rubella, smallpox and that it also served to treat diabetes and nausea.[838]

Traditional Medicine:
Yemenite Jews used the roots of the rhubarb to treat the eyesight, hemorrhages in the lungs, to regulate the functions of the kidney, stomach, breathing, and to dissolve kidney stones, to treat hemorrhoids both internally and externally, to purify the blood, and to cure skin diseases.[839] Various kinds of rhubarb such as: garden rhubarb, Hermon rhubarb, *Rheum rhaponticum* and *Rheum palmatum*, were used for medicinal purposes in different countries of the world, mainly in the East.[840]

General Uses:
The Arabs in Israel use the leaves of the rhubarb as food and to make tea. The stems of the cultivated variety are used to prepare a reddish soup.[841] The varieties *Rheum hybridum* and garden rhubarb serve in the production of confectionery, juices and wine. Hermon rhubarb grows in Iran, Afghanistan and Turkestan, its roots are sold in the markets of Iran and it is used to expel the intestinal worms of horses.[842]

Saffron

Scientific name: *Crocus sativus* (Iridaceae)
Hebrew: Karkom Arabic: Za'fran, Kurkama[843]

Description:
Saffron is a species of crocus. It is a small geophyte (up to 15 cm.) with lilac coloured flowers typical of irises. The floral stigmas are orange hued and are of high value. There are 70 varieties of saffron prevalent in holarctic regions. Nine varieties grow in Israel and the most commonly used is the winter saffron.[844]

History:
Saffron has been a seasoning plant since the 4th millennium BCE in Chaldea. It was used in Assyria and Babylon to cure urinary problems, stomach disorders and women ailments and also for disinfection during childbirth. Similar uses were also made in the framework of ancient Egyptian medicine.[845] In the Bible, saffron is mentioned only once (Song of Songs, 4:14). Dioscorides described the *Krpkos* which was a diuretic drug and was used for curing the eyes, for women ailments, womb disorders, skin diseases and ear inflammations. According to him, the *Krpkomagma* was a medication composed of saffron oil.[846]

During the Roman and Byzantine periods the plant was grown in Europe and was used as seasoning and for curative purposes. The Jewish Sages of the Mishna and Talmud also mention the plant occasionally: in connection with the incense for the Temple, as a medication for nose-bleeding, to cause infertility, and to strengthen the bowels.[847]

Medicinal Uses in Jerusalem:
Benevenutus mentions the use of 'za'fran' which was a component in a medication for cataract called the 'Jerusalem Electuary.'[848] Refael Malki refers to the "choice and select karkom" which was an ingredient in a general pill for the Jerusalem poor.[849] Moshe Poriat relates that he saw some cheap saffron sold in Jerusalem markets but it was of poor quality.[850] David de Silva asserted that the saffron is useful as a diuretic, for the treatment of lung diseases, heart ailments and to sweeten the breath.[851]

Saffron in the Levant:
Among the varieties of saffron, Yohana Ibn Masawayh mentions the 'shami' type currently used in his day.[852] The 'za'afran' is listed among the spices and seasonings which were used during the cultic rites performed at the Dome of the Rock on the Temple Mount during the early Arab period.[853] Physicians, geographers and writers of the 9th and 10th centuries described the cultivation of the 'jadi' - one of

[834] Amar, al-Baytar, p. 74, n. 71.

[835] Maimonides, Aphorisms, 9:88; 21:30, 75, 78; Maimonides, Regimen, 3:2.

[836] Ibn al-Baytar, al-Jami, II, p. 147; Leclerc, No. 1072.

[837] Ibn al-Baytar, al-Jami, II, p. 131; Leclerc, No. 1018. Cf. al-Antaki, p. 165 and Ibn Sina, p. 429.

[838] al-Qazwini, p. 250. Cf. Ibn Sina, p. 432.

[839] Reiani, p. 45, No. 103. Cf. Krispil, p. 1314.

[840] Uphof, pp. 448-449; Hill, p. 247; Hooper, pp. 163-164; Ducros, pp. 107-108, 163; al-Rawi & Chaakravarty, p. 81; Grieve, pp. 675-680; Krispil, p. 1315.

[841] Dafni, Edible, p. 111; Danin.

[842] Uphof, pp. 448-449.

[843] Identification and synonyms discussed in: Maimonides, Glossaire, p. 47, No. 135; p. 64, No. 205; Dinsmore & Dalman, No. 1653; Issa, Dictionary, p. 60, No.6.

[844] Plants & Animals, XI, p. 250. For other remedial uses see: Hill, pp. 131-132, 446-447; Uphof, p. 159; Dafni, Dudaim, pp. 41, 68.

[845] Levey, Chemistry, pp. 77, 105.

[846] Dioscorides, I.25, 26.

[847] In detail: Low, II, pp. 7-26; Feliks, World, pp. 249-251.

[848] Benevenutus, p. 37.

[849] Malki, p. 67.

[850] Ya'ari, Travels, p. 278.

[851] Amar, de Silva, p. 124.

[852] Ibn Masawayh, p. 15.

[853] al-Wasati p. 92.

the Arabic names for saffron[854] - which could be found in the al-Sham region especially in the village of Jadia located in present day Syria.[855] al-Biruni claimed that Damascus was one of the centers for the supply of the 'za'fran' in the area and he notes its medicinal uses.[856]

Cultivated saffron was imported into the region during the Middle Ages from Southern Europe. The 'za'fran' (zafferano) is listed among the products which residents of Italian cities traded in Acre, Beirut and Ramlah during the 13th and 14th centuries.[857] Hayim Vital described the use of 'za'fran' which was wrapped in onion skins and place upon the orifice of the sexual organ in order to open blockages in the urinary tract. It also served as a component in a medication for hemorrhoids.[858]

Medicinal Uses in the Medieval Period:
Assaph Harofe described the plant, indicating its names and listing its medicinal qualities: "Saffron is za'afran which has a hot and dry potency to release urine and cure women ailments, and its roots are effective in inhibiting urine ... even beneficial for the kidneys. If bandaged over a boil, it will dissolve and cure it."[859] al-Kindi reported that the 'za'fran' was an important component in many medications, mainly the 'Indian ointment' to improve the state of mind and to dispel headaches. Additional medicinal uses listed by him include the treatment of the liver, throat, mouth, teeth, gums, eyes and for epilepsy. He also described the use of 'za'fran' in spices and various mixtures.[860]

Maimonides quotes many medicinal uses for saffron, as for example: According to Ibn Zahar the 'za'fran' was a component in a mild purgative and according to al-Tamimi, it was a sexual stimulant and a component in various medications for curing intestinal ailments.[861] Ibn al-Baytar says that the 'za'fran' was a drug to strengthen the senses, to prompt the memory, to slow the heartbeat, improve the eyesight, relieve pains (of the ears, teeth, joints, feet and back). It stopped hemorrhages, strengthened the internal organs (stomach, liver and spleen), cured inflammations, women ailments and epilepsy, stimulated the appetite and prevented conception.[862] al-Qazwini also described the 'za'fran' and added that the crocus bulb was edible. He then quotes Ibn Sina who claimed that the seeds were sleep-inducing, improved the eyesight, while the plant itself was a sexual stimulant, a diuretic, and also accelerated childbirth, and strengthened the heart, but that high doses of it were poisonous.[863]

Traditional Medicine:
Saffron has many and varied medicinal uses among the inhabitants of this region and in Jewish communities. Yemenite Jews used the saffron stigmas to treat the eyes, earache, breathing difficulties and hemorrhages, to cure wounds, to strengthen the heart and eyesight, as well as to reduce fever and swellings, relieve pains and birth pangs, increase sexual potency and calm the mentally ill.[864] In Iraq and Iran, the 'za'fran' is used as a general and sexual stimulant, as well as to soothe and calm the stomach, nerves and nervous spasms. Extensive use is made of saffron in cases of high fever, melancholy and enlargement of the liver.[865] The Jews of Iraq use it to cure jaundice and urine retention, and Moroccan Jews use it for liver diseases. Indian Jews use the plant to treat chills, colds, and fever, while Persian Jews make use of it to treat infertility and eye pains.[866] Saffron stigmas serve as a perspirant, an emmenagogue, and to accelerate the process of recovery from jaundice.[867]

Savory of Crete

Scientific name: *Satureia thymbra* (Labiatae)
Hebrew: Zathra Arabic: Sa'tar parsi, Sa'tar al-hamir, Hasha[868]

Description:
Savory of Crete is an aromatic bush, growing mostly in the mountains on limestone earth. The plant is erect, up to a height of 30-50 cm. and has many stems. The whole plant gives off a strong scent of ethereal oils. The leaves are long and oval-shaped, and the lavender-pink flowers grow in clusters. In the Land of Israel there is one more wild varieties and one cultivated type: *Satureia hortensis*.[869]

History:
In Ancient Rome the cultivated plant was used to make a love potion. Classical physicians such as Pliny and others recommended the use of the plant for cancerous growths.[870] Dioscorides described the wild variety *Thumbra* and mentioned the cultivated one, asserting that it had limited potency.[871] The researcher Feliks identified the 'siah' which is mentioned in the Mishna in connection with hyssop and thyme, as Savory of Crete.[872] In the Jerusalem Talmud this

[854] Maimonides, Glossaire, p. 47, No. 135.

[855] For example: Yaqut, II, p. 5; al-Ya'qubi, p. 324.

[856] al-Biruni, I, p. 95.

[857] Pegolotti, pp. 64, 69, 90, 101; Ashtor, Levant, p. 52, n.134; Heyd, II, pp. 668-669.

[858] Benajahu, pp. 94, 102.

[859] Assaph, 4, p. 397.

[860] al-Kindi, p. 275, No. 127. Cf. Ibn al-Baytar, al-Jami, II, pp. 162-163; al-Antaki, pp. 178-179.

[861] Maimonides, Regimen, 3:2; Maimonides, Aphorisms, 9:46; 20:86; 21:76.

[862] Ibn al-Baytar, al-Jami, II, pp. 162-163; Leclerc, No. 1110. Cf. al-Antaki, pp. 178-179.

[863] al-Qazwini, p. 250.

[864] Reiani, p. 20, No. 36.

[865] Hooper, p. 107. For the content of substances in detail: al-Rawi & Chaakravarty, pp. 31-32.

[866] Krispil, p. 502. Collected references in: Ben-Yakov, p. 711.

[867] Reiani, p. 20, No. 36; Uphof, p. 159; Grieve, pp. 698-699.

[868] Maimonides, Glossaire, No. 319; Issa, Dictionary, p. 163, No. 10.

[869] Description: Plants & Animals, XI, p. 77.

[870] Hartwell, p. 278.

[871] Dioscorides, III.45

[872] Feliks, Shevi'it, p. 188.

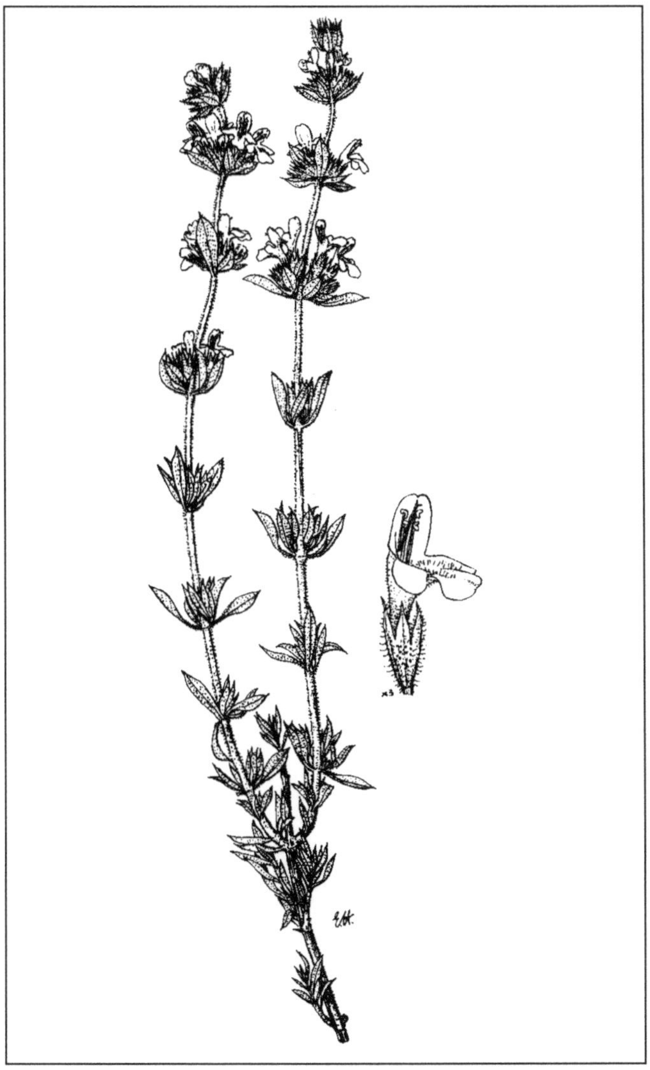

Figure 24 - Savory of Crete (*Satureia thymbra*)

identification is made explicit: 'siah' is savory, 'ezov' is hyssop, and 'koranit' is thyme.[873]

Identification:
The identification of the varieties of thyme is not a simple matter because, in different areas of this region, general names were give to plants that had similar features and qualities. Maimonides, for example, in his entry 'sa'tar' gave details about several varieties and tried to identify them.[874] Different condiment plants called 'za'tar parsi' and 'hasha' were mainly of the Labiatae family. However, according to the Arabic and Spanish names, the descriptions of the plants and the frequency of their use, they are one of the two varieties: Savory of Crete or Headed Thyme.[875]

Since there is some confusion among medieval writers as to the names and varieties of the Labiatae species - even among modern researchers - it seems impossible or perhaps mistaken to identify and distinguish between varieties that are closely related in form, habitat and usages. The two varieties mentioned above are therefore presented with their distinctive characteristics.

Medicinal Uses in Jerusalem:
Ibn al-Baytar described the 'hasha' which the inhabitants of Spain and herbalists knew as 'sa'tar al-hamir.' According to him, the plant grew widely in the 'lands of Bayt al-Maqdis" (Land of Jerusalem) and its suburbs.[876] Refael Malki says that 'the waters of sa'tar parsi' was a component in a syrup as a general medication for the Jerusalem poor. In his view, hyssop water was an effective substitute for the water of 'sa'tar parsi.'[877]

Varieties of Thyme in the Levant:
Ibn al-Baytar mentions elsewhere that the 'thymbra' is the 'za'tar al-farsi' - a well known plant among the Spaniards which they call 'shteria' and he goes on to say that "this type of thin-leaved za'tar is found in the cultivated areas of Egypt and in their orchards, as well as in al-Sham."[878]

Medicinal Uses in the Medieval Period:
According to Assaph Harofe, the plant is a "slender tree" called in Greek 'oregani,' in Aramaic 'zifa raba,' and in Latin 'shturiya - sturaya'. It is effective in treating pains in the kidneys and in dissolving kidney stones, for urine flow, for opening blockages in the ears, treating the intestines and eye diseases.[879] al-Kindi brings examples for various kinds of thyme: 'sa'tar parsi' served as a component in a medication for external treatment of growths on the neck;[880] 'hasha' was a component in a medication for the liver, stomach and swollen spleen;[881] while the drug 'hashi' was a component in an expectorant drink to cleanse the lungs as a result of asthma.[882] Ibn al-Baytar in his entry 'hasha' listed uses such as: an emmenagogue, diuretic, opening blockages, curing disorders in the respiratory system, elimination of intestinal worms, improving the eyesight, cleansing the liver and stomach and inducing diarrhea.[883] In the entry 'thuma' Ibn al-Baytar notes that this is a synonym for 'hasha.'[884] al-Qazwini described the plant in his entry 'hasha' and quotes Ibn Sina who described its use in straightening curly hair and improving the eyesight.[885]

Traditional Medicine and General Uses:
Throughout the world, wild and cultivated varieties of savory serve as well known condiments.[886] The Arabs of Israel

[873] Feliks, Yerushalmi, II, p. 120.

[874] Maimonides, Glossaire, pp. 90-91, No. 319.

[875] Issa, Dictionary, p. 163, No. 10; p. 180, No. 223; Dinsmore & Dalman, Nos. 1348, 1350; Maimonides, Glossaire, p. 52, No. 157; Witztum & Gruber; Amar, al-Baytar, p. 72, n. 65.

[876] Ibn al-Baytar, al-Jami, II, pp. 2-3; Leclerc, No. 548.

[877] Malki, p. 63.

[878] Ibn al-Baytar, Tafsir, p. 224.

[879] Assaph, 4, pp. 411-412.

[880] al-Kindi, No. 70. Cf. al-Biruni, I, pp. 205-206.

[881] al-Kindi, Nos. 6, 8.

[882] Maimonides, Asthma, 12:1,3.

[883] Ibn al-Baytar, al-Jami, II, pp. 2-3; Leclerc, No. 548. Cf. al-Antaki, p. 113.

[884] Ibn al-Baytar, al-Jami, I, p. 153; Leclerc, No. 456; al-Antaki, p. 113.

[885] al-Qazwini, p. 244. Cf. Ibn Sina, pp. 314-315.

[886] Loewenfeld & Back, p. 228; Uphof, p. 473.

usually use the 'sathra' to reduce swellings in the legs, to relieve arthritic pains, to disinfect open wounds and to cure palsy.[887]

The plant also serves as a general strengthener, purgative, to treat dizziness, tooth decay, pains in the heart, to open obstructions in the urinary and respiratory tracts, to cure colds, to relieve stomach pains[888] and also as immunization against snakebite.[889] Different varieties of savory are used around the world until today as drugs to dispel gases, induce perspiration and as expectorants.[890]

Scammony (Syrian Bindweed)

Scientific name: *Convolvulus scammonia* (Convolvulaceae)
Hebrew: Havalbal refui **Arabic: Mahmodia, Saqamuniya**[891]

Description:
Medicinal scammony is a perennial herb with a bare, winding stem, spear-shaped leaves, and large flowers (up to 4 cm.) which are funnel-like, of a pale yellow colour five violet stripes along their length. The fruits are rounded capsules.[892]

History:
The researcher, Zilberstein, thought that the name of the variety 'scammonia' which was retained in the Arabic language and in certain European languages as well, perpetuates the memory of a city called Shikmona which lies in ruins to the south of Haifa. In his view, it may be that this ancient port city was once a marketing centre for the scammony plant that grows in that area and was sent to neighboring countries and to Europe.[893] Other researchers think that the name is linked to the sycamore tree ('shikma'). Classical physicians considered the juice derived from the roots of the *Skammonia* as a medicinal substance. Dioscorides, for example, recommended the varieties from "Judea and Syria" and claimed that the plant was a purgative drug, an abortive and a remedy for leprosy and headache.[894] Various types of scammony were used as purgatives even in Europe. The scammony plant was imported from the region of Syria and extensive medicinal use was made of it, especially during the Middle Ages.[895]

Medicinal Uses in Jerusalem:
According to Refael Malki, scammony was a strong purgative and a component in various preparations such as a medication against headache and cold, and in a pill to strengthen the heart and brain.[896]

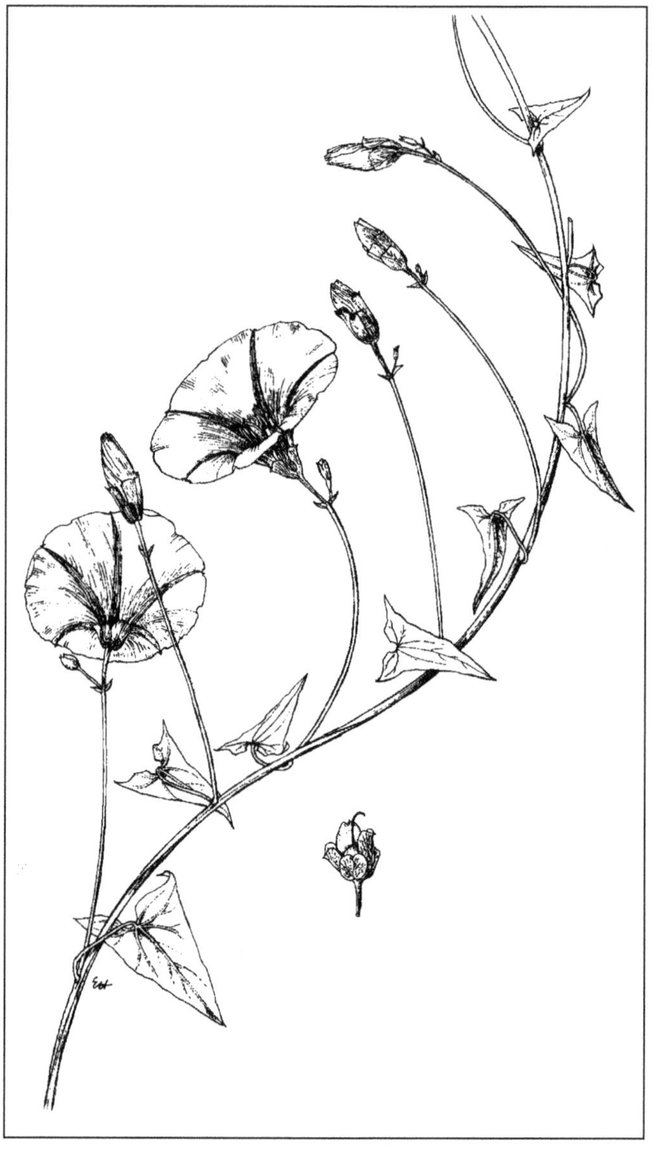

Figure 25 - Scammony (*Convolvulus scammonia*)

Scammony in the Levant:
Ibn al-Baytar noted in his entry 'saqamuniya' that he saw the plant in the region of al-Sham and in Falastin.[897] al-Dimashqi listed the 'saqamuniya' with the 90 varieties found in Mount Lebanon from which one could earn a living by harvesting it.[898] Evidence of trade in scammony in the Land of Israel during the Middle Ages can be found in Italian trading documents dated 1481 which describe the purchase of the plants sent to Italy.[899]

Rabbi Moshe Bassola who visited the Land of Israel in 1521, mentioned the 'skalmonia' - a kind of medication sold in Safed, "a city where many Jews deal in spices."[900] Frederick

[887] Dafni, Edible, p. 105.

[888] Palevitz et al, p. 141 which gives the content of active substances. Cf. Grieve, pp. 718-719.

[889] Dafni, Edible, p. 105.

[890] Uphof, pp. 472-473.

[891] Maimonides, Glossaire, p. 65, No. 207; p. 80, No. 281; Issa, Dictionary, p. 56, Nos. 8, 21; Dinsmore & Dalman, Nos. 1225-1226.

[892] Plants & Animals, XI, p. 37; Feinbrun-Dothan, p. 517.

[893] Zilberstein, pp. 79-80.

[894] Dioscorides, IV.171.

[895] Grieve, pp. 102-103; Uphof, p. 149.

[896] Malki, pp. 65, 67.

[897] Ibn al-Baytar, al-Jami, III, pp. 17-19; Leclerc, No. 1193.

[898] al-Dimashqi, p. 199.

[899] In detail: Ashtor, Trade p. 299.

[900] Ya'ari, Travels, p. 138.

Hasselquist relates that he saw the plants grown in the valley between Haifa and Nazareth (i.e. the Jezreel Valley).[901] Juice extracted from the root of the plant was used as a purgative and was exported from Syria to Europe even in modern times.[902]

Medicinal Uses in the Medieval Period:
According to al-Kindi, scammony was a component in a medicinal preparation to reduce fever, to calm the nerves, and to relieve pains in the stomach and liver.[903]

al-Biruni stressed the poisonous properties of the juice derived from the 'saqamuniya' and the 'turbid.'[904]

Ibn al-Baytar in his entry 'saqamuniya' described the use of the root juice to cause diarrhea and abortion and he also stated that it was a component in an ointment to cure wounds, to seal scars and to treat headaches. Other physicians quoted by him recommended mixing the root juice with other substances to dilute its harmful effects, and noted its long shelf-life. They mentioned other uses such as: to cure scorpion stings, to eliminate worms and to treat problems in urinating.[905]

Maimonides mentions several uses of the plant, but specifically emphasized that it was a purgative substance.[906] Saladino d'Ascoli claimed that the scammony was 'the most powerful purgative."[907] Daud al-Antaki in his entry 'saqamuniya' described the use of the plant to cure skin diseases, to open blockages, to expel worms, to cause diarrhea, to cure intestinal diseases, heart palpitations and insanity.[908]

Traditional Medicine:
Among the Sinai Bedouins the thorny scammony (*Convolvulus hystrix*) was used as a purgative, to induce vomiting and to counteract jaundice.[909] In Iraq, two varieties of scammony are used for remedial purposes: meadow scammony (*Convolvulus arvensis*) all parts of which are used as a cathartic substance, and medicinal scammony, the root extract of which serves as a cathartic drug.[910] The Jews of Iraq call the plant 'mahmoda' and they also consider it a cathartic drug.[911]

Medical Qualities:
The root contains the active substance *Convolvium*. This substance is isolated from the gum-resin which exudes from the fresh root, or it is a powder made from grinding the root. This is a very strong purgative and increases the secretion of bile juices.[912]

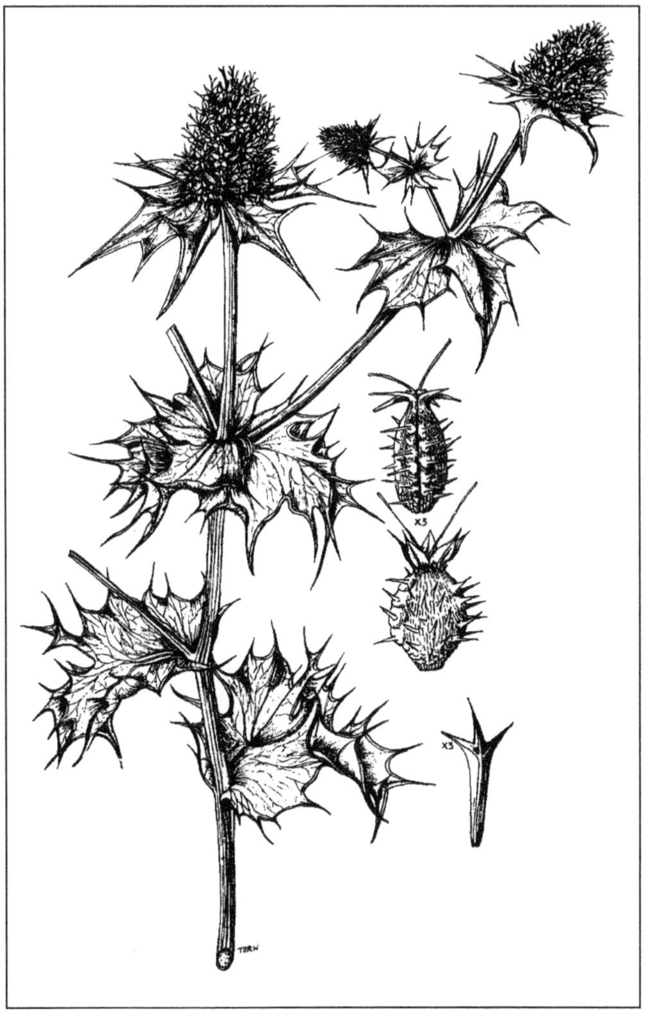

Figure 26 - Sea Holly (*Eryngium maritimum*)

Sea Holly

Scientific name: *Eryngium sp.* (Umbelliferae)
Hebrew: Harhabina

Description:
There are 230 varieties of sea holly, seven of which grow in the Land of Israel. The more prominent and widespread varieties will be described later.

Identification:
From medieval sources we learn that physicians and botanists of the region used three varieties of the sea holly. Ibn al-Baytar quotes Abu al-'Abas al-Nabati in describing several varieties of the plant 'qarza'na':

> White variety: "lies close to the ground ... has a very thin stem ... thorny... produces white flowers ... has long, sweet roots." This plant is identified as *Eryngium glomeratum* - a perennial plant, tall and erect (up to 80

[901] Hasselquist, p. 300.

[902] Uphof, p. 149.

[903] al-Kindi, p. 113.

[904] al-Biruni, II, pp. 58, 82.

[905] Ibn al-Baytar, al-Jami, III. Pp. 17-119; Leclerc, No. 1193. Cf. al-Antaki, pp. 193-194.

[906] For example: Maimonides, Aphorisms, 13:3; 21:80; Maimonides, Regimen, 2:6; Maimonides, Asthma, 9:9; 12:9.

[907] Saladino, p. 89.

[908] al-Antaki, pp. 193-194, and the entry 'turbid' on p. 91.

[909] Levey, Bedouins, p. 79.

[910] In greater detail, including content of substances in: al-Rawi & Chaakravarty, p. 30.

[911] Ben-Yakov, pp. 160, 616.

[912] Zilberstein, p. 80; al-Rawi & Chaakravarty, p. 30.

cm.) with rosette leaves from which many flowering stems emerge. The 'drakil' is described as a variety of the 'qarza'na' which is also called 'shandab.'[913] Modern researchers identify this plant with the *Eryngium glomeratum* and this seems to be an acceptable identification.[914]

Blue variety: "rounded leaves ... lies close to the ground in a circle ... produces a single stem covered with thorns and tends to be blue in colour." This plant is identified as *Eryngium creticum* - (field eryngo) a perennial herb which produces soft leaves in winter and in the summer it has thorny stems crowned with globular heads of blue blossoms.

Sea shore variety: "found along the seashore ... wider leaves ... with sweeter roots."[915] This plant is identified as *Eryngium maritimum* - (sea holly) a perennial plant which grows along the seashore, with large, thick, leathery leaves, broad and oblong-shaped, of a bluish green colour.[916]

History:
The Hebrew name for this species appears in the Mishna where it is listed with the type of vegetables permitted to be used as bitter herbs eaten at the Passover meal. The name is related to the root h-r-b (dry). The scientific name is derived from the Greek term for one of the varieties of this species.[917] According to Dioscorides, the *Erungion* is a food and medicinal plant which is used as: a heating drug, a diuretic, an emmenagogue, a cure for inflammations and for epilepsy, as well as to counteract poisons, bites and stings.[918]

Sea Holly in Jerusalem and the Levant:
Ibn al-Baytar quotes Abu al-'Abas al-Nabati who relates that he saw white 'qarza'na' in "the mountains of Lot's grave" (The Kingdom of Jordan) and in "al-Quds and its districts" (Jerusalem). Ibn al-Baytar also notes the colour of the stem and its use in these regions to treat backache, and goes on to report that he saw some white 'qarza'na' with large roots in the vicinity of 'Bayt al-Maqdis.'[919] In his entry 'drakil' Ibn al-Baytar describes a variety of the 'qarza'na' which the people of Mount Lebanon and Beirut recognize by the name 'shandab.'[920] Abu al-'Abas al-Nabati also described a variety called 'sahli' (sea shore)[921] with sweet roots which can give warmth and served to harden erection.[922] This use is also mentioned in popular medical books in Europe and is known till today among the Arabs of Israel.[923]

Medicinal Uses in the Medieval Period:
Maimonides described the medicinal use of the "water in which the 'qarza'na' is cooked" to treat abscesses and to reduce gases. The plant was considered a cold and dry drug.[924]

Traditional Medicine:
The Arabs of Israel are accustomed to eat various kinds of sea holly[925] and use the *Eryngium creticum* in their traditional medicine. They eat the leaves or smear the ground root to cure open wounds and scorpion stings. The seeds serve to cure stomach sores, cataract in the eyes, and to expel worms. The leaves are also eaten to strengthen the gums, and their juice is used to treat diabetes. The juice of the roots is drunk in order to treat kidney stones.[926] In Iraq, the leaves and roots serve as a medication for anemia, oedema and to protract menstruation.[927] In Jordan, the ash of the plant is spread over scorpion stings.[928] *Eryngium maritimum* used to be a diuretic and served as a digestive aid, to treat the womb and to accelerate the congealing of wounds.[929]

Seville Orange (Bigarade, Sour Orange)

Scientific name: *Citrus aurantium* (Rutaceae)
Hebrew Hosh'hash Arabic: Naranj[930]

Description:
This is a tall, evergreen citrus tree (up to 5 m.) with thorny branches, broad leaves, and highly fragrant white flowers. The fruit (approximately 10 cm. in diameter) has a hard, thick rind and the pulp is sour and bitter.[931]

History:
It is not clear when the Seville or sour orange appeared in the region. According to the researcher Tolkowsky, this type of orange has been known in the Land of Israel since the period of the Mishna and Talmud and should be identified with the "ball-shaped etrog" (citron).[932] Other scholars state that the 'naranj' (sour orange) was brought to the region from India in the 9th or beginning of the 10th century.[933]

913 Ibn al-Baytar, al Jami, II, p. 92; Leclerc, No. 865.

914 Dinsmore & Dalman, No. 721; Issa, Dictionary, p. 77, No. 22. Cf. Amar, al-Baytar, p. 63, n.41.

915 Ibn al-Baytar, al-Jami, IV, p. 12; Leclerc, No. 1754. Concerning identification see: Amar, Herbalist, pp. 238-239; Amar, al-Baytar, p. 63.

916 Description of varieties in: Plants & Animals, X, pp. 248-249.

917 On the identity of the sea holly and its uses in the sources see, in detail: Feliks, World, p. 194; Kislev.

918 Dioscorides, III.24.

919 Ibn al-Baytar, al-Jami, IV, p. 12; Leclerc,No. 1754.

920 Ibn al-Baytar, al-Jami, II, p. 92; Leclerc, No. 865.

921 This is apparently *Eryngium maritimum*.

922 Ibn al-Baytar, al-Jami, IV, p. 12; Leclerc, No. 1754. Cf. al-Antaki, p. 256.

923 Palevitz et al, p. 82; Grieve, pp. 408-409.

924 Maimonides, Aphorisms, 21:26, 73; 22:46.

925 Dafni, Edible, pp. 52-53; Uphof, p. 204.

926 Palevitz et al, p. 81.

927 al-Rawi & Chaakravarty, p. 41.

928 Dafni, Edible, p. 53.

929 In detail: Palevitz et al, p. 82; Grieve, pp. 408-409; Plants & Animals, X, p. 248. Cf. Dafni, Dudaim, p. 34; Dafni, Edible, p. 52.

930 Dinsmore & Dalman, No. 389; Issa, Dictionary, p. 51, No. 9. Discussion of the various species and their names in the Middle Ages in: Amar, Production, pp. 341-342.

931 Plants & Animals, XII, p. 127.

932 Tolkowsky, pp. 57, 195 ff. Because of insubstantial evidence, this should probably not be accepted.

933 al-Mas'udi, II, pp. 438-439; Watson, Innovation, pp. 45-48.

Medicinal Uses in Jerusalem:

Refael Malki described the medicinal use of 'mei zahar' in which the flowers of the 'naranjas' were steeped, and used as a component in a general medication for the Jerusalem poor.[934] According to him this was the "water which came from the 'naranja' blossoms" and was also a component in another general medication as well as being an additive to the 'sharupi' (syrup).[935]

Seville Orange in the Levant:

The 'naranj' was first mentioned by al-Muqaddasi at the end of the 10th century as being among the widespread agricultural products in the district of Palestine. Later it was said to grow in Greater Syria (Sidon and Tripoli).[936] There is considerable information regarding the cultivation of the sour orange during the Crusader, Mamluk and Ottoman periods and on its trade, including its export to Europe.[937] Hayim Vital recommended a medication for treating the tonsils which was made partly of fried 'naranja' and butter.[938]

Medicinal Uses in the Medieval Period:

Ibn Wahshiya described the production of 'naranj' oil and its use in reducing gases, and in strengthening the nerves and the joints.[939] Ibn al-Baytar described the tree and its fruit, and quoted other physicians who stated that the oil produced from the flowers was used among other things to reduce gases and strengthen the nerves. The fruit was a component in cathartic medications and in medicines to cure skin diseases as well as to cure intestinal inflammation and dysentery, and to cleanse the womb. The rind of the fruit was used to strengthen the heart, relieve stomach pains, expel stomach worms, treat stings and poisons and prevent fainting. The fruit was considered a cold and dry drug.[940] al-Qazwini noted that chewing the fragrant leaves of the 'naranj' eliminated the smell of garlic and onions, and he also mentioned that the fruit was beneficial for the head and strengthened the heart. In his view, it was the seeds that improved the scent, caused dryness and their smoke repelled ants.[941]

Traditional Medicine:

The dried peel was used in traditional medicine as a strengthening drug and a medication for stomach problems and to reduce gases. The flowers were used for a mixture of floral juices which also served as a remedy. The fresh fruit was extremely valuable as a source of Vitamin C.[942] The essential oil found in the blossoms and in the peel was used in the perfume industry and in the preparation of liqueurs. The fruit was used for making jams.[943]

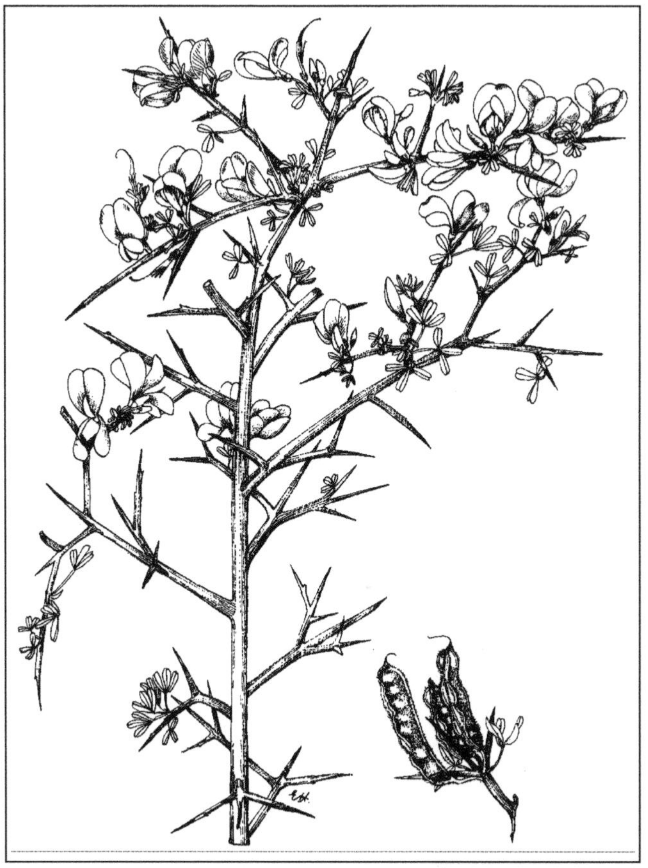

Figure 27 - Spiny Broom (*Calicotome villosa*)

Spiny Broom

Scientific name: *Calicotome villosa* (Papilionaceae)
Hebrew: Kida se'ira Arabic: Qandol[944]

Description:

The spiny broom is a tall, thorny bush (up to 15 cm.) with yellow, butterfly flowers, fragrant and intoxicating, and its fruit is an elongated hairy capsule (2-4 cm.) containing five or six seeds.[945]

History:

The 'kida' (spiny broom), translated in the English Bible as 'cassia,' is mentioned there as a merchandise exported from Tyre: "cassia and calamus were in thy market" (Ezekiel, 27:19) and also as one of the components the holy anointing oil (Exodus, 30:24). A few modern scholars identified this plant with the perfume scented tree (*Cinnamomum cassia*) imported from Ceylon, India and the Moluccas.[946] Feldman identified the spiny broom with the biblical 'ezrah' (Psalms, 37:35)

934 Malki, p. 61.

935 Ibid., pp. 61-62, 64.

936 al-Muqaddasi, p. 181; Khusraw, pp. 12, 18; al-Asfahani, p. 103.

937 In detail, with a list of sources in: Amar, Production, pp. 341-342.

938 Benajahu, pp. 106-107.

939 Ibn Wahshiya, I, p. 178.

940 Ibn al-Baytar, al-Jami, IV, pp. 174-175; Leclerc, No. 2204. Cf. al-Antaki, p. 327.

941 al-Qazwini, p. 235; al-Biruni, I, p. 320.

942 In detail, including the content of substances in: Uphof, p. 133. See Grieve, pp. 601-602 on the tree and its medicinal uses in Europe.

943 Plants & Animals, XII, p. 127; Uphof, p. 133.

944 Ibn al-Baytar,, al-Jami, IV, p. 32; Leclerc, No. 1830; Maimonides, Glossaire, p. 36, No. 88; Issa, Dictionary, p.37, No. 4; Dinsmore & Dalman, No. 417.

945 Plants & Animals, X, pp.154-155.

946 Feldman, p. 237; Feliks, World, p. 264.

because of its profuse yellow blossoms.[947] The 'aga' mentioned in the Tosefta was identified by the researcher, Feliks, with the spiny broom.[948]

Medicinal Uses in Jerusalem:
In his entry 'dahan nuar al-qandol' Ibn al-Baytar quotes al-Tamimi who wrote: "this is the oil from the buds of a tree called 'qandol' in al-Sham, and it is a large tree with sharp thorns along its branches ... and it grows mainly in the mountains of 'Bayt al-Maqdis' [Jerusalem]."[949]

Medicinal Uses in the Medieval Period:
Assaph Harofe stated that "the qindol tree which is called 'esplatos' is 'nushtila' resembling the spiny broom trees and some say it is of the same species. It is effective for boils in the mouth, and it grows on mountains. It is beneficial for one whose gums, palate and tongue are burning because the heat inside the body caused by extreme constipation makes the mouth constantly foul-smelling, and he will then be healed. It is worthwhile drinking it for liver and stomach pains, for snakebite and hemorrhoids, and also for most medications because of its high potency. It benefits one who vomits blood, it releases urine retention, and it will relieve all the spirits of the body."[950] al-Ghafiqi described the plant, quoting various physicians, and he noted especially its aromatic seeds and their use in reducing fever.[951] Ibn al-Baytar in his entry 'dahan nuar al-qandol' and in accordance with al-Tamimi, described the tree, its flowering and the process of plucking the blossoms and drying them on linen sheets.[952]

Traditional Medicine:
The flowers of the spiny broom are used by the Arab fellahin (farmers) in preparing perfumed liquids, food colouring (mainly for dairy products), writing ink and yellow dye for woven fabrics. The Arabs of Israel used the flowers to cure jaundice and in the Druse villages on the Golan Heights they are used to relieve stomach pains.[953]

Sugar Cane

Scientific name: *Saccharum officinarum* (Gramineae)
Hebrew: Kaneh sukar Arabic: Sukkar[954]

Description:
Sugar cane is a perennial, herbaceous plant, tall (2-4 m. or more), with multiple sections. Each stem is composed of 10 sections and each plant has ten sheath-like leaves wrapped around the sections. The stem is sealed and contains the sugar substance. It has a panicle with small seeds, but it reproduces mainly by its shoots. The plant ripens for use after a period of 8-24 months, preferably in regions where the temperature is above 20°C.[955]

History:
The plant was domesticated in Asia (probably in India) and already by the 4th century BCE it was considered an important agricultural crop in India.[956] Sugar is mentioned in classical Roman sources: Strabo refers to the honey produced from Indian sugar cane; Pliny wrote about sugar produced in Arabia and India and used as a remedy; Dioscorides desribed the *Sakcharon* made from sugar cane found in India and Arabia.

Among its medicinal uses, Dioscorides listed curing the stomach and intestines and relieving pains in the bladder.[957] The growing of sugar canes spread during the 7th century in the Near East in the wake of the Arab conquest. From India, the plant spread to Persia and from there to other countries.[958] Since this agricultural product was not known before the period of Islamic domination, halachic discussions arose during the period of the Geonim concerning the blessing to be pronounced upon it. Its cultivation spread to Europe (beginning with Spain) from 755 CE, but only from the 14th century onward was it used mainly for remedial purposes. At the beginning of the 16th century, after the discovery of America, it was taken over to the new continent.[959]

Medicinal Uses in Jerusalem:
In 1182 CE the general assembly of the Hospitallers instructed the head of their order in Tripoli (Monpelrin) to send sugar to their main headquarters in Jerusalem for the preparation of syrups and medications for sick patients.[960] Abu Zakri, the physician of several Ayyubid rulers was mentioned in a Genizah letter of 1196 CE written in Jerusalem. According to this letter, Abu Zakri noted that sugar with the addition of almonds was a medication.[961] Refael Malki stated that 'shukar' was a component in many medications and medicinal preparations in Jerusalem intended for a variety of purposes including its use as a purgative.[962] Moshe Poriat described the marketplace where thick and thin sugar canes were available and from which sugar was produced for sale.[963]

Sugar Cane in the Levant:
During the Middle Ages sugar can was included among the most important agricultural products in the Land of Israel. In Latin sources the sugar cane generally termed canameles (honey cane) and in Hebrew texts it was mainly called 'kaneh

947 Feldman, pp. 68-70.

948 Feliks, Yerushalmi, II, p. 108.

949 Ibn al-Baytar, al-Jami, II, p. 108; Leclerc, No. 918.

950 Assaph, 4, p. 396. Apparently in the second instance the reference is to a variety of cassia.

951 al-Ghafiqi, No. 233. Cf. al-Biruni, I, pp. 155-156; II, p. 92.

952 Ibn al-Baytar, al-Jami, II, p. 108; Leclerc, No. 918.

953 Krispil, pp. 1203-1205.

954 Maimonides, Glossaire, p. 82, No. 289; Issa, Dictionary, p. 159, No.6.

955 Plants & Animals, XII, p. 42.

956 Hill, p. 211.

957 Dioscorides, II.104.

958 Watson, Innovations, pp. 24-30.

959 Amar, Production, p. 246; Hill, p. 211. Regarding the role of Jews in the sugar trade, see: Shapira, Sugar.

960 Delaville, I, p. 427, Doc. No. 627.

961 Goitein, Jewry, p. 324.

962 Malki, pp. 58, 62.

963 Ya'ari, Travels, p. 280.

sukar.'[964] In the East the plant became a staple food. The sap of the plant was sucked or was purified to obtain a liquid honey or crystallized sugar. During the Middle Ages, the cultivation of sugar can became an important industry in the Near East.[965] al-Tamimi reported that the crystallized sugar was called 'ahowazi' in the al-Sham region.[966] Nasir Khusraw, a Persian traveller who visited the Land of Israel in 1047 CE, testifies that sugar cane was grown in abundance in Tripoli, and that they even produced sweet juice from it.[967] It appears from certain Genizah letters that the cities of Ashkelon, Ramlah and Tyre were centres of trade and export for sugar to Egypt and other places.[968] These letters indicate that Jews played a role in the sugar trade and in its process of production.[969]

After their conquest of the Land of Israel, the Crusaders found significant areas planted with sugar cane and in their sources they described its cultivation and processing which later continued during the Mamluk period mainly along the coastal plain, the Galilee, Lebanon (Acre, Achziv, Tyre and Sidon), in Caesarea, the Jordan Valley and the Kinneret (Sea of Galilee).[970] Hayim Vital tells of the use of 'sukar nabat' in a compound medication for asthma and in a medication to improve the appetite.[971] Daud al-Antaki in his entry 'sukkar' describes the sugar cane and its production process, and stresses its medicinal uses. In his view, sugar was a hot and dry drug manufactured in Egypt and in the al-Sham region at several levels of quality (according to the heat and duration of cooking).[972]

Medicinal Uses in the Medieval Period:
Assaph Harofe called the sugar cane[973] 'the sweet cane.' al-Kindi described the use of red sugar in a mixture for a clyster[974] and of pure sugar in several medications such as: a preparation for treating sore throat, for smelling salts, in toothpaste and in ointments and powders for the eyes to cure cataract.[975] Maimonides reported on the wide use of sugar as a remedy and on roasted sugar called 'sukkar roshdo'. He also described the use of sugar in which medicinal herbs such as violets were boiled.[976]

Sugar served as a component in purgative medications and in other medicinal preparations. It was recommended to eat it with various foods such as almonds and raisins, and to use it as a drink to strengthen the lungs.[977] In his letters to the Ayyubid Sultan, which dealt with other medical matters, Maimonides recommended dipping food in sugar.[978] al-Qazwini in his entry 'kasab' described medicinal uses such as: treating cough and chest pains, urine flow and draining mucus in the chest. A quotation from Ibn Sina shows that it was used to treat cough, oedema, and to improve the eyesight. The ash served to slow the heartbeat, to reduce eye swellings, strengthen the heart and to cure malaria.[979]

Saladino d' Ascoli wrote in his medical treatise: "Cane honey for cough and for furry throat, and 'Zuccarum' - red sugar - can be made of it, and it is very cleansing."[980] Daud al-Antaki reported in his entry 'sukkar' that sugar was beneficial for the body, it was fattening, and it strengthened the muscles, nerves and liver, it softened the cough, treated hoarseness and cured eye and skin diseases and sores.[981]

Traditional Medicine and General Uses:
Molasses (liquid sugar) was used for cooking, for the confectionery industry and to produce industrial alcohol, explosive materials, synthetic rubber, alcoholic beverages, animal feed, paper and petrol.[982] Yemenite Jews use sugar to regulate bowel movements, the liver and the kidneys, and to strengthen the eyesight, quench thirst and to treat backache.[983] The Jews of Iraq used to put different kinds of sugar in their compound medications to treat various illnesses.[984] It is considered a nutritionous substance, a diuretic, for food preservation and for medicinal preparations. It was also used to sweeten bitter medicines.[985]

Summary and Conclusions:
Apparently it was the Arabs who disseminated the use of sugar throughout the Western world and transmitted its medicinal uses which were: a medication against cold and cough, to strengthen the muscles, and as a sweetener for compound medications mainly in liquid preparations which were called in Arabic 'sharb' - an expression which was adopted in Western languages as 'Syrop.' The use of sugar as a remedy declined with development of modern medicine, mainly in the 20th century. During the course of the Middle Ages, in the area between Syria and Egypt, sugar cane was grown and sugar was manufactured. It was widely used as food among all social levels and also served extensively as a remedy. Indirect evidence for the prevalent use of sugar is revealed from a pathological test of human skeletons from the Crusader

964 Detailed sources in Amar, Production, p. 244; Shapira, Sugar, pp. 138-139.

965 Amar, Production, p. 246.

966 al-Tamimi, p. 10b.

967 Khusraw, p. 6

968 Gil, p. 187. No. 487; p. 272, No. 508.

969 For example: Goitein, Society, I, pp. 89, 366-367; IV, pp. 247-248.

970 Amar, Production, pp. 247-256. for the price and quality of sugar see: Ashtor, Trade, pp. 96-97; Amar, Production, pp. 256-258.

971 Benajahu, pp. 96, 111.

972 al-Antaki, p. 195.

973 Assaph, 4, p. 188

974 al-Kindi, Nos. 149, 215.

975 Ibid., Nos. 9, 15-16, 64, 77, 91, 99, 104, 109, 115-117, 157, 175.

976 Maimonides, Regimen, 2:9; Maimonides, Aphorisms, 22:55.

977 Maimonides, Regimen, 3:2, 4, 11; Maimonides Aphorisms, 13:6; 20:78; 21:69; 22:40.

978 Maimonides, Answers, 4:20.

979 al-Qazwini, p. 230. Cf. Ibn Sina, p. 417.

980 Saladino, p. 123.

981 al-Antaki, p. 195. Cf. Ibn al-Baytar, al-Jami, III, pp. 22-23; Leclerc, No. 1198; Ibn Sina, pp. 389-390.

982 Uphof, p. 463; Hill, pp. 210-214.

983 Reiani, p. 47, No. 109.

984 References in: Ben-Yakov, p. 737.

985 al-Rawi & Chaakravarty, pp. 84-85.

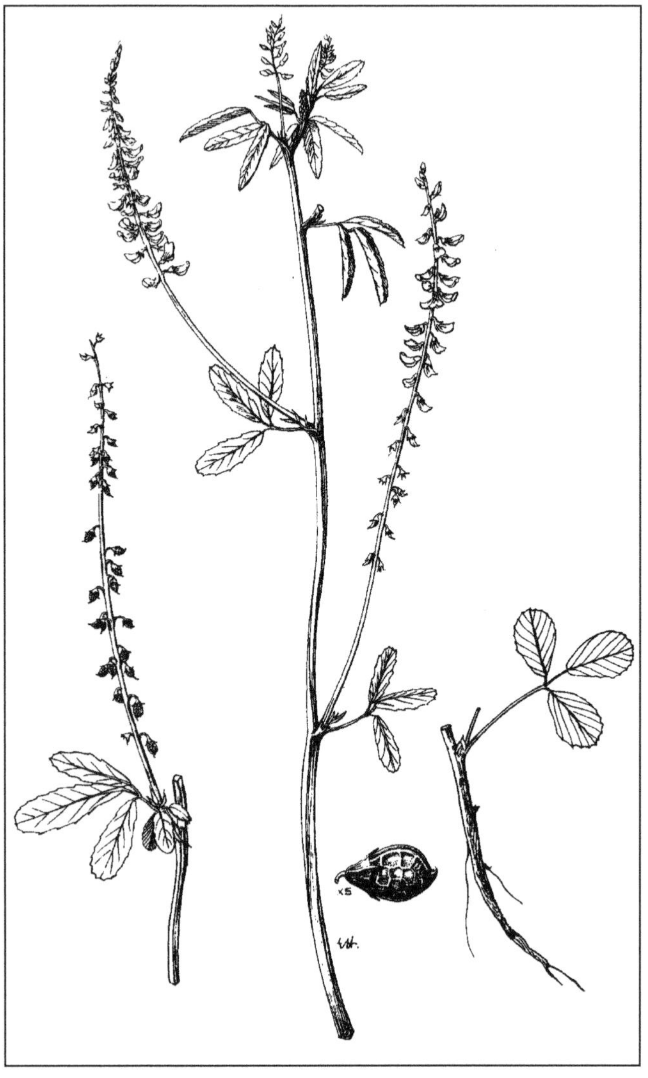

Figure 28 - Sweet Clover (*Melilotus albus*)

period in Tel Yizre'el which show a high frequency of tooth decay. Researchers link this with the increasing use of sugar by the general population.[986] A similar effect was revealed in a modern research conducted on certain tribes in Africa which habitually sucked sugar cane.[987]

Sweet Clover (White Melilot)

Scientific name: *Melilotus albus* (Papilionaceae)
Hebrew: Divsha levana Arabic: Iklil al-Malik[988]

Description:
Sweet clover is a wild, annual or biennial plant, tall and erect (up to 2 m.) that grows in damp habitats throughout the Land of Israel. Its leaves have triple leaflets with toothed margins, its flowers are white and the ripened fruit is black or brown. In Israel there are six species of clover, but only the white variety is a medicinal plant.[989]

[986] Mitchell, p. 70.

[987] Frencken et al.

[988] Maimonides, Glossaire, p. 18, No. 7; Issa, Dictionary, p. 166, No. 20.

[989] Feinbrun-Dothan, p. 351; Zohary, p. 445.

History:
The use of sweet clover for remedial purposes was known to classical physicians during the Hellenistic and Roman periods. Dioscorides described the *Melilotos* plant and noted its uses: to relieve pains and to treat swellings, inflammations, pains and wounds in all parts of the body, mainly in the ears, eyes, testicles and anus. An extract from the leaves served as a diuretic and emmenagogue.[990]

Medicinal Uses in Jerusalem:
In his entry 'Iklil al-Malik' Maimonides mentioned that sweet clover was a medicinal plant and noted the existence of two varieties. The fruits of one type resembled the tail of a scorpion and was called 'Iklil al-Malik al-mu'aqrab.' The roots of this plant were imported from Syria and used to prepare theriac[991] to counteract the bites of venomous creatures.[992] Elsewhere, Maimonides adds that 'arak al-heya' was the "root of the plant which surrounds Bayt al-Maqdis (Jerusalem) "and they have testified its value and confirmed its application." He supported his statement by explaining that he learnt about this matter from "those who know plants and recognized that this medicine was from the root of the variety 'makrona rial' called 'al-mu'akrabi.'[993]

Sweet Clover in the Levant:
Ibn al-Baytar in his entry 'iklil al-malik' quotes classical and medieval physicians from whom one learns of the argument concerning the identity of the plant, although there is general agreement as to its uses. Ibn al-Baytar summarised this argument and noted that this variety was widely used in Egypt and in the al-Sham region where it was grown, and that special use was made of the variety with fruits resembling ox horns.[994]

Medicinal Uses in the Medieval Period:
Assaph Harofe in his entry 'klila de-malka' described a plant with a good scent which was used to cure the wombs of women, snakebites and those affected by various poisons. According to him the 'handkoka' identified with 'melilotus' was effective in treating the liver, lungs, heart, womb, snakebites and scorpion stings, to dissolve kidney stones and to cure malaria. Elsewhere he describes this plant, noting that it was called 'taltan' and that it served also to treat head wounds, swollen eyes and earache.[995] According to Maimonides, sweet clover was a hot and dry drug.[996] He says that the method used to cure swollen eyes was by soaking a sponge in the water in which clover plants were cooked and placing it as a compress over the painful eyes.[997] A similar

[990] Dioscorides, III.48.

[991] Theriac is the accepted term for a compound medication against poison, snakebite and the bites of poisonous creatures. See the entry for Theriac in Chapter V and also in the entry for 'Adder' in Chapter II of this book.

[992] In detail: Maimonides, Glossaire, p. 18, No. 7.

[993] Maimonides, Poisons, p. 107, also n. 128.

[994] Ibn al-Baytar, al-Jami, I, p. 50; Leclerc, No. 128. Detailed discussion in Amar, al-Baytar, p. 60.

[995] Assaph, 4, p 403, 405, 415.

[996] Maimonides, Aphorisms, 21:69.

[997] Ibid., 9:22.

use was mentioned by Hunian ibn Ishaq.[998] al-Kindi reported on the use of the plant to treat the liver and stomach and to reduce fever.[999] Other physicians such as Ibn Sina, al-Biruni, and al-Ghafiqi, noted similar medicinal uses for different varieties of sweet clover.[1000] Daud al-Antaki in his entry 'iklil al-malik' described a commonly found plant similar to 'hulbah' (*Trigonella feonum-gracum*) which was used to reduce swellings, to relieve headaches, eliminate kidney stones, to treat wounds, inflammations, backache, liver, spleen, stomach and the womb.[1001]

Traditional Medicine:
Among the Jews of Iraq the 'iklil al-malik' was a component in a medication against insanity.[1002] In Europe, two varieties of sweet clover were known by traditional medicine: *Melilotus albus officinals* which is the common yellow melilot, and white melilot. The leaves are used as a poultice or ointment to treat inflammations, cuts and abrasions, as well as an expectorant and to cure diseases of the digestive tract.[1003]

Chizik described the use of the stems to produce the drug 'herba meliloti' which he says was used "as plasters for abscesses and also as a smelling powder for diseases of the breathing organs"[1004]

General Uses:
Various kinds of sweet clover were used as fodder[1005] and as a source for good honey.[1006] The flowers of the white melilot and the yellow melilot serve to scent clothing and improve the taste of cheese.[1007]

Identification:
Many researchers have dealt with the questions of the various names and identifications of this plant.[1008] Most of the sources so far mentioned describe varieties of the sweet clover species. Some of them describe the varieties used as remedies.[1009]

In his dictionary, Issa identified the 'rei'an' with the white melilot[1010] while the 'iklil al-malik' and 'melilotos' were identified with the yellow melilot.[1011] The researchers, Crowfoot and Baldensperger, identified the 'handkok' with certain types of clover and indicated that the white melilot was rare in the Jerusalem area.[1012] It should be noted that trefoil and clover were similar varieties and closely related from a scientific point of view. Moreover, according to some of the sources which describe the fruit as having horns, the plant may probably be identified with Jerusalem trefoil (*Trigonella hierosolymitana*).

Summary and Conclusions:
It appears that the use of different kinds of clover, especially white and yellow melilot, was well known since Hellenistic times. The medicinal uses were varied and centred mainly on treating poisons and attacks by venomous creatures, to cure eye diseases and various kinds of inflammation. Considerable evidence for the use of clover during the Middle Ages is found in Arabic medical literature in which the plant is connected with Jerusalem (from the 12th century). Maimonides also notes the connection with Jerusalem in his report on the plant growing in Bayt al-Maqdis.[1013] The tradition of the medicinal use of the plant has been preserved among Arabs and Jews until today, especially in Iraq.[1014] The connection of the plant with Jerusalem was retained by traditional medicine until the beginning of the 20th century.[1015]

Sweet Violet

Scientific name: *Viola odorata* (Violaceae)
Hebrew: Sigal reihani Arabic: Banfsaj[1016]

Description:
Perennial with long-stemmed roots, heart-shaped leaves and small, purple coloured and sweet scented flowers (2 cm.), which bloom in spring. Four wild varieties grow in the Land of Israel and are closely related to the cultivated species such as the pansy.[1017]

History:
The violet species consists of 300 varieties that grow in gardens throughout the world. The perfume produced from the scented, purple flowers is mentioned in the Talmud as 'sigali.' Dioscorides reported on the use of the plant *Ion* to treat epilepsy and throat inflammation.[1018]

---

998 Hunian, p. 181.

999 al-Kindi, Nos. 8, 36, 47, 59 and also p. 235.

1000 For example: Ibn Sina, p. 243; al-Biruni, I, p. 41; II, p. 75; al-Ghafiqi, No. 30.

1001 al-Antaki, p. 55.

1002 Ben-Yakov, pp. 295, 434.

1003 Loewenfeld & Back, p. 179.

1004 In detail: Chizik, p. 728.

1005 Zohary, p. 445; Chizik, p. 710. In detail: Hill, p. 344 where he also describes the use of medicinal clover.

1006 Uphof, p. 340; Chizik, p. 728; Plants & Animals, X, p. 177.

1007 Loewenfeld & Back, p. 179. In this connection Crowfoot & Baldensperger note that the inhabitants of the Land of Israel preferred the white melilot for this purpose.

1008 For example: Ben-Yakov, p. 445, who identified 'iklil al-malik' with the species growing in Iraq and called 'Crown imperial'; Dietrich, pp. 47-49; Amar, al-Baytar, p. 60, expecially n.33.

1009 For example: Maimonides, Glossaire, p. 18, No. 7; Loewenfeld & Back, p. 179.

1010 Issa, Dictionary, p. 116, No. 14.

1011 Ibid., No. 20.

1012 Crowfoot & Baldensperger, p. 62. In this connection see also the research by Hooper (p. 90) who identified the 'iklil al-malik' with *Astragalus hamosus* and reported that the source for the name of the medicine was those varieties of clover and trefoil which had unciform fruit.

1013 Maimonides, Glossaire, p. 18, No. 7.

1014 Ben-Yakov, p. 295, 434; Hooper, p. 90.

1015 Crowfoot & Baldensperger, p. 62. Iklil al-Malik

1016 For discussion of identification in medieval and Jewish sources, see: Amar, Production, pp. 224-225; Synonyms in: Issa, Dictionary, p. 189, No. 18; Dinsmore & Dalman, No. 212.

1017 Description in: Feinbrun-Dothan, p. 339; Plants & Animals, XII, p. 216; Kohen & Shemid'a.

1018 Dioscorides, IV.122.

Medicinal Uses in Jerusalem:
Refael Malki recommended the use of "the leaves of the violet that is called violash" to treat fever.[1019] David de Silva asserted that the roots were used to treat fever and the leaves as a component of enema.[1020]

Sweet Violet in the Levant:
al-Muqadassi mentions the 'dahan al-banafpsaj' (violet oil) which is produced in Damascus and is of low quality.[1021] 'Abd al-Latif al-Baghdadi, who was active in the region during the Ayyubid period, noted that the 'banafsaj' which grew in Egypt had an exceptionally sweet scent, but the people in Egypt did not know how to produce oil from it in the proper way and to preserve it.[1022] During the Mamluk period the sweet violet was listed among the perfume plants of Greater Syria[1023] especially the region of Beaufort and the Litani River.[1024]

Medicinal Uses in the Medieval Period:
al-Kindi claimed that the 'banafsaj' was used to treat the breathing tracts, intestinal disorders, mumps, toothache, hemorrhoids and night blindness.[1025] Maimonides told the Ayyubid Sultan that he recommended rubbing 'banafsaj oil' - purified violet oil - on the skin, and it was mentioned as a component in a sleeping drug.[1026] It was said of the 'violash' that it was a cold and moist drug and a mild purgative. 'Violash oil' was used as protection on "the lips of one who had sucked poison."[1027]

Ibn al-Baytar notes in his entry 'banafsaj' that the substance was used as a medication for the stomach, for the cough, to cure eye diseases, relieve pain, reduce fever and dispel gases.[1028] In his entry 'dahan al-banafsaj' Ibn al-Baytar described the violet oil and listed its medicinal uses.[1029] al-Qazwini relates that the plant grew in shady areas and served as a medication for severe eye inflammation, to treat colds and various skin diseases.[1030]

Traditional Medicine:
Yemenite Jews called the three-coloured violet (*Viola kitaibeliana*) 'banpasaj' and used it medically as an eye bandage for inflammation and sores. It was used internally to treat fever, swellings in the body and to regulate the digestive tract, cleanse the stomach, cure jaundice and severe cough, to soothe and induce sleep.[1031] Various types of violet, especially the sweet violet, were used in Iran to reduce fever, relieve headache, as a mild purgative, a medication for constipation, a soothing drug and to induce perspiration.[1032] The use of this plant is widespread in the East until today for treating cough.[1033]

Modern Medicine and General Uses:
Violet is a perfume - one of the most widely known - which is produced from the sweet violet that grows in Europe. Essential oils are derived from it that are used also to give flavor to liqueurs.[1034] Violet oil is an expectorant and a diuretic, and is used for treating skin diseases and cough.[1035]

Toadflax

Scientific name: *Kickxia (Linaria) sp.* (Scrophulariaceae)
Hebrew: Kicksia Arabic: Mah'lasa[1036]

Description:
This species contains 25 varieties which used to be included among the flax species (Linaria). Five perennial desert species and four annual Mediterranean species grow in the Land of Israel. The flowers are yellow, double-lipped, with a long spur projecting from the lower lip. The fruit is capsulated.[1037]

History:
The species was given the name of an 18th century Belgian pharmacist and botanist.[1038] According to Disocorides, *Elantine*, which is identified with *Linaria spuria* (round-leaved toadflax), was a plant used to cure inflamed eyes and dysentery.[1039]

Toadflax in Jerusalem and the Levant:
Ibn al-Baytar in his entry 'mah'lasa' described two varieties of plants: "the herb with the square stem and leaves similar to those of the plant, which is 'reihan' except that it has no smell but has a bitter taste and it is ineffective. It can be found in abundance in 'Jabal Nablus' [mountains of Shechem] and in other places in 'Balad al-Sham' .... And there is another herb known in Eastern parts especially in the land of Horan by the name of 'kinafsha' ... which was also mentioned by al-Tamimi in connection with the 'mah'lasa' and it is an elongated and stiff plant, with a gray stem, and is very bitter to the taste. It

1019 Malki, p. 78.

1020 Amar, de Silva, p. 114.

1021 al-Muqadassi, p. 181; al-Badri, p. 79.

1022 It seems that the writer intended making a comparison with the high quality scented violet in Greater Syria: al-Baghdadi, p. 76. In detail: Amar, Production, p. 225.

1023 al-'Umari, p. 26; al-Qalqashandi, p. 87.

1024 'Uthmani, p. 481.

1025 al-Kindi, Nos. 9, 60, 78, 125, 169. For additional uses by physicians of that period, see: Ibid., p. 247, No. 47. Cf. Ibn Sina, p. 266.

1026 Maimonides, Answers, 5; Maimonides, Sexual, 18:1.

1027 Maimonides, Regimen, 2:7, 9, 20; 3:4; Maimonides, Poisons, p. 97; Maimonides, Aphorisms, 21:74.

1028 Ibn al-Baytar, al-Jami, I, pp. 114-115; Leclerc, No. 353.

1029 Ibn al-Baytar, al-Jami, II, p. 107; Leclerc, No. 912.

1030 al-Qazwini, p. 242.

1031 Reiani, p. 51, No. 123. The Jews of Iraq made similar use of the plant and other closely related varieties: Ben-Yakov, pp. 462-463.

1032 Hooper, p. 185. In detail, including content of these substances: al-Rawi & Chaakravarty, p. 97.

1033 al-Kindi, p. 247, No. 47.

1034 Hill, p. 185; Uphof, p. 545.

1035 Uphof, p. 545; Chizik, p. 730; Reiani, p. 51, No. 123; Grieve, pp. 834-839.

1036 Ibn al-Baytar, al-Jami, IV, p. 163; Leclerc, No. 2163; Issa, Dictionary, p. 109, Nos. 11, 13-14.

1037 Plants & Animals, XI, pp. 95-96; Zohary, p. 536.

1038 Plants & Animals, XI, pp. 95-96.

1039 Dioscorides, IV.40.

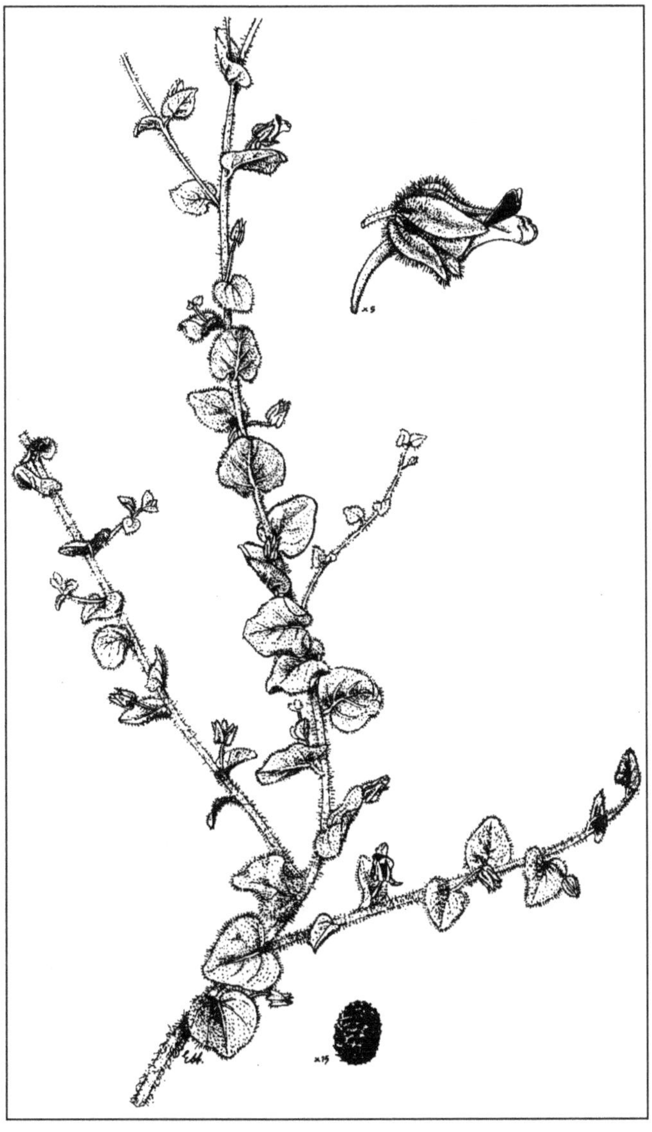

Figure 29 - Toadflax (*Kickxia spuria*)

has few leaves ... and from its roots medicinal substances are produced. It is also gathered in the land of al-Sham and I saw it in Majdal Yaba [Migdal Sedek] near Kever Kalba and I picked it there. Much of it can also be found in those other lands and in Tahar Ghaza [the Gaza area], al-Hasi, as far as Jabal Khalil [Hebron mountains] and up to Jabal al-Maqdis [Jerusalem mountains] in great abundance, as well as in the regions of Halab [Aleppo, Syria] known as ....where there is plenty of it."[1040]

Identification:
The researcher, Amar, identified the 'mah'lasa' with the round-leaved toadflax (*Kickxia spuria*) and the 'kinafsha' with *Kickxia sieberim var. bombycina*.[1041]

Medicinal Uses in the Medieval Period:
The main medicinal use of the two varieties which Ibn al-Baytar described in his entry 'mah'lasa' was as a medication against snakebite (on his own personal evidence). An added source for this medicinal use was derived from a respectable person on which the writer relied implicitly: "The man whom I trust for his reliability is one of the important personages in al-Sham, Kadi Fahr al-Din the qadi of Shechem, may Allah bless him, who said that anyone who is bitten or stung should drink from it and be cured ... and this has been proved by experience."[1042] Daud al-Antaki in his entry 'mah'lasa' described the different varieties of the plant and listed its medicinal uses: a hot and dry drug, giving immunity against poisons, strengthens the heart and cures joint pains.[1043]

Medical Qualities:
Many flax species growing in Israel contain glycoside which breaks down into a harmful acid, and therefore animals refrain from eating these plants.[1044] The species called *Kicksia elatine* serves as a constricting substance, stops internal hemorrhaging and nosebleeds, and is also a strengthening substance.[1045]

Summary and Conclusions:
The toadflax plants are known mainly for their beauty. Their characterisation as medicinal plants is not well noted except by Dioscorides and Ibn al-Baytar. Because of limited medieval sources and also those of traditional medicine, it appears that its use was confined to the locality of Syria and Israel.

Tragacanth

Scientific name: *Astragalus gummifer* (Papilionaceae)
Hebrew: Keded ha-saraf Arabic: Kathira[1046]

Description:
Tragacanth is a thorny bush, conic-shaped and lowly, with long, yellow spikes. Its many branches diverge from the neck of the root, its composite leaves are pinnate and pointed, its flowers are white or yellow. A scentless gum is produced by slashing the neck of the root or stem. It grows on Mt. Hermon and other mountains in the Middle East, in Asia Minor and in Southern Europe.[1047]

History:
The Bible describes a caravan of Ishmaelites on the road from Mt. Gilead to Egypt, with camels "bearing spicery ['nekho'at'] and balm and myrrh" (Genesis 37:25), and elsewhere it mentions the "best fruits of the land" which the sons of Jacob brought down to Joseph in Egypt: "a little balm, a little honey, spices ['nekho'at'] and myrrh, nuts and almonds" (Genesis 43:11). The Hebrew word 'nekho'at' is identified with the gum of the tragacanth.[1048] According to Dioscorides, the *Tragakanthe* (identified with *Astragalus aristatus*) was a lowly, prickly bush spread along the ground. This name was

1040 Ibn al-Baytar, al-Jami, IV, p. 142; Leclerc, No. 2094; Sickenberger, pp. 12, 18-19.

1041 Amar, al-Baytar, pp. 73-74, n. 69; Feinbrun-Dothan, p. 602.

1042 Ibn al-Baytar, al-Jami, IV, p. 142; Leclerc, No. 2094.

1043 al-Antaki, p. 292.

1044 Chizik, p. 737.

1045 Uphof, p. 314.

1046 Maimonides, Glossaire, p. 61, No. 191; al-Antaki, p. 267; Issa, Dictionary, p. 26, No. 7; Low, II, pp. 419-424.

1047 Zohary, p. 439; Feinbrun-Dothan, p. 309; Uphof, p. 57.

1048 Discussion in: Feliks, World, p. 274.

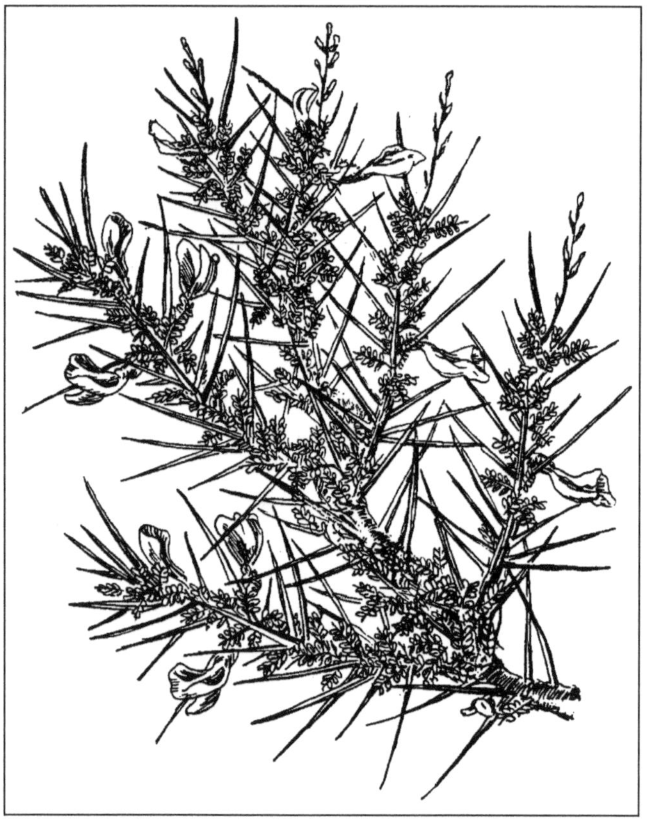

Figure 30 - Tragacanth (*Astragalus gummifer*)

also given to the jellified sap that dripped from the slashed plant. The gum is translucent, smooth, and has a sweet taste, and its characteristics resembles acacia gum. It serves as a component in eye medications for chest diseases, cough, kidney pains and glandular problems.[1049] The Talmud mentions the word 'kashritha' which probably means 'kathira.'

Medicinal Uses in Jerusalem:
According to Refael Malki, the 'dragaranti' is the 'electira' - a component of equal value to the 'samaj ha-arabi' (see the entry for Gum Arabic in this chapter) - which is a pill for strengthening the heart and brain.[1050]

Tragacanth in the Levant:
The export of tragacanth from the region was done regularly during the Middle Ages. The gum was sent to various countries where medications were made from it, mainly for diseases of the eye, stomach, intestines and for smallpox.[1051] In a Genizah letter dated 1060, Ya'akov ben Yosef of Ashkelon asks Naharai ben Nissim of Fustat for the price of the 'kathira' in Egypt. This probably shows that he intended supplying the gum to Egypt.[1052] Ibn al-Baytar in his entry 'kathira' says that "there is a lot of it in the mountains of Beirut and Lebanon in the al-Sham region."[1053] al-Dimashqi listed the 'kathira' with 90 other varieties of medicinal plants growing in Lebanon which could be a source of livelihood by their harvesting.[1054]

Medicinal Uses in the Medieval Period:
According to Assaph Harofe the substance was the gum of a plant called in Aramaic 'ankat ayla' and in Greek 'drakkanti' and its medicinal uses were: a perspirant, to cure cough and diseases of the breathing tracts, throat pains, diseases of the intestines and the eyes, elimination of kidney stones, to stop bleedings and to treat wounds.[1055]

According to al-Kindi, tragacanth gum was used to strengthen the limbs, to treat cough, legs and eyes diseases and it was a component in ointments.[1056]

Maimonides claimed that the 'dragaman' was added to strong purgatives in order to prevent vomiting and damage to the intestines.[1057] In his entry 'kathira' Ibn al-Baytar described the use of the gum to prevent 'moisture issuing from the head, to relieve bad feelings, to strengthen the intestines, to effectively treat abscesses in the eyes and lung diseases, to cure cough, burns, eye diseases, smallpox and to stop hemorrhages.[1058]

Traditional Medicine and General Uses:
The gum of this plant is used in the process of dyeing fabrics and in the cosmetic industry. In Iraq the gum is used in making ice-cream and to paint walls. In Iran medicinal uses are being made until the present day.[1059] The Jews of Tripoli use the substance to treat cough[1060] while the Jews of Iraq called it 'kathira biza' and report on its use in treating disorders of the urinary tract.[1061] Tragacanth gum is marketed today in the form of drops or thin flakes, and serves as an adhesive in pills and tablets, as a suspension for non-soluble powders and to produce an emulsion for oils and other gums.[1062]

Turpeth (Turbith / Indian Jalap)

Scientific name: *Ipomoea turpethum* (Convolvulaceae)
Hebrew: Lefofit ha-turbit Arabic: Turbud[1063]

Description:
Turpeth is a tropical, perennial climber and the resinous extract from its roots is used for medicinal purposes.[1064]

[1049] Dioscorides, III.23.

[1050] Malki, p. 67.

[1051] On trading in tragacanth gum, see: Heyd, pp. 623-624; Amar, Substances, p. 52.

[1052] Gil, No. 487, p. 18a.

[1053] Ibn al-Baytar, al-Jami, IV, pp. 52-53; Leclerc, No. 1889.

[1054] al-Dimashqi, p. 199. Cf. al-Nuwayri, p. 298.

[1055] Assaph, 4, p. 415.

[1056] a-Kindi, Nos. 55, 111, 115, 134, 173. Cf. Ibn Sina, p. 340.

[1057] Maimonides, Aphorisms, 3:112; 21:78; Maimonides, Asthma, 12:8.

[1058] Ibn al-Baytar, al-Jami, IV, p. 52; Leclerc, No. 1889. Cf. al-Antaki, p. 267.

[1059] Uphof, p. 57; Hooper, p. 90; Ben-Yakov, p. 523; Howes, pp. 39-44; Morton, p. 145.

[1060] Krispil, p. 1192.

[1061] Ben-Yakov, p. 330.

[1062] Hill, p. 152; Uphof, p. 57. For the contents of active substances in tragacanth gum see: Chopra et al, p. 76. Medicinal uses in: Beach; Morton, pp. 143-144.

[1063] Issa, Dictionary, p. 100, No. 9.

[1064] Description: Grieve, p. 823; Hooper, p. 130.

Medicinal Uses in Jerusalem:
Benevenutus described the use of *Spurge* which was a component in the 'Jerusalem pill' - a medication against cataract.[1065] According to Refael Malki the 'turbith' was a component in a general pill to treat the Jerusalem poor.[1066]

Turpeth in the Levant:
Italian trade documents dated 1481 CE describe the trading of packages of turpeth bought in Acre and sent to Italy.[1067] According to Hayim Vital the 'turbid majzuf' (rinsed turpeth) was a component in a medication for asthma.[1068]

Medicinal Uses in the Medieval Period:
According to al-Kindi the 'turbud' was a component in a general medicinal preparation.[1069] Ibn al-Baytar quotes Abu al-'abas al-Nabati who reported that the plant grew in Iraq.[1070] Maimonides claimed that the 'turbid' was a hot and dry purgative drug.[1071] Saladino d'Ascoli relates that the 'turbit' was a 'herb root' and detailed its qualities and uses.[1072]

Traditional Medicine:
In Iran today the plant is called 'turbud' and is imported mainly from India and Ceylon (Sri Lanka). In the Near East and India it is used as a purgative as well as to treat backache and diseases of the kidney.[1073] In Egypt the 'turbud nabati' also serves as a purgative substance and to treat hemorrhoids.[1074] The roots of the turpeth were used as a purgative drug in Europe during the past centuries.[1075]

Watercress

Scientific name: *Coronopus squamatus* (Cruciferae)
Hebrew: Shahlil saru'a Arabic: Rajal al-gharab[1076]

Description:
Watercress is a spreading annual plant with its under-leaves dissected and pinnate. It blooms briefly with white blossom and its fruit is a small seedpod that does not open when ripe.[1077]

History:
Disocorides in his entry *koronopus* described a plant that the editor identified with *Lotus ornithopodidoides* which was used mainly to treat diarrhea.[1078]

Medicinal Uses in Jerusalem:
Ibn al-Baytar in his entry 'rajal al-gharab' quotes al-Tamimi who mentions in his book *al-marshad* the name of a plant in al-Sham - 'rajal al-za'a' and in the Jerusalem environs as 'wadis.' According to al-Tamimi, the inhabitants of Jerusalem and that region used an oil, produced from the plant as an astringent. They also used to eat the plant.[1079] In his entry 'rajal al-gharab' Daud al-Antaki says that this was the name of a plant in 'Bayt al-Maqdis' (Jerusalem).[1080]

Identification:
The plant 'rajal al-gharab' was identified by Leclerc with *Lotus ornithopodidoides*[1081] and by other researchers with *Plantago cornopus*.[1082] This plant has rosette leaves with a leaf-structure very similar to that of the watercress and to bird-feet. Because of this leaf shape and as a result of the description by Ibn al-Baytar, the researcher Amar identified the plant with 'shahlil saru'a' (watercress) - a widespread plant in this region which also grows in the Jerusalem mountains.[1083] Chizik noted that the Arabic name for the 'shahlil saru'a' was 'rashad bari.'[1084]

Traditional Medicine:
The plant is commonly found in the markets of Iraq and serves as an appetizer.[1085]

White Water Lily

Scientific name: *Nymphaea alba*
Hebrew: Nimfe'a Arabic: Nilofar
Additional names: al-Nahal, al-'arus, Bashin

Description:
White water lily is a perennial water plant. Its root stem is buried in the mud, and the round leaf blades floats on the water. The white flowers are large and resplendent, floating in the water or protruding from it. Two other similar species are known in this region: *Nymphaea nauchali* (Blue water lily) and *Nymphaea lotus*.[1086]

History:
In his entry 'numphaia' Dioscorides described the *Nymphaea alba* and noted its uses such as: to treat dysentery, intestinal

[1065] Benevenutus, p. 33; The editor, Wood, identified this with turpeth.

[1066] Malki, p. 67. The editor mistakenly identified this as mineral.

[1067] Ashtor, Trade, p. 298.

[1068] Benajahu, p. 97.

[1069] al-Kindi, No. 214; Ibn Sina, p. 446.

[1070] Ibn al-Baytar, al-Jami, II, pp. 136-137; Leclerc, No. 407. Cf. al-Antaki, p. 91.

[1071] Maimonides, Aphorisms, 21:80; Maimonides, Regimen, 2:11. Cf. al-Biruni, I, p. 89.

[1072] Saladino, p. 85.

[1073] Hooper, p. 130. Cf. Uphof, p. 283.

[1074] Ducros, p. 50.

[1075] Grieve, p. 823 where the content of substances is given.

[1076] Issa, Dictionary, p. 58, Nos. 10-12. Cf. Dinsmore & Dalman, No. 149.

[1077] Feinbrun-Dothan, p. 258.

[1078] Dioscorides, II.158.

[1079] Ibn al-Baytar, al-Jami, II, pp. 136-137; Leclerc, No. 1031.

[1080] al-Antaki, pp. 166-167; Ibn Sina, p. 413.

[1081] Leclerc, No. 1031.

[1082] Issa, Dictionary, p. 146, No. 113.

[1083] Amar, Traditions, p. 31, n.39

[1084] Chizik, p. 852.

[1085] Ben-Yakov, p. 607.

[1086] Description: Feinbrun-Dothan, p. 203; Plants & Animals, X, p. 86.

diseases, illnesses of the spleen, and problems of the urinary bladder.[1087]

White water lily as a Medicinal Plant in Jerusalem:
From an 18th century document in the Jerusalem court archives it seems that nuphar water was used to cure pregnant women in Jerusalem.[1088] The document describes a lawsuit brought by an Arab from the village of Silwan (Siloam) against a Jewish physician, Salmon ben ha-Yehudi, which was presented at the Shari'a law court in 1711. From this document it appears that the physician (who was acquitted) had recommended the use of nuphar water and chicory water to cure a pregnant woman, but her husband had given her cassia water which caused his wife to abort the fetus and to die.

White water lily in the Levant:
In a description of the Safed region during the 14th century, al-'Uthmani notes that in the Kadesh lake (Lake Hulah) 'nilofar' plants were growing.[1089] al-Ghazi described the 'nilofar' with all its varieties (red, white and blue) and also emphasized the yellow Damascus variety. The seeds of different varieties were used for medicinal purposes.[1090]

Identification:
During the Middle Ages and in modern times the terms 'nufar' and 'nilofar' as well as 'al-arus' 'bashinin' and 'lotus'[1091] were used to describe two varieties of waterlilies - nuphar and nymphea which were similar in form and habitat. A description of both plants is presented in this book.

Medicinal Uses in the Medieval Period:
According to Maimonides, the 'nilofar' was one of the plants that strengthened the appetite and the spirit, and was a medicinal substance for skin diseases. The flower was used as a purgative drug and a component in a preparation to sweeten the breath. The leaves served as a component in an anaphrodisiac preparation to "suppress sexual desire."[1092] al-Qazwini reported that the 'nilofar' was a water plant that grew in the region and was used as a soporific, to relieve headache and to treat leprosy and baldness. Its use also inhibited sexual desire.[1093] According to Daud al-Antaki the 'nilofar' plant was used to reduce fever, to cure inflammations, and to prevent thirst. It was also used in medicinal preparations to cure wounds, treat heart palpitations, headaches, cold, diseases of the spleen, hemorrhages, swellings, to remove freckles and inhibit the appetite.[1094]

[1087] Dioscorides, III.148.

[1088] Cohen, 18 century, p. 325, No. 279.

[1089] 'Uthmani, p. 480.

[1090] Hamarneh, Plants, p. 256.

[1091] Maimonides, Glossaire, p. 74, No. 252; Issa, Dictionary, p. 125, No. 15; Dinsmore & Dalman, Nos. 42-43; Plants & Animals, p. 86; Hooper, pp. 144-145; al-Ghafiqi, Nos. 129-130.

[1092] Maimonides, Regimen, 2:20; Maimonides, Aphorisms, 9:106; 13:51; 21:74; Maimonides, Sexual, 5:5; 7:1.

[1093] al-Qazwini, p. 261.

[1094] al-Antaki, pp. 333-334. Cf. Ibn Sina, p. 375; al-Biruni, I, pp. 323-324. This description conforms with the plant *Nymphaea nauchali*.

Traditional Medicine:
A powder derived from the root stem of the *Nymphaea lotus* serve as a medication for digestive or intestinal problems and the powder of the crushed seeds are used in the Sudan to treat skin diseases.[1095] In Iraq and Iran the *Nymphaea alba* is called 'kol nilofar.' Flowers of various types of the white water lily are sold in India where they are used as a medicinal drug, mainly as an astringent to stop hemorrhages and to serve as a component in a preparation to reduce fever and cure lung diseases in children.[1096]

Yarrow

Scientific name: *Achillea millefolium* (Compositae)
Hebrew: Achilea Arabic: Hazanbal

Description:
The Achilea genus consists of 200 species. Five wild varieties grow in the Land of Israel. The most common varieties growing in this region are: *Achillea santolina* (Santolina-Leaved Sneezewort), *Achillea fragrantissima* (Lavender Cotton), and *Achillea biebersteinii* (Yellow Milfoil). The common domesticated species is called *Achillea millefolium* (Yarrow) - a perennial dwarf shrub (up to 80 cm.) that grows in temperate climates. Its many leaves are feathery and split into narrow lobes.[1097]

Identification:
The Arabic name 'hazanbal' is the common name for one of the yarrow varieties growing in the Middle East.'[1098] Medieval sources apparently use the name 'hazanbal' to describe the local yarrow species such as *Achillae santolina* and *Achillea fragrantissima* which grow in the Land of Israel and other Middle Eastern regions. These varieties may have been a local substitute for the yarrow (*Achillae millefolium*) that appears in classical texts but is not a natural plant of the Levant.[1099] Until now we have not found any evidence that this domesticated plant was grown in the region. It may therefore be assumed that the local physicians and botanists who mentioned the 'hazanbal' in their writings, were referring to the local species, but they were actually describing the *Achillea millefolium* - the most famous variety of the yarrow which is mentioned in many classical sources.[1100]

History:
The name for the Achillea species commemorates Achilles, the legendary warrior of the Trojan War. According to the legend the centaur Chiron (who was half-man half-horse)

[1095] Uphof, p. 363.

[1096] Hooper, pp. 144-1145. For the medicinal uses of the nuphar and nymphea varieties in Europe see: Grieve, p. 484.

[1097] Plants & Animals, XI, pp. 147-148; Feinbrun-Dothan, pp. 699-700. Arabic names also in: Issa, Dictionary, pp. 3-4.

[1098] Dinsmore & Dalman, p. 158.

[1099] According to modern research, the plant grows wild near Damascus. See: Post & Dinsmore, II, p. 45; Chizik, p. 643.

[1100] In this connection se also: Amar, al-Baytar, p. 55.

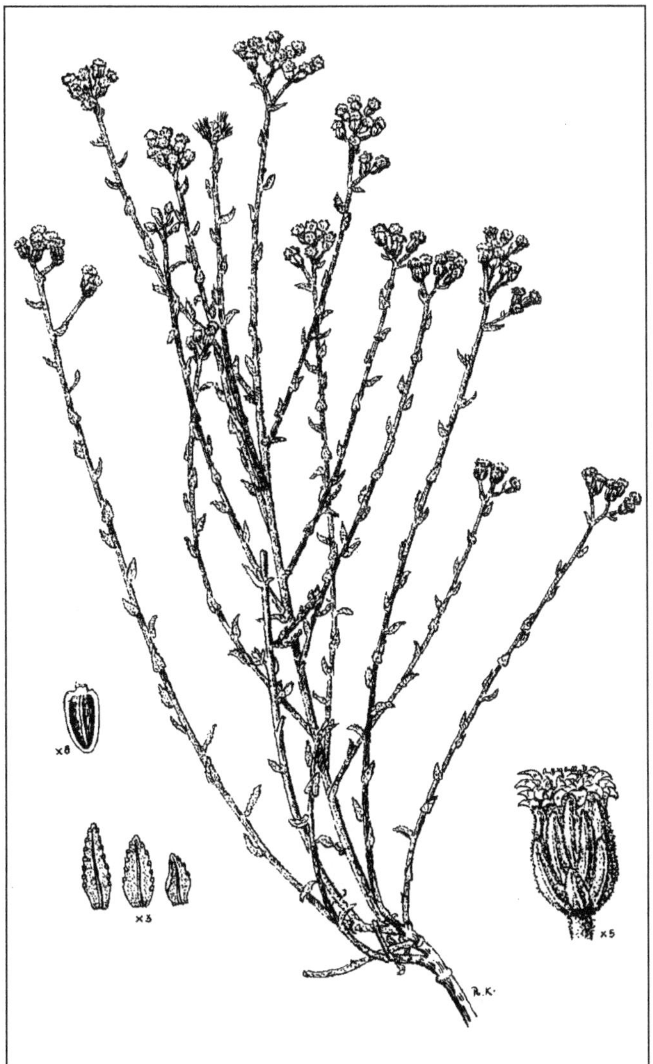

Figure 31 - Yarrow (*Achillea fragrantissima*)

taught Achilles the medicinal qualities of the plant.[1101] The yarrow was mentioned as a medicinal plant by Dioscorides who claimed that the *muriophullon* was used to treat heart diseases and inflamed ulcers.[1102] Yarrow is mentioned in many medical treatises in Europe from early times till today. Its medicinal applications were common among soldiers and warriors in different cultures and periods in the ancient world, in the medieval period and even among the Indian tribes in America as well as the soldiers fighting in the American Civil War.[1103]

Medicinal Uses in Jerusalem:

Ibn al-Baytar in his entry 'hazanbal' quotes al-Tamimi who describes the plant and its habitat. In his book al-murshad, al-Tamimi noted especially the thick root and its taste. Regarding its habitat, he said that "... it grows in Tarsus and in other places such as the al-Sham region, in Tiberias, and in the mountains of Jerusalem where it is found in abundance." Among its medicinal applications, al-Tamimi listed its ability to counteract the venom of poisonous snakes and scorpions.[1104] Daud al-Antaki mentioned the 'hazanbal' and noted the good variety that grew in Jerusalem and Tarsus.[1105] It seems that al-Antaki as usual quotes earlier writers regarding medicinal applications.

In his entry 'murifilon acher' Ibn al-Baytar quotes al-Kindi who claims that "it is a remedy brought from al-Sham and its root is similar to that of the autumn mandrake" (*Mandragora autumnalis*). He also discusses the argument among the physicians of al-Sham regarding its medicinal applications, identification and similarity with the 'hazanbal.'[1106]

Traditional Medicine:

Lavender cotton (*Achillea fragrantissima*) is used by the Arabs of Israel as an analgesic and for the treatment of ailments such as joint and heart pains, sand in the kidneys, renal obstructions, weakness, diabetes, and menstrual disorders.[1107] The plant is also used by the Bedouins of the Negev and Sinai to disinfect wounds, to cure eye inflammations, relieve stomach pains and constipation, expel intestinal worms, and reduce fever.[1108] Santolina-leaved sneezewort (Achillea santolina) is used by the Arabs in Israel to relieve stomach pains, severe cough and chest colds.[1109] The Bedouins use it to cure intestinal disorders.[1110] The plant is well known among many traditional societies in the Middle East and North Africa as a remedy for chest diseases and as a strengthening drug. In Iran it is also used to cure respiratory disorders,[1111] in North and East Africa it serves as an expectorant, and in Iran and Iraq to treat diseases of the lungs and intestines.[1112]

Medical Qualities:

Recent research shows that all parts of the *Achillea millefolium* species of the yarrow contain essential oils. Other varieties contain different components that have anti-inflammatory and analgesic effects, while other components have anti-bacterial, anti-cancerous and cytotoxic qualities. The plant also contains substances which have spasmodic and alkaloid with haematic efficacy.[1113]

Modern Medicine:

The dried leaves and flowers of the yarrow are mentioned in pharmacopoeia compendiums in the United States, Poland, Switzerland, and Hungary. The main internal applications are: as a general stimulant, to accelerate menstruation, and as a medicinal tea, while external applications are: as a cream or a bandage, and also as a cure for gynecological disorders.[1114]

[1101] Palevitz et al, p. 27.

[1102] Dioscorides, IV.115.

[1103] In detail: Chandler et al, pp. 205-207; Palevitz et al, pp. 28-29.

[1104] Ibn al-Baytar, al-Jami, II, p. 20; Leclerc, No. 668.

[1105] al-Antaki, p. 123.

[1106] Ibn al-Baytar, al-Jami, IV, p. 147; Leclerc, No. 2104.

[1107] Palevitz et al, p. 27.

[1108] Levey, Bedouins, p. 76; Plants & Animals, XII, p. 148; Dafni, Dudaim, p. 14.

[1109] Palevitz et al, p. 27.

[1110] Abu-Rabia, p. 15.

[1111] Dafni, Dudaim, p. 14.

[1112] Hooper, p. 80.

[1113] In detail: Chandler et al.

[1114] Uphof, pp. 8-9; Chandler et al, pp. 203-205.

General Uses:
Different species of Achillea are used as an incense, as a substitute for spices such as cloves and cinnamon, to add flavour to beer, as a hair dye and as a remedy to prevent baldness.[1115] Among the local varieties, the Bedouins use the *Achillea fragrantissima* as a fragrance[1116] while the strong smell of the *Achillea santolina* is used to expel insects and stinking bugs.[1117]

Yellow Pond Lily

Scientific name: *Nuphar lutea {luteum}*
Hebrew: Nufar zahov Arabic: Nufar

Description:
This is a perennial plant that grows in still or running water, with a creeping root stem and large oval-shaped leaves which are immersed, floating or protruding from the water. Its yellow flowers bloom in spring and its fruit is a grape-like capsule.[1118]

History:
According to Dioscorides the yellow pond lily which described in his entry *Nymphaia alle* is a species of nymphea and is used as an emmenagogue.[1119]

Yellow pond lily as a Medicinal Plant in Jerusalem:
From an 18th century document in the Jerusalem court archives it seems that nuphar water was used to cure pregnant women in Jerusalem.[1120] The document describes a lawsuit brought by an Arab from the village of Silwan (Siloam) against a Jewish physician, Salmon ben ha-Yehudi, which was presented at the Shari'a law court in 1711. From this document it appears that the physician (who was acquitted) had recommended the use of nuphar water and chicory water to cure a pregnant woman, but her husband had given her cassia water, which caused his wife to abort the fetus and to die.

Yellow pond lily in the Levant:
In a description of the Safed region during the 14th century, al-'Uthmani notes that in the Kadesh lake (Lake Hulah) 'nilofar' plants were growing.[1121] al-Ghazi described the 'nilofar' with all its varieties (red, white and blue) and also emphasised the yellow Damascus variety. The seeds of different varieties were used for medicinal purposes.[1122]

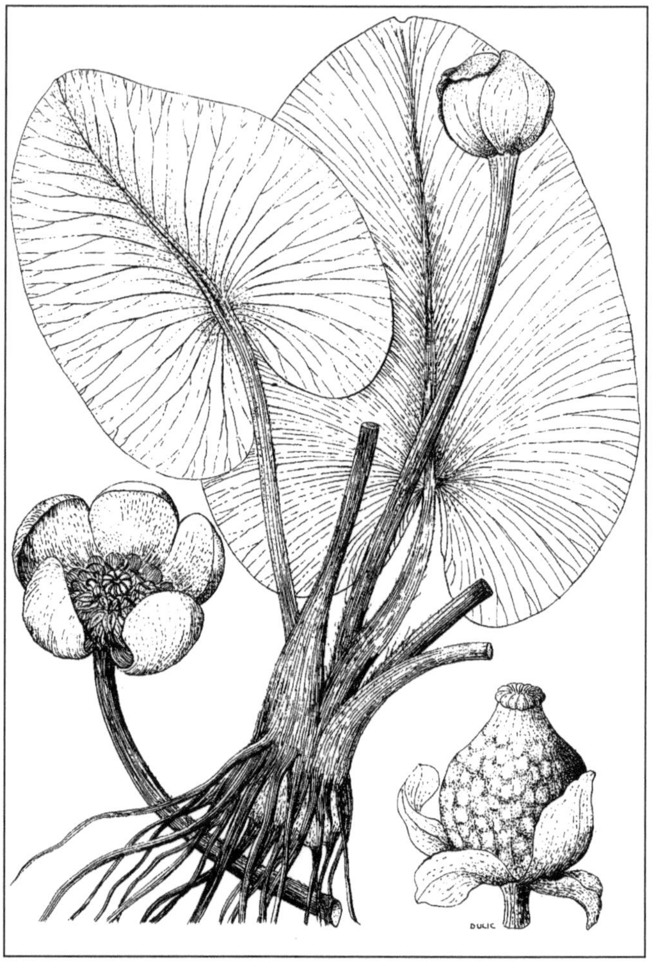

Figure 32 - Yellow Pond Lily (*Nuphar lutea*)

Identification:
During the Middle Ages and in modern times the terms 'nufar' and 'nilofar' as well as 'al-arus' 'bashinin' and 'lotus'[1123] were used to describe two species of waterlilies - nuphar and nymphea which were similar in form and habitat. A description of both species is presented in this book.

Traditional Medicine:
The yellow pond lily contains tannin and gallic acid, and was once used to cure skin diseases.[1124]

1115 Ibid.

1116 Plants & Animals, XI, p. 148.

1117 Hooper, p. 80; Dafni, Dudaim, p. 14.

1118 Description: Plants & Animals, X, pp. 86-87; Zohary, p. 314; Feinbrun-Dothan, p. 203.

1119 Dioscorides, III.148.

1120 Cohen, 18 century, p. 325, No. 279.

1121 'Uthmani, p. 480.

1122 Hamarneh, Plants, p. 256.

1123 Maimonides, Glossaire, p. 74, No. 252; Issa, Dictionary, p. 125, No. 15; Dinsmore & Dalman, Nos. 42-43; Plants & Animals, p. 86; Hooper, pp. 144-145; al-Ghafiqi, Nos. 129-130.

1124 Plants & Animals, X, p. 86.

Chapter V
Medicinal Substances of Other Origins

This chapter presents medicinal substances which do not fall into the categories set out in the earlier chapters. They are of mixed or unclear origin. The table below present six substances and remedies of mixed or unclear origin, these represent 2.6% of the total number of medicinal substances found in the historical sources.

Table 4 - List of medicinal substances of other origins

Name	Selective References
Balsam of Jerusalem	FH
Flower Water	RM, DS
Manna	MU, TA,
Mummy	AN, FH
Oxymel	DS
Theriac	MU, TA, MA

Sources
AN – Daud al-Antaki
DS – David De Silva
FH – Frederick Hasselquist
MA – Maimonides
MU – al-Muqaddasi
RM – Refael Malki
TA - al-Tamimi

Three substances of this category, had been chosen to be presented here in detail: Jerusalem Balsam, Mummy and Theriac.

Jerusalem Balsam

Description:
Jerusalem balsam is a fluid smearing substance which was invented, compounded and marketed in Eastern countries and even in Europe by Franciscan monks in a Jerusalem pharmacy.

Jerusalem Balsam in the Levant:
The production of Jerusalem balsam began at the end of the 17th century. The discovery of this medication is ascribed to the monk Antonio Manzani di Cuna who was a physician and pharmacist in the East. This unique medication became famous throughout the Eastern world and served to cure wounds, to treat stomach pains, pustules and boils. According to the sources, successful applications of Jerusalem balsam were carried out in Jerusalem, Ein Kerem, Acre and Beirut and even in Constantinople and Palermo.[1] At the beginning of the 18th century Franciscan chronicles reported on cases of its application in the treatment of heart illnesses and pus-infected wounds.[2] The exact composition of the medication was a guarded secret. Later sources relate that it was prepared from many kinds of medicinal substances (40 substances) including four types of root, myrrh, frankincense, roses and lemons.[3] Later on additional ingredients of European production were added to the medication.[4]

A description of Jerusalem balsam is preserved in the official archives in Venice. It lists the names of 40 components that were melted together in wine and water. After the liquid evaporated, a sticky substance remained which served as a plaster to disinfect and heal wounds.[5] Frederick Hasselquist informs us that "Jerusalem Balsam is famous in all these countries and it is prepared from various curative products and a few spices melted in wine. Its great importance lies in the curing of external wounds but it is not to be used for internal wounds because of its pungency. This medication is used when the patient vomits blood and also to treat whiplashes and wounds."[6]

An interesting description of the pharmacy and the Jerusalem balsam produced in it, is given by Elazar Horn, a monk who was active in the Holy City during the first half of the 18th century, a short while after the death of the monk Antonio.[7]

Summary and Conclusions:
The Franciscan Order which had originated among the European poor, did not engage in the healing arts in Europe. But in this

1 Bagatti, p. 355.
2 Cirelli, p. 219.
3 Bagatti, p. 355.
4 Ibid., p. 354.
5 Schittny, p. 44.
6 Hasselquist, p. 136.
7 Horn, pp. 176-181.

region, especially in Jerusalem, the monks of this order were the only representatives of the Catholic Church during the Mamluk and Ottoman periods, and therefore they were forced to include medical services as part of the general services they offered to Catholic pilgrims visiting the Holy Land.[8]

In time, the monks became expert in concocting medications especially in the production of Jerusalem balsam which became famous in the East and also in Europe for its unique effectiveness as a medicine. Apparently, specialisation in the production of compound medications was a tradition in Jerusalem among the different religious groups. It may be that the sanctity of Jerusalem was no less important in this instance than the quality of the substance and the medical knowledge which resulted in the composition of such medications.

Mummy

Scientific name: ***Rissasphalt***
Hebrew: Mumia **Arabic: Kafar al-Yahud, Mumiat al-Kaboria**[9]

Identification and Description:
Mummy has been a common medical substance for ages and there are several theories about its identification and source:

a. Mummy comes from the mummified bodies found in Egypt. In the mummification process, different herbs, oils, resins and medicinal minerals were used in order to preserve the body. This substance was found in the desert sands of Egypt and in sealed graves and was exported all over the East and even to some Western countries.

b. Mummy is a black mineral substance composed of carbon and hydrogen (similar to asphalt) which is formed from organic materials in a natural chemical process. This substance was collected in the mountain areas of Iran and Iraq.

c. The substance comprises the concentrated urine of mountain goats which subsequently underwent chemical processes over a long period of time.[10]

History:
Mummy is one of the most ancient drugs in Iran and Northern India.[11] In the Eastern Mediterranean, recent research proved that asphalt from the Dead Sea had been used in the mummification process commonly practiced in Egypt during the Hellenistic period (2nd cent. BCE).[12]

Medicinal Uses in Jerusalem:
Frederick Hasselquist asserted that he had seen mummy (a mineral he claimed was from Iran)[13] among the many medical substances in the Franciscan pharmacy in Jerusalem. In addition, he described mummy which had been brought from Iran to Egypt, and was impressed by its high cost and its application as an important component in several remedies for the treatment of wounds and broken bones.[14]

Mummy in the Levant:
Daud al-Antaki explained the meaning of the Greek word *Mumie* which he claimed meant: "That which preserved bodies." Antaki adds that it originated from Iran although "it was seen on the shores of Morocco and inside trees in Andalusia, Yemen and Syria (al-Sham)."[15]

Medicinal Uses in the Medieval Period:
Muslim physicians such as Ibn Sina, Al-Razi and al-Biruni claimed that mummy was a black substance similar to asphalt which slid down to the sea from high mountains. According to their writings, mummy was a component in various remedies for the treatment of headache, ear and throat pains, coughs, paralysis and heart and stomach disorders. Mummy was used externally to mend broken bones, cure wounds of the sex organs and for internal uses such as renal disorders.[16]

Ibn al-Baytar reported that 'Mumiat al-Kaboria' originated in Egypt and asserted that: "this name was also given to the black stone" found in San'a (Yemen) which was easily broken and contained black fluid used for the treatment of broken bones.[17]

al-Qazwini wrote about the similarity he found between mummy and asphalt, and claimed that mummy, which was brought from Iran and Iraq, had the best medicinal qualities. The medicinal uses he mentions are similar to those by other physicians.[18]

Mummy was also used for medicinal purposes in medieval Europe.[19]

Traditional Medicine:
Babylonian Jews use mummy to treat wounds, bruises, dislocations and back pains. It has also been used to treat panic and internal wounds.[20] Both mineral mummy and other kinds of mummy can be found in the markets of countries such as Israel, Jordan, Syria, and Egypt. Some of its applications are similar to medieval ones, including bone-mending. Other uses such as the reduction of sugar and cholesteral levels in the body are modern.

Conclusions:
Ancient and medieval physicians made use of at least two different kinds of mummy for medicinal purposes. Many medicinal substances such as beeswax, aromatic components

---

8 Schur.

9 Maimonides, Glossaire, No. 234.

10 Hooper, pp. 198-199; Ben-Yakov, pp. 534-535.

11 Hooper, pp. 198-199.

12 Nissenbaum, Mummies, pp. 5-6.

13 Hasselquist, pp. 199-200; Horn, p. 6.

14 Ibid., pp. 303-304.

15 al-Antaki, pp. 325-326.

16 Ibn Sina, pp. 367-368; al-Biruni, I, pp. 310-311.

17 Ibn al-Baytar, al-Jami, IV, pp. 169-170.

18 al-Qazwini, p. 214.

19 Gordon, Medieval, p. 665.

20 Ben-Yakov, pp. 94, 234, 236, 266, 268, 349, 355, 414, 533.

of plants and asphalt from the Dead Sea were involved in the mummification process in Egypt.[21] These substances contained disinfectants, purifying and sealing qualities that were crucial for the preservation of bodies. It seems that these qualities explain the use of mummy by ancient physicians to treat wounds, to mend broken bones and as a painkiller. The use of mummy of mineral origin mentioned in historical sources was probably due to its medicinal qualities similar to that of bitumen.

Theriac

The word theriac is similar in Latin, Hebrew and Arabic. In English theriac was once known as 'treacle' but this word is now used in a different sense - as a kind of molasses.

Description:
Theriac is a preparation (serum) which used to made of the venom of snakes and scorpions and other poisons derived from medicinal plants and animal parts. During the Middle Ages special and complex kinds of theriac were known.[22]

History:
Man has always been exposed to attack by fatal poisons from animals, plants and minerals.[23] In view of this, the need arose to discover antitoxic medications which were known in the ancient world by the name of theriac - which comes from the Greek word *theriakon* meaning a wild or venomous monster.

There were two well known types of theriac: one was ascribed to Andromachus, the physician of the Emperor Nero, and the other to Mithridates VI, King of Pontus in Asia Minor. These two types differed from each other in their composition of medicinal herbs and especially in the amount of opium they contained. Later on, theriac served as a medication for various illnesses.[24]

From the writings of Jewish Sages it appears that they too made medical use of theriac.[25] During the Middle Ages a great deal of medical literature was written on this subject and one of the famous ones was the book by Maimonides: *Poisons and their Antidotes*. This book was written by order of the Muslim ruler because of the numerous cases of people harmfully affected by poisonous drugs in Egypt and the lack of adequate medical services.[26]

In medieval times and the Renaissance period theriac was traded internationally in Europe until the 18th century. In France, the use of theriac reached its peak in the 17th century, while in other countries its use was limited because of its addictive influence. The preparation of theriac involved 40-60 kinds of medicinal substances including minerals such as: bitumen, clay and sulphur; animal parts such as: the flesh of the lizard and snake, and beaver testicles; resinous gums such as: ferula gum, myrrh resin, gum arabic (acacia gum) opium and aloe; condiments such as: cardamon, aniseed, fennel, lemon, and saffron; medicinal herbs such as aristoloche, deer balls, valerian and iris.[27]

Theriac in Syria and the Land of Israel:
al-Muqaddasi described the theriac produced in the Land of Israel.[28] al-Tamimi reported on the 'excellent Jewish asphalt which was produced from the Dead Sea and served as a component "in the great theriac compound called al-faruk."[29]

Maimonides noted that the important ingredient in theriac was 'arak al-haya' which the root of the plant which grows around the Temple Mount ..."[30]

Many Christian and Islamic sources of the medieval period have indicated that the region of Jericho was the source for the snakes and scorpions used in making theriac. Especially well known was hunting in that region for the striped adder (*Echis coloratus*).[31] During the Mamluk period, theriac was considered a highly valued medication produced under the monopoly of the ruling authorities. Many pilgrims visiting the Dead Sea region described the adder in detail, the method of its capture, and the milking of its venom. For example, in the 15th century, the traveller Felix Fabri described the Dead Sea area and especially the adder and its uses: "From this snake they made theriac, this great and most precious medicine..."[32]

Medicinal Uses in the Medieval Period:
al-Kindi called theriac 'darik' and described its use in the treatment of stuttering.[33]

al-Biruni, as did other Arab physicians and pharmacists, described seven varieties of theriac and their uses.[34] According to Maimonides, the 'great theriac' served as the recommended medication for treating illnesses such as ulcers, gout, and malaria. He says that the medication was prepared by using snakes, especially the adder, after removing the head and tail.[35]

Elsewhere Maimonides noted that wine served as an important component in theriac to counteract snakebite and scorpion stings which causes a feeling of coldness. However,

21 Nissenbaum, Mummies.

22 Detailed history and medical description in: Watson, Theriac.

23 Matossian.

24 Schreiber, pp. 23-26; Berman, pp. 5-7; Thompson, Art, pp. 58-66.

25 In detail: Preuss, pp. 436-437.

26 Maimonides, Poisons. On theriac, its cost and difficulties in its preparation, see: Ibid., p. 93.

27 Schreiber, pp. 23-26; Berman, pp. 5-7; Earles & Pharm.

28 al-Muqaddasi, p. 181; Le Strange, p. 17.

29 al-Tamimi, p. 25.

30 Maimonides, Poisons, p. 107. This plant was identified in this study with white melilot (sweet clover). See the entry for 'Sweet Clover' in Chapter IV above.

31 For example: Jacques de Vitry, PPTS, Vol. 10, p. 676; Arnoul, PPTS, Vol. 12, p. 136; Frescobaldi, p. 42.

32 PPTS, Vol. 2, pp. 151-153; Suriano, p. 255.

33 al-Kindi, No. 94.

34 al-Biruni, I, pp. 88-89; II, p. 81.

35 Maimonides, Aphorisms, 9:86, 103; 10:56; 21, 52-53, 55.

when concocting this medication for a Muslim, the wine could be substituted by anise which is "effective for all the poisons of living creatures." In concocting theriac against snakebite which causes a feeling of extreme heat, milk and vinegar are used. Additional substances recommended by Maimonides as components for this medication were: the seed of the citron, gallstone, stomach of the hare, spikenard, myrrh, balsam, garlic, ginger, aristoloche, honey and cinnamon.[36]

Traditional Medicine:
Among the Jews of Iraq it was the practice to use various kinds of theriac. It was compounded of 42 medicinal plants and animal parts, and served as a remedy for removing fatty nodes dispelling gases, curing skin diseases, colds, hemorrhoids, epilepsy and typhus. Overdosage causes a weakening of the eyesight and poisoning.[37]

Summary and Conclusions:
Medications against poisons were used by mankind since early times. Because of the wealth of unique medicinal substances in the region, the sanctity of Jerusalem for the different religions, and the expertise of the physicians and pharmacists, the theriac preparations in the Land of Israel and in Jerusalem in particular became famous throughout the East until the end of the Middle Ages, and it was also exported to other countries.[38] The use of theriac with all its different names was widespread in both East and West until the development of modern medicine. Since then, the use of theriac has been confined solely to traditional medicine.

[36] Maimonides, Poisons, pp. 107-120. Cf. al-Antaki, pp. 95-96.

[37] Ben-Yakov, pp. 98, 103, 108, 143, 161, 182, 204, 210, 228, 316.

[38] In detail: Amar, Theriac.

Chapter VI
Summary and Conclusions
(10th to 18th Centuries)

After a review of the written sources from the 10th to the 18th centuries and the lists presented in chapters 2-5, a complete list of the medicinal substances used in Jerusalem at this period was compiled (see Appendix 3). These substances had been scientifically identified and then historically researched for their medicinal uses until the present day. Special emphasis was placed upon the description of their uses throughout the generations in Jerusalem and in the region of the Land of Israel and Syria.

This study is primary and unique in the range of substances that have been examined and the variety of sources that were reviewed and which are of multilingual origins. In earlier historical records, especially those written in medieval times, there existed a science which was clearly understood to the writer dealing in this field, but which is unclear to the contemporary reader. This study helps in understanding the historical and medical information regarding the identity of substances and medications.

The importance of the list of substances lies in the fact that it is the first time that all the medicinal substances used in Jerusalem until the beginning of the 19th century have been included in a single listing, constituting a basis for understanding the use of natural medicinal substance in the Land of Israel in general and in Jerusalem in particular. Unfortunately, there are hardly any sources that deal with medicinal substances in Jerusalem prior to the early Islamic period. On the other hand, a large quantity of source material has been amassed from the examination of medieval texts that provide the scientific basis for this study.

The list, which contains 218 substances, is part of a more comprehensive listing of medicinal substances now being studied in detail by the author of this book, which covers the whole region of Greater Syria and includes 286 substances.[1] It should be noted that both lists contain only those medicinal substances mentioned in direct connection with the region under research. For example, where there is no mention of other medicinal substances specifically related to Jerusalem, even though they were clearly known to have been in use during the period under research, such substances were not included in the listing.

Table 5 - Division of Medicinal Substances According to their Origins

Origin of Substances	Number	Percentage
Plants	175	80.2
Minerals	14	6.7
Animals	23	10.5
Others	6	2.6
Total	218	100%

According to Table 5 it appears that the composition of the list resembles the lists of other medicinal substances in the Land of Israel and in the world.[2] From this study and other research works on the subject it seems that local plants were the main components in the inventory of medicinal substances. The reasons for this are as follows:

- The availability of wild plants, the ability to ensure their quality and the possibility of supplying them at the appropriate time.
- The low cost of the plants gathered by the physicians and their assistants or by 'plant gatherers.'
- The relatively high cost of minerals, animals products and imported substances bought from traders or manufacturers.
- Practical experience and knowledge handed down through the generations.

Most of the medicinal substances which were in use in Jerusalem was available because they were wild plants that were cultivated and utilised for the local agriculture or were part of the natural fauna or the mineral deposits in the Land

1 Lev, Materials, pp. 338-344.

2 Ibid., p. 325.

of Israel and the region. Asphalt is one example for a mineral produced in the region and used for curative purposes in Jerusalem.

Table 6 - Division of Medicinal Substances According to their Derivation

Origin	Number of Substances	Percentage
Local – wild	82	37.8
Local – agricultural	73	33.6
Imported	62	28.6
Total	217	100%

The medicinal substances derived from agriculture can be divided according to the following criteria:

- Agricultural crops grown in the Land of Israel such as Marjoram, Grape Vine, Seville Orange, Chicory, Sugar Cane, Plum and Garden Cress.
- Animals as part of the agricultural economy: Bees (Honey).

Imported substances that appear in the list throw light upon the trade in the Land of Israel and in Jerusalem in particular during the period under research, and it is sometimes possible to even learn about the origin of the product imported or its final destination. From an analysis of the list we can conclude the following:

- Most of the imported products were spices such as: Cloves, Ginger, Pepper, and Cinnamon.
- Other products were prominent medicinal substances such as: Yarrow, Aloe, Myrolaban, Quinine and Turpeth.
- The most expensive products were the substances for perfumes and incense such as Balsam oil and Myrrh.
- Other imported products were: Zinc, Alum, Kohl and Mummy.

Conclusions

As a result of the research on the medical materials and an analysis of the sources it may be concluded that the inhabitants of Jerusalem did not suffer from any lack of medicinal substances because the overwhelming majority of these were of local origin. The imported medicinal substances were more expensive and were not always available, but the curative methods of the Byzantine and Muslim periods that were practiced in the Land of Israel and in the region included a list of substitutes for every one of these substances so that it was possible to concoct medications even when the patient could ill afford to purchase these expensive materials, or when it was not available in the markets of Jerusalem and the surrounding region. It seems that state or political events had no special effect on the trade or use of natural medicinal substances. The trade flourished during peace time and did not cease altogether even during times of war.

To sum up, the list of medicinal substances reflects the medical and pharmacological knowledge found in the sources in connection with Jerusalem, which was a holy city of cosmopolitan character. Apparently this international atmosphere also had an influence on the inventory of medicinal substances in the city during the Middle Ages, and contributed to its variety. One of the characteristics of Jerusalem in the past as well as in the present was its status as a place of pilgrimage for all members of the monotheistic faiths in the East and West, and for the immigrants of different races. The international ambience is felt through the babel of languages spoken there, the various dialects in which people wrote, in the different kinds of coinage they used and the variety of merchandise sold in the markets. This wealth is reflected in the relative abundance of materials that arrived from the East and the scarcity of materials from the West which supplemented the local medicinal substances.

The high esteem given the city was due to the fact that certain medieval sources claimed that Jerusalem was the source for certain medicinal substances or for a specific medication. This apparently was due to its holiness and its name gave added distinction to the substance in question. Perhaps this is the reason that Islamic sources use the term 'Bayt al-Maqdis' (Jerusalem) and sometimes even note that the plant grew in the 'Haram' (Temple Mount). Quite probably, Benevenutus Grassus called some of the medications mentioned in his book 'Jerusalem Medicines' because he used them or concocted them during his stay in the city, or in order to give them additional curative powers in the name of the Holy City.[3]

This phenomenon of strengthening the power of a medication by mentioning its place of origin is well known in medieval scholarly medicine as well as in the traditional medicine of various cultures.

It should be remembered that this information is derived from all the available sources that can be obtained at present, but which may be enriched when new sources are found in the future. Hopefully, this list of substances will be expanded and updated in the course of time through archaeological excavations in Jerusalem and the discovery of manuscripts and new historical sources on the subject of medicine.

[3] Lev, Jerusalem.

PART B

Chapter VII
European Island in Jerusalem - The Franciscan Pharmacy

The medical institution of the Franciscan order in Jerusalem developed during the Mamluk period (1260-1517). Though there is some historical evidence of the medical activity of Franciscan monks in Jerusalem under Mamluk rule, there is no concrete information about a special hospital in Jerusalem for the Christian community. The Franciscans did operate a hostel on Mount Zion at the end of the Mamluk period, but this institution was mainly used to serve pilgrims and for purposes of grace and charity.[1]

The historian Arce, a Franciscan monk, claimed that the Franciscans begun to practice medicine and pharmacy in Jerusalem as early as 1342, with the settlement of twelve monks in the sacred city.[2] Another historian, Wadding, indicated that medical activity began in the middle of the 14th century.[3] The Franciscan chronicler, Calahorra, mentions the year 1477 as the beginning of medical activity.[4]

It seems that most of the Christian population of Jerusalem used either the services of the municipal hospital of Jerusalem or private medical aid or social-medical treatment given at the monasteries and other Christian institutions in the city and its vicinity. The lack of proper Christian medical institutions in Jerusalem, and the formal Christian ideology which had acquired formal authorisation from Pope Gregory XIII in his letter dated 1581 stating that Christians should avoid getting Jewish[5] or Moslem medical care, were some of the main factors for the development of the Franciscan hospital and pharmacy in Jerusalem.[6]

The Franciscans, who did not deal with medical care in Europe, were "forced", while staying in Jerusalem, to supply medical care to Catholic pilgrims in the Holy Land. At first, monks who were qualified as physicians, pharmacist, surgeons and nurses were sent to Jerusalem. Most of them came from Italy, and only a few arrived from other European countries such as France, Spain and even Czechoslovakia.[7]

The patients were treated and hospitalised at the boarding house for the poor, located in the Christian quarter of the Old City, separate from the monastery. This location was called "Dar Isthak Bek" in Arabic and "Casa dei Principi" in Italian. According to Dr. Titus Tobler, it contained about twenty rooms by the mid-19th century, and accommodated an indefinite number, never exceeding one hundred, of poor and sick Catholic pilgrims. Only a few patients were housed in the monastery.[8]

An impressive medical library and a big and modern European style pharmacy were at the disposal of the medical staff. The Franciscan researcher, Bagatti, claims that the pharmacy was first mentioned in 1620.[9] Other scholars, such as Arce, claimed it was mentioned even earlier.[10] The pharmacy continued to develop during the 17th century and it is worth mentioning one of its famous workers, the monk Antonio Menzani di Cuna, who served as physician and pharmacist in Jerusalem for 43 years (1686-1729). This monk is said to have been the inventor of "Jerusalem Balsam".[11]

A large number of medical practitioners served in the Franciscan medical institutions in Jerusalem until the 19th century, most of them having been sent from Italy where they returned at the end of their period of service. They had access to a richly stocked medical library and a dispensary.[12] The dispensary, which served the members of all communities and religious faiths in Jerusalem, developed rapidly into one

1 Schein, p. 144.

2 Arce, p. 123.

3 Wadding, pp. 309-310.

4 Calahorra, pp. 297-298.

5 Arce, pp. 12, 23.

6 Amar & Lev, Jerusalem, p. 78.

7 See for example: Arce, pp. 117-120, 324-325; Schur, pp. 99-101.

8 Tobler, Denkblatter, pp. 403-404.

9 Bagatti, pp. 138, 353.

10 Arce, pp. 122-123, 136-138.

11 See Chapter V.

12 Schittny; Schur, Franciscan, pp. 99-105.

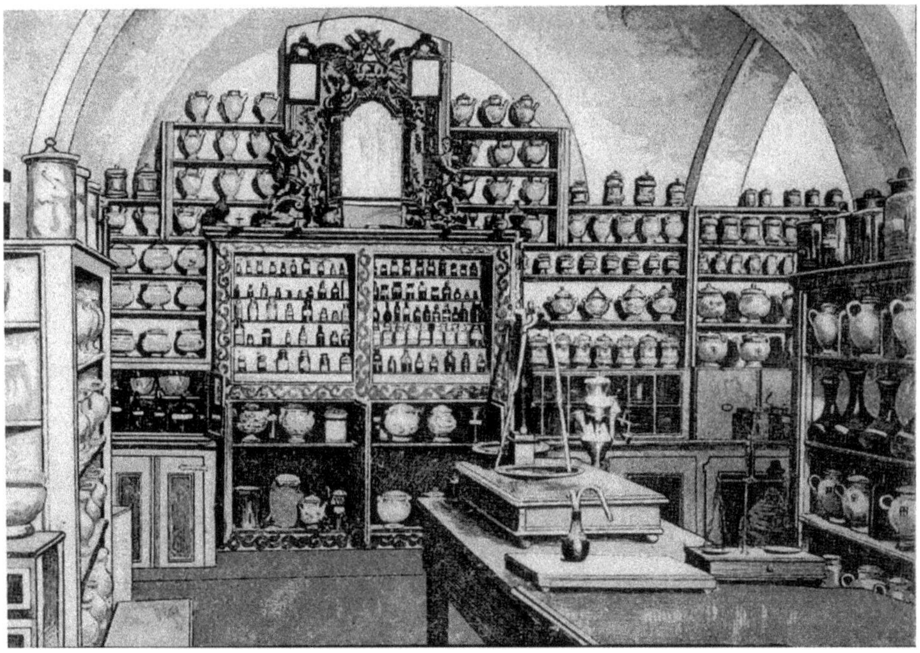

Figure 33 - The Franciscan Pharmacy – reprint of the 19th century

of the largest of its kind in the East. It contained a large variety of medications and was run by a staff trained in modern European institutions.[13] The dispensary became famous for its innovative medicines, especially for the "Jerusalem Balsam" concocted by secret formula and containing forty different medicinal ingredients.

Jerusalem Balsam, which was the subject for many articles,[14] is under intensive research until the present day at the School of Pharmacy, the Hebrew University, Jerusalem. Recent investigation includes: collection of different recipes, choosing the most original one, laboratory manufacture of this formula and clinical tests for its medical effects.[15]

The stocks of the Franciscan pharmacy were a mystery, and very little information could be gathered from the testimonies of its visitors throughout the years, from the Franciscan writings and from the Franciscan historians. The most interesting descriptions are presented below.

A reliable description of the contents of the dispensary at the beginning of the 18th century is given by the monk, Elazar Horn, who lived in Jerusalem during the years 1724-1744: "The dispensary in Jerusalem is one of the best in the Christian world. The storehouses contain medications of all kinds which were purchased with donated funds, and especially with funds contributed for this specific purpose by the Venetian Republic".[16]

The Swedish botanist, Frederick Hasselquist, who visited the institution in 1750, reported that: "It was amazing to see the quantities of expensive medications stored there. [...] Here they prepare the Jerusalem Balsam so famed in these countries [...] it is very effective for all fresh external wounds. [...] The whole pharmacopoeia (dispensary stock) is valued at several hundred thousand piasters."[17]

In 1806 the German traveler, Jasper Ulrich Seetzen, was impressed by the monks' garden where these medicinal substances were produced, and noted that he received "two bottles of real Balsam with written indications of its qualities."[18]

After visiting the pharmacy in 1835, Dr. Titus Tobler wrote in his notebook:

> 'the place looks ancient... the laboratory is strange, unmatched by any European competitor for being so strange...the instruments have old-fashioned shapes, like the traditional tools of mystic alchemy and astrology.... Together with those instruments were some skeletons, surgical instruments, threatening monsters covered with mould...different type of amulets... and all in ancient dark rooms. Yet the storeroom of the medicinal substances was exceptionally fine'.[19]

Two of the most interesting and unique materials of the Franciscan pharmacy, Jerusalem Balsam and Quinine, were described at previous chapter.

New documents, which were found and loaned for research by the Franciscan monks in Jerusalem, shed new light on the Franciscan pharmacy and its library. The documents including lists of the books in the monastery medical library in the 18th and 19th century and lists of the contents (stock) of the pharmacy. Among the lists (inventories) found, two are

[13] Bagatti; Cirelli, p. 219.

[14] See: Bagatti, p. 355; Schittny, pp. 43-44; Cirelli, p. 219; Schur, pp. 100-101.

[15] Moussaieff.

[16] Horn, pp. 176-181.

[17] Hasselquist, p. 135.

[18] Seetzen, II, pp. 205-206.

[19] Tobler, Beitrage, pp. 14-15.

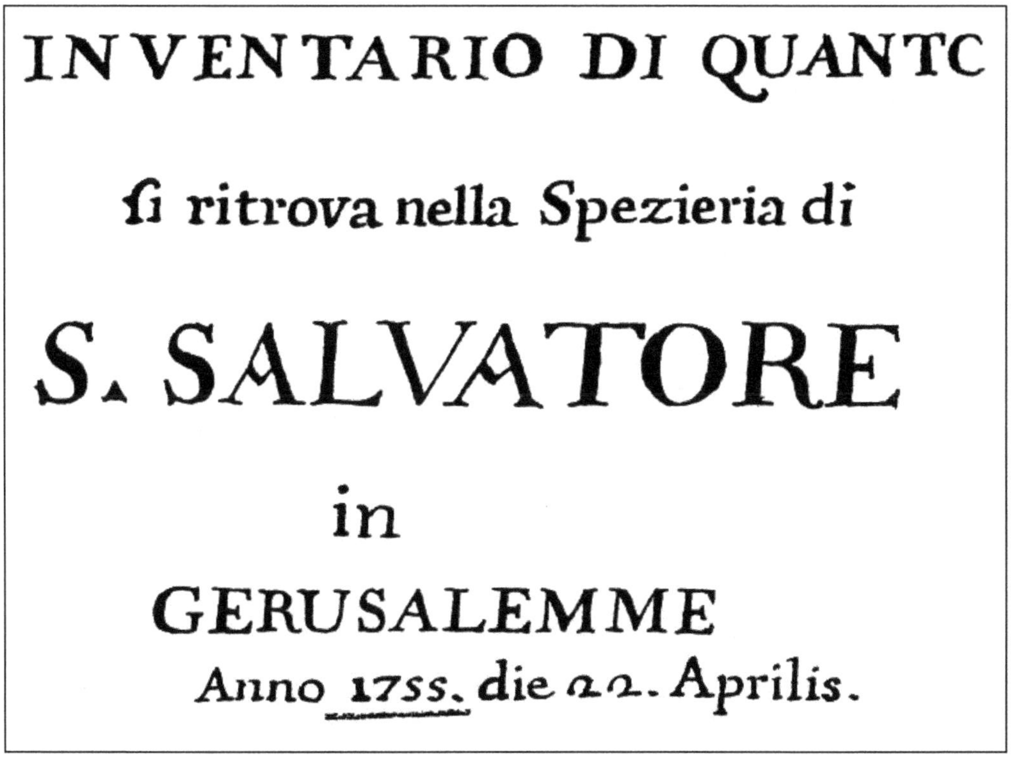

INVENTARIO DI QUANTC

ſi ritrova nella Spezieria di

S. SALVATORE

in

GERUSALEMME

Anno 1755. die 22. Aprilis.

Figure 34 - Front Page of the Franciscan List of 1755

complete and can be researched - the list of 1755 and the list of 1798.

Transcription and identification of the materials mentioned in the list are being done intensively, but this will take a long time due to its complexity. The work is done by an interdisciplinary team, headed by the author and including Arie Mosayof, of the School of Pharmacology at the Hebrew University, Jerusalem and Dr. Zohar Amar of the Department of Land of Israel Studies at Bar Ilan University.

A first decipherment of the 1755 list shows that the pharmacy had 679 medical materials in stock. It seems that the list is special since it contains materials which were used in 18th century Europe, some of which were brought from Asia, Africa and from the new world - America.

The lucky patients, who were admitted to the Franciscan medical facilities during the 17th and the 18th century, were well treated by European trained physicians, and were provided with the newest medications, all at European standards.

We hope soon to publish a complete monographic work about the Franciscan medical activity in Jerusalem. This work will include the lists of the drugs, their identification and an analysis of the Franciscan phenomena in Jerusalem from sociological, economical and pharmacological points of views.

Chapter VIII
Medical Substances Used in Jerusalem in the 19th Century

Introduction: Medical Conditions of 19th Century Jerusalem

Palestine, which once experienced a glorious era of medical progress, had by the end of the 18th century descended to an unprecedented nadir in this field. The main reason for this lowering of medical standards in the region was the prolonged and continuous decline of the Ottoman Empire, which forced the inhabitants of Palestine to rely mainly upon folk medicine. This deficiency in adequate medical services, which lasted until the mid-19th century, was also the result of the seriously deficient sanitary conditions, poverty, and ignorance, as well as a lack of public health facilities. In the prolonged absence of sufficient medical care over several generations, the outbreak of diseases and plagues was seen as inevitable, fated by heavenly decree.

The poor sanitary conditions in Jerusalem at the beginning of the 19th century require a separate discussion. This situation resulted mainly from overcrowded and unventilated quarters, excessive garbage deposits, sewage flowing through the streets, disregard for personal hygiene, and water drawn from untreated wells. These harsh conditions caused infectious diseases, and plagues broke out, claiming many victims. Among the diseases that afflicted the inhabitants most frequently were malaria, eye infection, headaches, and dysentery, as well as other infectious maladies and contagious child illnesses. Among the plagues we note cholera, bubonic plague, typhoid fever, smallpox, and meningitis.[1]

In the course of time, a variety of popular folk remedies were developed, based on old medical treatises and on medicinal substances in use since ancient times. Alongside these were remedies, cures, charms, amulets, incantations and superstitious beliefs. These curative methods were often applied with the assistance of minor religious functionaries of all three faiths reciting passages from their scriptures and sending their flock of worshippers to prostrate themselves on the graves of saints buried in the Holy Land.

[1] A detailed description of this situation is given by the Dr. Tobler. See Tobler, Beitrage, pp. 24-63. Also see, Chaplin and Masterman.

Amulets and curative remedies were commonly used as the solution for incurable diseases, mainly mental illnesses.[2] The terrible symptoms that accompanied such illnesses led those in contact with the patient to believe that magical powers and demons caused them, and that magical cures would therefore relieve the distress. Folk medicine of this type, which is common among most cultures of the world, began to lose its standing in Europe with the development of modern medicine. Yet its use was deeply rooted among the inhabitants of the Middle East in the period under study. Such curative methods are in fact still characteristic of a few countries in the region. Some of their elements are in use still today in the popular folk remedies of various Jewish communities and minority groups in Israel, as of those in more or less developed cultures around the world.

The level of medicine can be measured by a number of standards. The main ones are a system of public health, medical training, and medicinal substances. Medical science in Palestine generally and in Jerusalem particularly exemplified the continuation of classical Hippocratic-Galenic medical methods, but adopted and improved by the Muslims during the Middle Ages. In the regions under their rule, important centeres arose where physicians of repute engaged in the art of healing, research, writing, and teaching. During the 18th century and the first half of the 19th century, Palestine and the outlying areas lacked such centers for prominent physicians to practice medicine, so that region produced no trained medical practitioners. For most of the Ottoman period, Palestine was considered an area of marginal importance, far away from the centers of culture and government, and eminent physicians stayed away from it.

The situation portrayed above gives a general view of medical realities during that period. However, the practice of medicine in Jerusalem merits more detailed examination since it was made up of three main strata: public medicine, communal medicine, and private medicine. A fourth stratum, voluntary medicine, gained ground only in the course of the 19th century, and this will be dealt with later on.

[2] See Nahmias.

In Jerusalem, as in other large cities of the Ottoman Empire, there were minimal medical services, which were meant to supply the needs of the general population without distinction of religion or nationality. But by the nature of things only the Arab population benefited from these services. The general public hospital in Jerusalem, which functioned throughout the Ottoman period, was the continuation of the medical institution dating from the period of the Ayyubid caliphate of the 12th and 13th centuries, and it belonged to the charitable endowment trust named for the donor. Physicians who served in this hospital, which was also supported by the central government, had received official appointments by the government, which paid their salaries and premiums. These physicians were not allowed to leave the city without providing a good reason, obtaining a permit, and finding a replacement. The physical condition of the institution deteriorated in time, and despite all attempts to repair it, the building remained partially in ruins. The institution had different sections: the general hospital, the hospital for the mentally ill, and the eye clinic. The standard of this institution, as in other similar institutions, fell to the same low level to which the Ottoman Empire itself was gradually descending.[3]

Only in 1886 did the Jerusalem municipality set up a clinic, which functioned three times a week, and in 1891 the municipal hospital was built in Sheikh Bader (today 86 Jaffa Street, in the heart of Jerusalem).[4] The residents of Jerusalem were therefore obliged to make do with the medicinal substances in use throughout the region for centuries. As time passed, the variety of medications decreased because of disruptions in the trade routes. The harsh economic conditions suspended the demand for exotic and expensive substances, and there was a lowering of standards among physicians and caregivers.[5] Among the scores of substances mentioned in the various historical sources concerning the medical situation in Jerusalem until the beginning of the 19th century, only quinine is listed as a medicinal compound introduced from the new world of modern medicine. This medication was prescribed in the dispensaries of the Franciscan community in Jerusalem during the first half of the 18th century.[6]

In that same century, new substances from Africa, Asia, and America became important components in the reservoir of medications, as testified in the volumes of *Materia Medica*.[7] Most of the materials traded in Palestine and Jerusalem for use by authorized physicians are definable as traditional medicinal substances. As indicated by their plant, mineral, and animal origins, these were derived mostly from local sources during the period under discussion.[8]

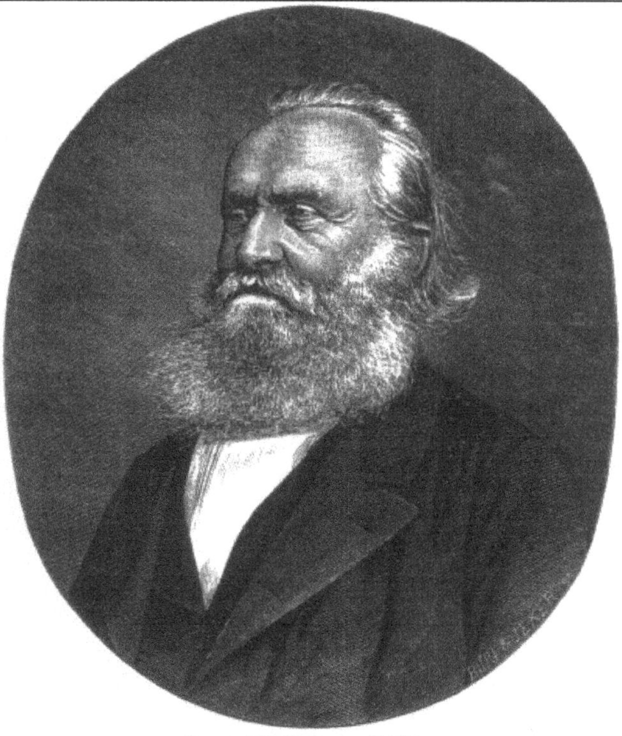

Figure 35 - Dr. Titus Tobler

Key testimony to the medical conditions of Jerusalem during the 19th century is found in the writings of Dr. Titus Tobler. He was born in 1806 in the village of Wolfhalden in the Swiss canton of Appenzell. He studied and practiced medicine in Zurich, Vienna, and Würzburg (Germany), and in 1827 was awarded his doctorate. Tobler made his living by practicing medicine, but he was also a linguist and a writer. He died in 1877 in Munich and was buried in his native village.[9] Titus Tobler's legacy is particularly his contributions to knowledge of Jerusalem in the 19th century. He may well be considered 'the father of the German scholarship on the land of Israel'. He made four visits to Jerusalem (1835, 1845-6, 1857, 1865), each of which yielded articles and books reporting his researches and his intellectual experiences.[10]

Tobler's first visit to the Holy Land in 1835 was prompted by his natural curiosity. On that occasion he concentrated on the Holy City of Jerusalem; the chief purpose of his second journey, in 1845-6, was to study the Holy Land generally. Tobler lodged at the home of Dr. Shimon Frenkel (1809-1880). This was first Jewish physician of modern Jerusalem,[11] sent by Sir Moses Montefiore primarily to establish a Jewish hospital there[12] as a proper substitute for the British mission hospital established some years before by the London Society for Promoting Christianity Amongst the Jews.[13] The two physicians became friends and Tobler found the information given by Frenkel reliable and useful. In 1853 Tobler published

3 Amar & Lev, Jerusalem, pp.74-93.

4 Levy, Medicine, pp. 133-135. For further details on the Municipal Hospital see Greenberg.

5 On the medicinal substances, which were used by the inhabitants of Jerusalem until the beginning of the 19th century, see Lev, Jerusalem.

6 Regarding quinine, see Horn, p. 189; Amar & Lev, Jerusalem, p. 189.

7 See for example Lewis.

8 In this connection, see Amar & Lev, Tobler.

9 Heim; for more information see Goren, pp. 191-208.

10 Stern, Tobler; Stern & Goren.

11 Levy, Frenkel.

12 Kass, Montefiore.

13 Perry & Lev.

his book *Denkblatter aus Jerusalem (*Recollections of Jerusalem*)*, which was based on his last visits to the city.[14] One chapter of the book gives a detailed description of the medical institutions in Jerusalem at the time, together with an account of the establishment of the modern medical institutes. Two years after his second and longest visit he wrote *Beitrage zur Medizinischen Topographie von Jerusalem (*A description of medical conditions in Jerusalem*)*.[15] This volume draws a unique picture of that aspect of life, one almost totally neglected by the majority of descriptions of the Holy Land written during the 19th century, which numbered in the hundreds. This volume has recently been partially translated into Hebrew.[16]

The book deals with the prevailing medical conditions in Jerusalem, the major diseases, and the licensed physicians. It contains important information about the common traditional medical methods, local traditional 'pharmacies' and medicinal substances, medical facilities, medicaments, fertility and mortality rates of the population, and other aspects of the medical conditions prevailing in Jerusalem at the time of Tobler's visit. The author also provides details about medical conditions of earlier periods, according to written documentary material, and about the opinions of the few Jewish and Christian doctors who worked in Jerusalem until the second half of the 19th century. This chapter includes Titus Tobler's contribution to our knowledge of the medical conditions of Jerusalem shortly before the penetration of the modern medicine.

Communal Medicine and Hospitals

Communal medicine, which gained adherents in Jerusalem, was an essential need of the various ethnic groups in order to provide an alternative for the defective public health system. For religious reasons, the Jews and Christians, with the permission of the Ottoman government, preferred to use the medical services of their own community. However, in all probability Muslim almshouses also existed, which offered limited medical care.[17]

The centre of communal medicine for the Jews of Jerusalem from the 16th to the 18th century was its own hospital located in the Jewish Quarter, where patients stayed until their recovery. This hospital, apparently belong to the Oriental Jewish (Sephardi) community, while the European Jewish (Ashkenazi) community, which was recognized as a separate minority group, sometimes operated their own hospital.[18] A trustworthy description of the Jewish hospital, which was called Bikur Holim, can be found in the writings of the physician, Rabbi Refael Mordecai Malki who received his medical education in Italy, went to Palestine in 1667, and served as the community physician until his death in 1702. From his description, the hospital seems to have been headed by the community treasurer, who in the absence of a doctor was the supreme medical authority. The institution was supported mainly through contributions from the Jewish community in Amsterdam, and with these funds the treasurer bought food and medicine for the patients. One of his main duties was to prepare a drink containing sugar, almonds, and rosewater, mixed with various condiments as could be afforded, and to distribute it to patients in their homes.[19]

Dr. Tobler added information and wrote about the **Jewish hospital**, which was built by Sir Moses Montefiore in 1843; as noted, Dr. Frenkel was its director.[20] By the time Tobler's book was published (1855) this hospital no longer existed and Dr. Frenkel was practicing medicine privately in Jerusalem. In 1854 the Rothschild family established a new hospital in the Jewish quarter. This was an important institution, although it was the subject of an internal dispute within in the city's Jewish community.[21] Tobler did not mention the effort regarded by some scholars as the first to establish a Jewish hospital in Jerusalem, made by Rabbi Israel Baeck in 1844.[22]

The center of Christian community medicine was the Franciscan Order in Jerusalem, the most prominent Christian institution in the Holy Land during the Mameluke period and the first half of the period under Ottoman rule. The Catholic monks, who took possession of holy sites and supplied services for the pilgrims, also provided medical care. By the 14th century, a Franciscan hospital had already begun to function alongside the monastery on Mount Zion. Later on, Christian patients were treated at the Franciscan hostel set up in the Christian Quarter. It contained 16 to 28 beds and in effect became a hospital.[23]

A large number of medical practitioners, nurses, pharmacists, physicians, and even surgeons served in the Franciscan medical institutions in Jerusalem until the 19th century. Most of them had been sent from Italy, whither they returned at the end of their period of service. They had access to a richly stocked medical library and dispensary, which were probably founded at the beginning of the 17th century.[24] The dispensary, which served the members of all communities and religious faiths in Jerusalem, developed rapidly into one of the largest of its kind in the East. It contained a large variety of medications and was run by a staff trained in modern European institutions.[25] The dispensary became famous for its innovative medicines, especially for the "Jerusalem Balsam", combined by secret formula out of 40 different medicinal ingredients.[26]

---

14 Tobler, Denkblatter.

15 Tobler, Beitrage.

16 Stern, Description.

17 Several sources from the 18th century refer to "the Hospital of St. Helena" which was a hostel for the poor and a "thekia" (a sort of soup-kitchen). See Horn, pp. 191-193 and Hasselquist, p. 135.

18 Freidin.

19 Malki, pp. 58-68.

20 Tobler, Denkblatter, pp. 410-411.

21 Shvarts, pp. 137-138.

22 Kottek & Schwake.

23 Schur.

24 Schittny.

25 Bagatti; Cirelli, p. 219.

26 See chapter V.

Another Catholic medical institution was described by Dr. Tobler, namely the **Catholic Church Institute for the Poor**, known as *Dar Isthak Bek.* It was located near the Church of Helena. This institute had about 28 rooms and operated as a hospital. Another Catholic institute was the French hospital, founded in 1851, perhaps to compete with the English hospital, having 22 beds and a clinic (dispensary).[27] Modern scholars such as Schwake agree with this, and have described its founding in detail.[28]

According to Tobler there were a number of hospitals in the city, including the following:

The Prussian hospital was not far from the Anglican Church. It was established in 1851, having been designed by the architect Conrad Schick, the renowned German scholar and pioneer in Palestine who spent over 50 years in Jerusalem. Dr. Macgowan administered the medical treatment.[29] One of the first directors of this hospital was Dr. Samuel Hoffman, son of the founder of the German colonies in Palestine. Note that Dr. Shimon Frenkel, being a Prussian citizen, was one of the first nominated physicians of the hospital.[30]

The hospital for the blind, situated near the Western Wall of Temple Mount. Tobler mentioned that only ten patients were treated there during the time of his visit.[31] Conrad Schick has well described the medical situation in Palestine and Jerusalem. Towards the end of the 19th century he wrote: "Philanthropic organisations and wealthy individuals who had an interest in the Holy Land [...] can function in various spheres in Palestine: There is a lack of hospitals, qualified and experienced physicians and pharmacists in cities and in large population centres such as Hebron, Gaza, Shechem, Jenin, Tiberias, Safed, etc. It is necessary to promote the construction of hospitals and clinics manned by young doctors. It is very important to set up a central institution or hospital and clinic for eye-disease patients in the centre of the country - preferably in Jerusalem".[32] Several years later the ophthalmic hospital of St. John began to operate and treated hundreds of patients every month.[33]

The lepers of Jerusalem had no hospital. They dwelt in hovels near Zion gate, where they lived apart in wretched conditions.[34] Twenty-four years after Tobler's account, on 30 May 1867, a leper hospital called the Jesushilfe was inaugurated in Jerusalem. In 1887 a better appointed hospital was opened near the German colony.[35]

The only hospital of European standards, according to Tobler, was **the English hospital** of the London Society for Promoting Christianity Amongst the Jews. This hospital, established it 1844 in the Syrian quarter, had 16 beds. As it belonged to the English mission the Jews placed a ban on it, and a Jew who died in that hospital could not buried in a Jewish cemetery. Their clinic was very busy, supervised by Dr. Macgowan .[36] The medical records of the hospitals and the physician have recently been reviewed and will soon be published in detail.[37]

Another aspect of the medical situation in Palestine was the existence of private medicine. A small number of patients in Jerusalem preferred to use the services of private physicians who received them in clinics generally set up in rented shops in the city quarters. During the 17th and 18th centuries a few Muslim and Jewish physicians served in a private capacity, most of them being public physicians who engaged in private medicine in their spare time.

Physicians and Healers in 19th Century Jerusalem

The title of physician in this period needs explanation. Generally speaking, there were two types of physicians in Palestine and Jerusalem, namely popular physicians and qualified physicians.

1. Popular physicians. These did not undergo professional training in a medical institution. They also included eye healers who were not mentioned in government listings and therefore worked with the semi-official permission of the authorities.

Tobler describes his meetings with many healers of different faiths, Jews, Christians, and Muslims. He was impressed by their numbers and amazed by their methods of cure. He censured the treatment administered by the old Jewish women, which, he wrote, "created major damage, especially in the treatment of eye inflammations". Another method of treatment that was very popular, according to Tobler, was bloodletting. He reported that Jewish, Christian, and Muslim men had been in the practice of opening blood vessels with a wide variety of contrivances and special instruments. He added that in the past they had performed this treatment on the streets, but later it was practiced indoors. It was done gratis for the poor and for a small fee for the rest of the patients.[38] Tobler denied the rumor about Muslim objection to bloodletting,[39] which, he asserted, his own experience proved unfounded.[40]

Barbers too engaged in "bloodletting", or more accurately "blood sucking". Tobler describes several Arab barbers, and even a Jewish one, who practiced a different method of blood release. They scratched the skin, placed the base of an animal's horn over the wound, and sucked the blood from the cut top of the horn. That way they did not touch the

27 Tobler, Denkblatter, pp. 403-404.

28 Schwake, pp. 241-244.

29 Tobler, Denkblatter, pp.409-410.

30 Schwake, pp. 238-241.

31 Tobler, Denkblatter, p.397.

32 Schick. A good description of the Western medical activity see Kass, Western. About the political aspects of such activity see Schwake.

33 Bedford & Holbeche, pp.154-158.

34 Tobler, Denkblatter, pp.412.

35 Schwake, pp. 252.

36 Tobler, Denkblatter, pp. 405-409.

37 Perry & Lev.

38 Tobler, Beitrage, pp. 4-5.

39 D' Arvieux, p. 309.

40 Tobler, Beitrage, p. 6.

blood. Suction lasted about thirty minutes and the barbers used a piece of leather to preserve the vacuum pressure when they had to breathe. "This method, which is well known all over the East, was once common in our land (Switzerland) and is still in practice in some spa sites". The scratching and sucking was done on the arms and the neck. The use of a cupping glass for blood letting was reported as well.[41] Medicinal superstitions were very common. People would empty their houses for nine days in order to be cured. "Amulets were a preferred means of cure; you could hardly find an Arab inhabitant in Jerusalem without an amulet. And Jerusalem was full of magicians...". Tobler described cases in which orthodox Jews sought help from Arab sheikhs (old religious men).[42] The treatment with fire (burns) was widespread: 'They warmed a stone or an iron and placed it on the skin; they frequently set light to cotton for the same treatment". Bathing in a spring was a common traditional treatment, as well as the use of leeches, which were bought in Jaffa or Bethlehem. The leeches were cheapest in the summer.[43]

2. Qualified physicians. These were professionally trained at a medical institution or a hospital, or were accredited by well-known physicians. They obtained written authorization from the institution in which they studied or from the government, with explicit indication as to the area of their specialization. The physicians in Jerusalem were members of a professional association headed by the Chief Physician of Jerusalem, who was charged by the government to supervise medical standards and professional training. Qualified physicians from Europe, both Christians and Jews, had received their training at various universities, especially in Italy.[44]

Tobler's portrayal brings to mind other medical reports sent from the East to London some years previously. These reports, which were published in important medical journals of the time, *Lancet* and the *London Medical Gazette*, and also in the *British and Foreign Medical Review*, in 1842-1843, drew similar pictures of the medical conditions prevailing in Syria and Palestine. Jerusalem was an important city in that region, which attracted the attention of millions of people in Europe and developed countries elsewhere. The lack of physicians was described: "There has not been a single resident practitioner to be found from Gaza to Antioch, from Hebron to Horan, or from Beyrout to Damascus, Homs and Hamah".[45] As for the inferior medical conditions:

> The poor people all over the country are in sad misery, for want of medical advice; and they flock to such travellers as are in the company of a physician. There is no such thing as a medical man in all Syria; nor do the people appear to have any local knowledge even of herbs. No hospitals, dispensaries, infirmaries, or public charities exist, to receive the diseased, the mendicant, the orphan, or the helpless widow.[46]

Tobler wrote about the first physicians active in the Holy City in his time. He praised the British mission, which was the first to send qualified physicians to Jerusalem. However, he criticized its members' excessive zeal. According to Tobler's writings, Dr. Albert Wilhelm Gerstmann (1815-1841), a converted Jew, was the first European physician (of the 19th century) to practice medicine in Jerusalem.[47] He arrived in 1838 and was assisted by his pharmacist, Dr. Melville Peter Bergheim (1815-1890). After the death of Dr. Gerstmann, Dr. Edward Macgowan (1759-1860) was sent to take his place. He arrived in Jerusalem in 1842 and had to work hard, curing hundreds of Jews.[48] Tobler lauds Dr. Macgowan's manners and medical skills, but questions his reports on the number of patients he treated.[49]

The first Jewish physician arrived in Jerusalem on 11 April 1843. As noted above, this was Dr. Shimon Frenkel who was sent by Sir Moses Montefiore, at his own expense, at the request of the Jewish community of Jerusalem. According to Tobler, many Jews, being mainly people on a lower social and economic level, did not appreciate Dr. Frenkel's manner.[50] After some years of communal medical service among the Jews, Dr. Frenkel left this position and engaged in private practice in the city.

The Greek community of Jerusalem had its own physician, Dr. Giovani (Joannes) Assuani, a prominent physician from Capelonia, who acquired his medical education in Italy and arrived in the city in1844. For a short period, from 1862 to1863, Dr. Assuani served as a physician of the Rothschild hospital.[51]

In contrast to his warm words about the Greek physician, Tobler repeatedly berates the Franciscan "so-called physicians". He criticizes their wasting of money, their attempts to convert patients, and the low level of their medical skills. He also observes that very few patients went to the Franciscan institute in search of medical help.[52]

A critical change in level and characteristics is evident with the first signs of modern European medicine in the Holy Land in the mid-19th century. The penetration of modern medicine was slow and laborious over the years, until at last it became partly established around the end of that century.[53]

The Pharmacies of Jerusalem

According to Tobler's observations, there were four European pharmacies functioning in Jerusalem at 1846:

41 Ibid.

42 Tobler, Beitrage, pp. 7-10.

43 Tobler, Beitrage, p. 63.

44 Amar & Lev, Jerusalem, pp. 71-74. See also the list of physicians in Jerusalem, Ibid., pp. 103-116.

45 Yates & Kerns, Lancet; Yates & Kerns, Gazette.

46 Medical Report.

47 Tobler, Beitrage, p. 2.

48 Perry & Lev.

49 Tobler, Beitrage, p. 2.

50 Ibid., p. 3.

51 Schwake.

52 Tobler, Beitrage, p. 3.

53 Kass, Western.

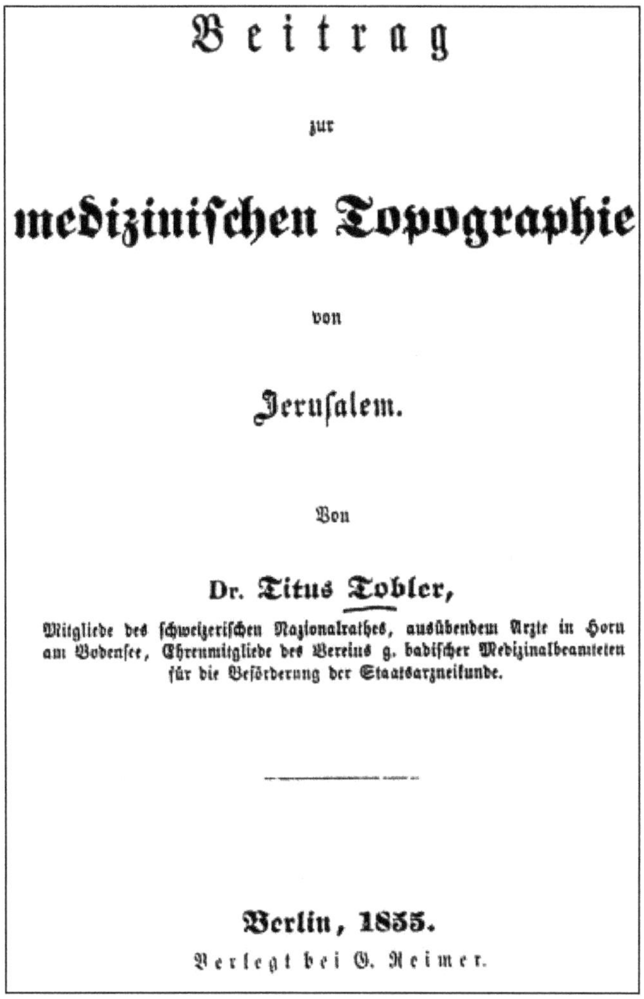

Beitrag

zur

medizinischen Topographie

von

Jerusalem.

Von

Dr. Titus Tobler,

Mitgliede des schweizerischen Nationalrathes, ausübendem Arzte in Horn am Bodensee, Ehrenmitgliede des Vereins z. badischer Medizinalbeamteten für die Beförderung der Staatsarzneikunde.

Berlin, 1855.

Verlegt bei G. Reimer.

Figure 36 - Tobler's Book "Beitrag fur Medizinifchen Topographie von Jerusalem"

A. The Franciscan pharmacy, the best known in the city, was located in the Franciscan monastery. Being the longest standing European pharmacy in Jerusalem, it was highly thought of through the ages. Travellers and visitors to Jerusalem, such as Troilo at the beginning of the 18th century,[54] Hasselquist[55] in 1750, and Seetzen[56] in 1806, have left us their impressions. All visitors were impressed by the famous medication Jerusalem balsam, which was manufactured and sold at the place, by the wide variety of medicinal substances, and by the large quantities of drugs in stock.[57] Tobler wrote in his notebook, after visiting the pharmacy in 1835: "The place looks ancient... the laboratory is strange, unmatched by any European competitor for being so strange...the instruments have old-fashioned shapes, like the traditional tools of mystic alchemy and astrology.... Together with those instruments were some skeletons, surgical instruments, threatening monsters covered with mould...different type of amulets... and all in ancient dark rooms. Yet the store room of the medicinal substances was exceptionally fine".[58]

B. The Greek Orthodox pharmacy, situated in Dier al-Rum al-Kabbir. According to Tobler, "This was the cleanest of all, it was bright and well designed. The names of medicines were written in magnificent Greek lettering. The Greek Orthodox inhabitants and pilgrims received the medication free of charge".[59]

C. The English pharmacy located in their hospital. A detailed study on English medical activity in 19th-century Jerusalem will published soon.[60]

D. The Jewish pharmacy which was located in Dr. Frenkel's house. Tobler recalled some medicine sellers whose "pharmacies" were in the Jewish quarter and were better equipped than those of the Arab drug sellers. Two of these were "of importance; the names of the medicines were written in Hebrew and cleanliness was non-existent". Tobler added that he found there the "Kalomel" and opium decoction that he could not find in the Arab drug market. He also found theriac and other materials. Tobler concluded this subject thus: "Other than at the Christian pharmacies, physicians could find the most essential substances here, as long as they could read the drug's name".[61]

Traditional Substances in 19th Century Jerusalem According to the Swiss Physician Titus Tobler

Tobler gives an exceptional account of a visit to *Suk al-Attarin*, the drug market of Jerusalem, in the northwest of the city. He made a list of the substances he saw in one shop, which in the event proved to be the only list, as far as we know, of medicinal substances ever compiled or published in the entire history of Jerusalem until the present. It was written as a distorted transliteration in German script of the Arabic names, and it has subsequently been translated and studied. It contains 81 substances and is similar to lists drawn up in the same market in the last few years.[62]

Among the 57 substances of plant origin we find herbs such as rosemary (*Rosmarinus officinalis),* camomile *(Matricaria aurea),* spices such as cinnamon (*Cinnamomum zeylanicum*), ginger (*Zingiber officinale*), and clove (*Eugenia caryophyllata*). The list also contained resins and gums such as tragacanth (*Astragalus gummifer*), sarcocolla (*Astragalus sarcocolla*) and myrrh (*Commiphora myrrha*), roots such as spikenard (*Nardostachys jatamansi*), rhubarb (*Rheum officinale*), sweet-violet (*Viola odorata*), seeds and fruits such as myrobalan (*Terminalia citrina*) and bitter-vetch (*Vicia ervilia*), and different oils: black pepper oil (*Piper nigrum*), caraway oil (*Carum carvi*), nutmeg oil (*Myristica fragrans*), and many others.

As for minerals, Tobler describes nine mineral substances in his list, most of which were different kinds of salts such as

54 Troilo, p. 762.

55 Hasselquist, p. 135.

56 Seetzen, II, p. 205.

57 Horn, pp.176-181.

58 Tobler, Beitrage, pp. 14-15.

59 Ibid.

60 Perry & Lev.

61 Tobler, Beitrage, pp. 12, 17.

62 Lev & Amar.

Table 7 - Traditional substances used in 19th Jerusalem according to Dr. Titus Tobler

Plants

Scientific name	Part used	English Name
Alhagi camelorum	Sugar secretion	Alhagi manna
Aloe sp.	Resin	Aloe
Arbutus andrachne	Fruits	Strawberry Tree
Aristolochia sp.	Roots	Birthwort
Artemisia sp. (or Eryngim sp.)	Seeds	Wormwood
Asarum europaeum	Root	Wild Ginger
Astragalus gummifer	Resin	Tragacanth
Astragalus sarcocolla	Resin	Sarcocolla
Balanites aegyptiaca	Oil	Jericho Balsam
Carum cervi	Oil	Caraway
Cassia absus	Leaves	Cassia
Cassia acutifolia	Leaves, fruits	Senna
Cephaelis ipecacuanha	Resin	Ipecac
Cinchona sp.	Bark	Quinine
Cinnamomum camphora	Leaves	Camphor
Cinnamomum zeylanicum	Bark	Ceylon Cinnamon
Citrus limon	Juice	Lemon
Commiphora myrrha	Resin	Myrrh
Convolvulus scammonia	Roots	Scammony
Cordia myxa	Fruits	Sebesten
Dornonicum scorpioides	Root	Panther Strangler
Elettaria cardamomum	Seeds, oil	Malabar Cardamom
Eugenia cartophyllata	Flower buds, oil	Cloves
Ferula galbaniflue	Resin	Galbanum
Glycyrrhiza glabra	Juice	Liquorice
Gossypium herbaceum	Seeds	Cotton
Hyoscyamus sp.	Seeds	Hebane
Jalappa sp.	Root	Jalappa
Lepidium sativum	Oil	Garden Cress
Linum usitatissimum	Seeds	Flax
Lycium sp.	Juice	Boxthorn
Malve sp.	Leaves	Mallow
Matricaria sp.	Flowers	Chamomile
Myristica fragrans	Seeds, oil	Nutmeg
Nardostachys jatamansi	Roots	Spikenard
Orchis sp.	Bulbs	Salep
Papaver somniferum	Resin	Poppy Head ,Opium
Pimpinella anisum	Seeds	Anise
Piper nigrum	Oil	Black Peper
Pistacia lentiscus	Resin	Lentisk Pistachio
Plantago sp.	Seeds	Fleawort
Prunus armeniaca	Seeds	Apricot
Prunus mahaleb	Seeds	Perfumed Cherry
Pterocarpus santalinus	Leaves	Red Saunders
Rheum sp.	Roots	Rhubarb
Rosmarinus officinalis	Leaves	Rosemary
Ruta sp.	Leaves	Rue
Salvadora persica	Stem	Toothbrush Tree
Sarsaparilla officinalis	Juice	Sarsaparilla
Sassafras officinale	Root	Sassafras
Tamarindus indica	Fruits	Indian Date
Terminalia citrina	Fruits	Myrobalan
Terminalia horrida	Fruits	Myrobalan
Triticum sp.	Seeds	Wheat
Vicia ervilia	Seeds	Bittervetch
Viola odorata	Roots	Sweet Violet
Zingiber officinale	Roots	Ginger

Minerals

Name
Armenian Earth
Borax
English Salt
Hematite
Magnesia
Sulphur
Tartaric acid
Tartrate Salt
Verdigris

Animals

Scientific name	Part used	English Name
Castor fiber	Glands	Common Beaver
Castor fiber	Oil	Common Beaver
Hirudu medicinalis	Animal body	Leech
Homo sapiens	Urine	Human urine
Homo sapiens	Mummified Body parts	Mummy
Lytta vesicatoria	Insect body	Spanish Fly, Cantheridis
Tubipora musica	Coral parts	Coral
Unidentified	Insect body	Kermes

Different substances

English Name
Jerusalem Balsam
Manna
Theriac
Pine resin
Kali
Kalomel
Mineral Mummy

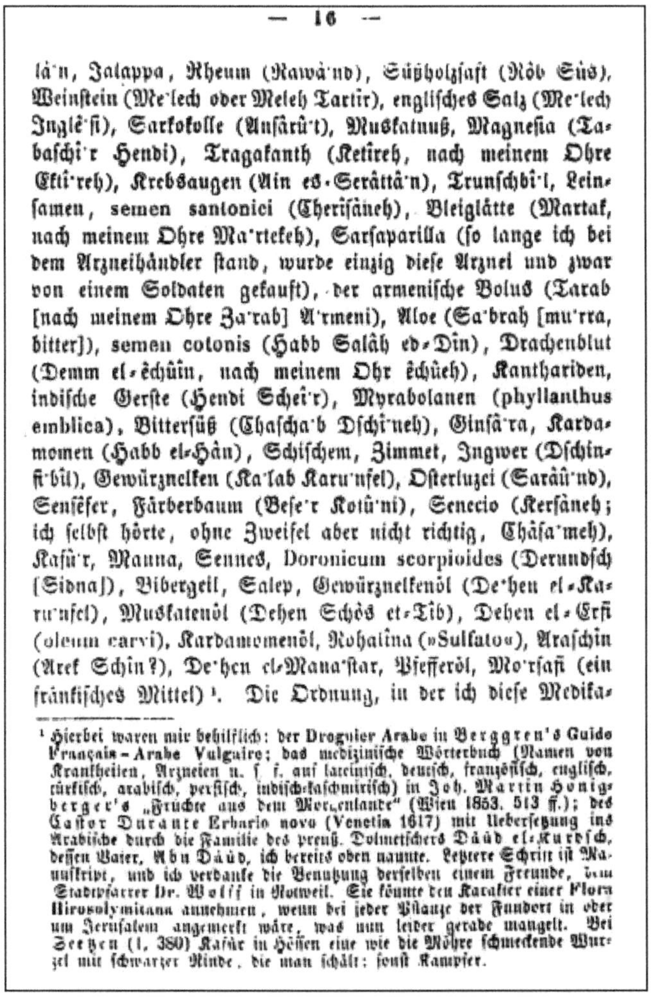

— 16 —

lâ'n, Jalappa, Rheum (Rawâ'nd), Süßholzsaft (Rôb Sûs), Weinstein (Me'lech oder Meleh Tartîr), englisches Salz (Me'lech Inglê'si), Sarkokolle (Ansârû't), Muskatnuß, Magnesia (Tabaschî'r Hendi), Tragakanth (Ketîreh, nach meinem Ohre Ektî'reh), Krebsaugen (Ain es-Serâttâ'n), Trunschbî'l, Leinsamen, semen santonici (Cherîsâneh), Bleiglätte (Martak, nach meinem Ohre Ma'rtekeh), Sarsaparilla (so lange ich bei dem Arzneihändler stand, wurde einzig diese Arznei und zwar von einem Soldaten gekauft), der armenische Bolus (Tarab [nach meinem Ohre Za'rab] A'rmeni), Aloe (Sa'brah [mu'rra, bitter]), semen colonis (Habb Salâh ed-Dîn), Drachenblut (Demm el-êchûin, nach meinem Ohr êchûeh), Kanthariden, indische Gerste (Hendi Schei'r), Myrabolanen (phyllanthus emblica), Bittersüß (Chascha'b Dschi'neh), Ginsâ'ra, Kardamomen (Habb el-Hân), Schischem, Zimmet, Ingwer (Dschinsi'bîl), Gewürznelken (Ka'lab Karu'nfel), Osterluzei (Sarâû'nd), Sensêfer, Färberbaum (Bese'r Kotû'ni), Senecio (Kersâneh; ich selbst hörte, ohne Zweifel aber nicht richtig, Châsa'meh), Kafû'r, Manna, Sennes, Doronicum scorpioides (Derundsch [Sidnal]), Bibergeil, Salep, Gewürznelkenöl (De'hen el-Karu'nfel), Muskatenöl (Dehen Schôs et-Tîb), Dehen el-Ersi (oleum carvi), Kardamomenöl, Rohalîna (»Sulfato«), Araschin (Arek Schîn?), De'hen el-Mana'star, Pfefferöl, Mo'rsasi (ein fränkisches Mittel) ¹. Die Ordnung, in der ich diese Medika-

¹ Hierbei waren mir behilflich: der Droguier Arabe in Berggren's Guide Français-Arabe Vulgaire; das medizinische Wörterbuch (Namen von Krankheiten, Arzneien u. s. f. auf lateinisch, deutsch, französisch, englisch, türkisch, arabisch, persisch, indisch-kaschmirisch) in Joh. Martin Honigberger's „Früchte aus dem Morgenlande" (Wien 1853, 513 ff.); des Castor Durante Erbario novo (Venetia 1617) mit Uebersetzung ins Arabische durch die Familie des preuß. Dolmetschers Dâûd el-Kurdsch, dessen Vater, Abu Dâûd, ich bereits oben nannte. Letztere Schrift ist Manuskript, und ich verdanke die Benutzung derselben einem Freunde, dem Stadtpfarrer Dr. Wolff in Rotweil. Sie könnte den Karakter einer Flora Hierosolymitana annehmen, wenn bei jeder Pflanze der Fundort in oder um Jerusalem angemerkt wäre, was nun leider gerade mangelt. Bei Seetzen (I, 380) Kafûr in Hessen eine wie die Möhre schmeckende Wurzel mit schwarzer Rinde, die man schält; sonst Kampfer.

Figure 37 - Page 16 of Tobler's book "Beitrag fur Medizinifchen Topographie von Jerusalem" – List of Traditional Medicinal Substances

borax, English salt, and tartar, pure minerals such as sulphur, and other substances of mineral origin such as the 'der armenische Bolus', which is Armenian earth.[63] Of the eight substances of animal origin, two were derived from the beaver (*Castor fiber*). Tobler describes *Bibergeil*, meaning beaver gland, and the Arabic term *Dehen el-Mannasar*, which is the oil of beaver gland.[64]

"Medical superstitions were very common in Jerusalem: the magic cure included spells, amulets and the use of magical substances", wrote Tobler.[65] Another physician and ethnobotanist working after the First World War wrote similarly on this subject. This was Dr. E.W.G. Masterman, who furnished a detailed description of the different superstitions and traditional cures current among the inhabitant of the Holy City.[66] His book concluded more than 25 years of medical work in Jerusalem. A local experienced physician, Dr. T. Canaan, published some works on this subject too, [67] as did the two English scholars, G. M. Crowfoot and L. Baldensperger.[68]

"One of the most unique substances was the 'Mumie' (local name); the inhabitants believed it has an exceptional curing power".[69] This material was the remains of bodies, mainly of Egyptian mummies, which was sold in the markets of Jerusalem.[70] It still may be purchased at one shop in the Old City of Jerusalem. The mummies were used by members of all faiths to cure people who were dying.

Tobler added that he heard about the oil of the 'Zaqum', which cured wounds within a day. "A Venetian traveller who fell off his horse felt a worrying ache in chest, rubbed his body with 'Zaqum' oil and drank some, and within some days the wound was scarred over and the internal aches were eased".[71] *Zaqum* is the Arabic and the Hebrew name for Egyptian balsam *(Balanites aegyptiaca)*, a tropical tree growing wild in the Judean desert. The oil pressed out of its fruit has been used as a medicine since early history.[72] Tobler also mentioned the frequent use of "Theriak", (theriac).[73] Theriac is a mixture of many medicinal substances: plants, poisonous minerals, and extracts of animals, generally poisonous such as snakes

63 Amar & Lev, Tobler

64 Tobler, Beitrage, p. 16.

65 Ibid., p. 62.

66 Masterman, pp. 24-30.

67 Canaan, Plant-lore; Canaan, Saints.

68 Crowfoot & Baldensperger.

69 Tobler, Beitrage, p. 62.

70 Lev, Materials, pp. 316-317.

71 Tobler, Beitrage, p. 62.

72 Lev, Materials, pp.152-153.

73 Tobler, Beitrage, pp. 17,45,62.

and scorpions.[74] The manufacture of theriac was a well-kept secret kept throughout history. Medieval Muslim medicine made use of a different kind of theriac. Jerusalem theriac was famous for its medicinal qualities and was even exported to other countries.[75] The composition of Tobler's list is shown in Table 2.

Table 8 - Composition of Dr. Tobler list of Medical Materials

Origin / Source	Number of substances	Percentage
Plants	57	70.4%
Minerals	9	11.1%
Animals	8	9.9%
Other	7	8.6%
TOTAL	81	100%

The Penetration of Modern Medicine into Jerusalem: The British Missionary Society and its Medical Activities

Britain showed very little interest in Palestine during the 19th century. In those days it was of lesser importance for the British Empire to take over Palestine and to precipitate the demise of the "Sick Man on the Bosphorus", as the Ottoman Empire, ruler of Palestine, was then called, than to take the necessary steps to prevent other powers from carrying out any actions that might jeopardize British interests in the East. The loss of the British Crown Colonies in North America several decades earlier had no doubt cast its shadow over British foreign policy, resulting in priority being given to India and the route that led to it. In addition, the underlying interest of Protestant England was not the holy sites in Palestine but the idea of the "Restoration of the Jews". The main tenets of faith that had taken hold among the Protestants told of the imminent Second Coming of Christ, and his advent would herald the utopian epoch of the Millennium. An important factor in this body of faith and a condition for the fulfillment of this apocalyptic vision was the return of the Jews to the land of their fathers and their immediate conversion, or alternatively their recognition of the Messianic claims of the Christian Savior.

On the basis of this belief, many missionary groups formed around the world with the aim of spreading the Christian gospel among the Jews. The most prominent was the London Society for Promoting Christianity amongst the Jews (known as the London Jews' Society, or LJS). The society was established in May 1809 by a German-Jewish apostate, Christian Friedrich Frey.[76]

First, LJS decided to send out a missionary to determine at first hand the possibility of expanding missionary work in Palestine. The medical enterprise of the LJS in Palestine had been abandoned when most of the missionaries left Jerusalem during the second war between Mohammed Ali and the Ottoman Empire in 1840. Aware that the work of the missionary doctors had left an impression on the Jews of Jerusalem, and realizing how essential it was to continue this enterprise in order to achieve the society's goals during the 1830s, its leaders were encouraged to implement their decision of March 1841 to renew their activities after the imposed cessation of hostilities. It was resolved to execute the plans for founding a hospital for the Jews; next to it "a School [is to] be established in Jerusalem under the immediate direction and management of the Head of the Medical department, and in which Surgery and Pharmacology is to be taught". Also, Dr. Edward Macgowan was to be informed that his offer to go out and serve as a doctor at the Jerusalem mission was accepted, and that "His professional character stands too high to make it necessary for him to transmit his Testimonials".[77]

The aforementioned Dr. Bergheim, the first of those who left England to rehabilitate the medical department, arrived in Jerusalem in the summer of 1841, while Macgowan joined him in January 1842. At the end of his first month of work Macgowan sent a detailed report describing the poor state of health of the Jerusalem Jews, his activities among them, and his recommendations for the construction of a hospital and dispensary by the LJS. He urged the London Committee to arrive at some practical decision on this matter and hinted that it would be possible to economize on the expenses of the medical department by growing medicinal herbs. Macgowan even exhorted the society to let him lease some land for this purpose and to employ a local worker. While still awaiting permission from London, he began to renovate a small building for use as a dispensary to render first aid to Jewish patients and as a center for the sale of medicines. Assisted by Bergheim, Macgowan even conducted a few simple operations, using equipment he had bought in England.[78]

On December 12, 1844 the Jews' Hospital in Jerusalem was opened, and within days was full to capacity. The new institution filled the hearts of the missionaries with pride, which found expression in the frequent reports to London.

In the mid-1870s rumors began to spread in Jerusalem and London concerning the need for a new hospital because of the dilapidated state of the old hospital building and the increasing rate of occupancy in that period.

The new hospital for the Jews in Jerusalem, the flagship of LJS in Palestine and the institution in which most of the funds and attention were invested, was dedicated on April 13, 1897. Taking part in the festive ceremony were some of its leaders from England, Thomas Chaplin, the hospital director for 25 years, consuls of foreign countries, heads of churches in Jerusalem, representatives of the Turkish

74 Watson, Theriac.

75 Amar, Theriac.

76 On the London Society see mainly Norris; Gidney and Perry.

77 ITAC, London Committee Resolutions, Nos. M1329, M1330, M1337 (26.3.1841).

78 Archive of the L.J.S. at the Bodleian Library, Department of Western Manuscripts, Oxford (Bodleian), Dep. Cmj, c.125: Lease agreements and the purchase of parts of the pharmacy building.

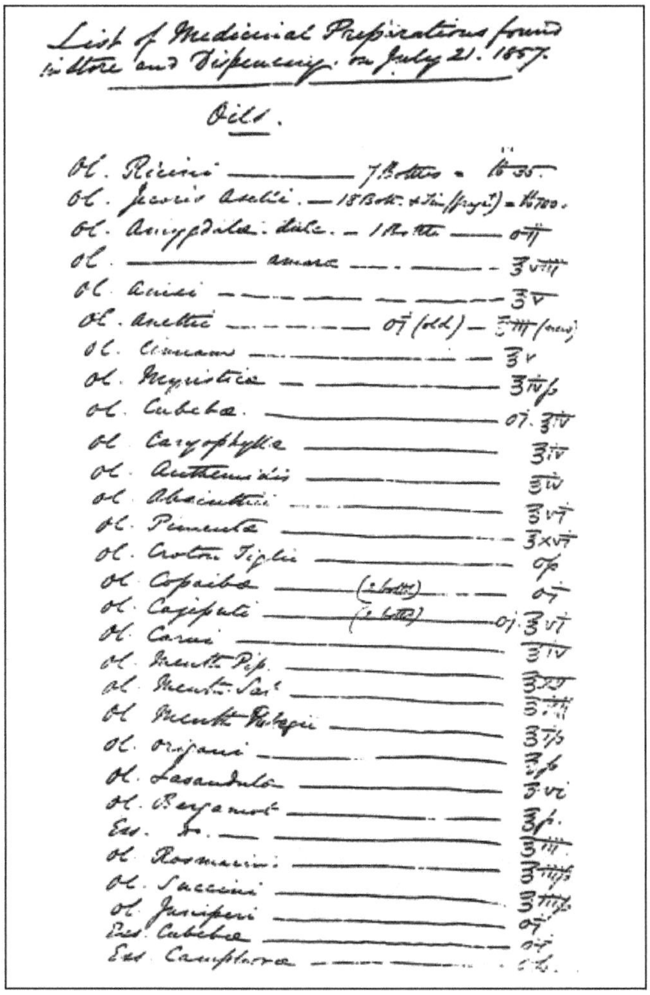
List of Medicinal Preparations found in Store and Dispensary. on July 21. 1857.

Oils.

Figure 38 - "List of Medicinal Preparations"... of the British Hospital of Jerusalem 1857

government, all the LJS members in Palestine; but not a single Jew was present![79]

The Pharmacological and Medical Aspects of the British Hospitals in Jerusalem

Clinics and hospitals in distant lands and underdeveloped countries were not a unique or exceptional phenomenon in the 19th century. As a colonial power, Britain provided advanced medical services for its citizens who were stationed as government officials, military personnel, or merchant traders in every corner of the globe. As proof of this, the medical press in England ran regular features on British medical activities around the world, advertisements to enlist doctors and pharmacists for medical work in the colonies, and even reports on military medicine in the world. Detailed and accurate reports were part of the culture of governing which made the existence of a colonial empire possible. This remained an ingrained feature of British colonial practice for centuries and the medical staff serving in the Jerusalem hospitals acted accordingly. Although the hospital functioned as a private institution belonging to a philanthropic organization, strict regulations regarding the keeping of records and drawing up reports were observed.

Below is a chart showing the list of medicinal substances in the British Hospital for the Jews in Jerusalem in 1857 (Table 3).

Table 9 - list of medicinal substances in the British Hospital for the Jews in Jerusalem in 1857.

Original Text (handwritten)	Scientific/English Name
Oils	
Ol.Ricini	*Ricinus communis*
Ol. Jecasis ?	--------
Ol. Amygdale dulc.	*Amygdalus communis*
Ol. Amygdale amara	*Amigdalus communis*
Ol. Anici	*Pimpinella asnisum*
Ol. Cimettic	--------
Ol. Cinmomm	*Cinnamomum zeylanicum*
Ol. Myristica	*Myristica fragrans*
Ol. Cubeba	*Piper cubeba*
Ol. Caryophylata	*Eugenia caryophyllata*
Ol. Cantheridis	Cantharis sp. or Mylabris sp.
Ol. Absinthum	*Artemisia absinthium*
Ol. Pimenta	*Eugenia pimenta*
Ol. Croton tiglum	*Croton tigilium*
Ol. Cosuibo	
Ol. Cajeputi	*Melalrua minor*
Ol. Carui	*Carum carvi*
Ol. Menth pip.	*Menth piperita*
Ol. Menth sat.	*Menth sativa*
Ol. Menth pulegi.	*Menth pulegium*
Ol. Origani	*Origanum vulgare*
Ol. Lavendula	*Lavandula vera*
Ol. Bergamot	*Monarda didyma*
Ass. Bergamot	*Monarda didyma*
Ol. Rosmarini	*Rosmarinus officinalis*
Ol. Succini	*Physeter catodon*
Ol. Gumiperi	*Acacia arabica ?*
Ess. Cubebe	*Piper cubebe*
Ess. Camphorra	*Cinnamomum camphora*

Preparation ??fr. .....

Extract Sarse (fluid)	*Sarsaparilla sp.*
Dec. Aloei co.	*Aloe vera*
Glycerine	Glycerine
Lquid?? Lobelia ather	Liquid *Lobelia inflata*
Lquid?? Cydto ather	--------
Lquid?? Ferri liquidilis	Solution liquid Iron
Liquid?? Arsenicalis	Arsenical Sol.
Liq. Ars. Sod. Et hydr.	Sol. Ars. Sod. Hydr.
Liq. Potasse	Sol. of Potash
Liq. Plumbi Diac.	Sol. of Lead
Liq. Ammonia fort.	Sol. of Ammonia
Sol. Soda Chloride	Sol Soda Chloride
Sol. Calci Chlorinati	Sol. Calcium Chloride

[79] Bodleian, Dep. Cmj, d.25: Invitation to the inauguration events of the new hospital, signed by the head of the Jerusalem Mission, Hastings Kelk and Percy d'Erf Wheeler, director of the hospital; Ibid.: Program of the inauguration ceremony.

Acids

Acidi Sulphurici fnt.	Sulfuric Acid
Acidi Hydrochlnic fnt	Hydrochloric Acid
Acidi Nitric fnt	Nitric Acid
Acidi Sulph aromatic	Sulfuric Aromt. Acid
Acidi Oxymuriatici	---------
Acidi Acetic. Fort	Acetous Acid
Acidi Tartar (cryst)	Tartaric Acid (Crystal)
Acidi Tartar (polv)	Tartaric Acid (Powder)
Acidi Oxalici	Oxalious Acid
Acidi Citrici	Citron Acid
Acidi Benzoici	Benzoic Acid
Acidi Gallici	Gallic Acid
Acidi Boracic	Boric Acid
Acidi Tannic	Tannic Acid
Acidi Hydrocyanic (schab)	Hydrocyanic Acid
Acidi Arseniosi	Arsenic Acid

Alkali and Salts

Magnesia Cale Oft.	Cacium of Magnesia
Magnes. Carbonate	Carbonate of Magnesia
Magnes. Sulphatis	Sulfate of Magnesia
Potassa Sulph.	Sulfate of Potash
Potassa Tartrat	Tartrate of Potash
Potassa Bitart	Acid Tartrate of Potash
Potassa Chlorate	Chlorate of Potash
Potassa Carbonet	Carbonate of Potash
Potassa Carbonat (cryst)	Carbonate of Pot. (cry.)
Potassa Acetatis	Acetate of Potash
Potassa Jodidi	Iodine of Potash
Soda Tartratis	Tartarted Soda
Soda Carbonat cryst.	Carbonated Soda (cry.)
Soda Sulphatis	Acetate of Soda
Soda Pot. Tart.	Soda Potassium Tartrate
Ammmmonia?? Carb	Carbonate of Ammonia
Ammonia Hydrochlis	Chloride of Ammonia
Creta perparata	Prepared Chalk

Alkaloides

Quinine Disulphatis	*Cinchona lancifolia*
Chinchonia	*Cinchona condaminea*
Atropine	Belladonna sp.
Morphia Hydrochlis	Mercury of Morphia
Morphia Acetatis	Acetate of Morphia
Morphia Sulphatis	Sulfate of Morphia
Morphia Citratis	Citrate of Morphia
Quinine Citratis	Citrate of Quinia
Piperine	Piper sp.
Bebeerin Sulph.	Sulfate of Beberia
Strychnine	*Strychnos nux-vomica*
Strychinine Sulph.	Sulfate of Strychnia
Veratrini	Verateria

Metallic Salts

Ferri Sulphatis	Sulfate of Iron
Ferri Cyanide	Cynaic of Iron
Ferri Carbonat Sacchar.	Carbonate of Iron (Sug)
Ferri Tartarizata	Tartrate of Iron
Ferri Carbonatis	Carbonate of Iron
Ferri Sesquioxidi	Hydrated Peroxidum of Iron
Ferri Tartratis	Tartrate of Iron
Ferri Iodusetic	Iodine of Iron
Ferri Ammoniaca chlor.	Ammon. Chlo. of Iron
Ferri Ammonia tartrat	Ammo. Trat. of Iron
Ferri Ammonia Citrat	Ammo. Citr. of Iron
Ferri Citrat e Quinie	Citrate of I. E Quinine
Ferri Percitrate	Ctr. Peroxide of Iron
Ferri Pot. Tartratis	Tartrated Iron
Plumbi Acetatis	Acetate of Lead
Plumbi Oxide	Oxide of Lead
Plumbi Carbonat	Carbonate of Lead
Hydrogyri chloride	Carbonate of Mercury
Hydrogyri bichloride	Perchloride of Mercury
Hydrogyri binioxide	Oxide of Mercury
Hydrogyri nitro-Oxide	Red Oxide of Mercury
Hydrog. Nit.-Ox. Living	Red Oxide of Mercury
Hydrogyri Peroxidi	Peroxide of Mercury
Hydrogyri Jodide	Iodine of Mercury
Hydrogyri Bisulph.	Bisulphate of Mercury
Hydrongyrum metallic	Metallic Mercury
Hydrog. e crita	Mercury with Chalk
Zinci Oxide	Oxide of Zinc
Zinci Chloride	Chloride of Zinc
Zinci Jodidi	Iodine of Zinc
Zinci Sulphate	Sulfate of Zinc
Zinci Acetat	Acetate of Zinc
Zinci Valerianatic	Valerianate of Zinc
Arsenici Jodidi	Iodine of Arsenate
Arsenious Acid	Acid of Arsenate
Antimon Pot. Tart.	Trat. Pot. of Antimon
Antimonalis Pulv.	Antimon Powder
Iodininum	Iodine
Sulphuris Jodidum	Sulfate Iodine
Strontia Carb.	Carbonate of stronia
Barri Sulphanti	Sulfate of Barium
Manganese Oxidi …..?	Oxide of Magnisum
Bismuthum Oxide	Oxide of Bismuth
Bismuthum Trisnitr…?	Nitrate of Bismuth
Cupri Acetatis	Acetate of Copper
Cupri Sulphatis	Sulfate of Copper
Argenti Nitrate	Nitrate of Silver
Potassa pura.	Pure Potash
Potassa e Calc.	Potash and Calcium

Gums

Gum Opii	Papaver somniferum
Gum Gambogia	*Garcinia morella*
Gum Galbani	*Ferula galbaniflua*
Gum Kino	*Pterocarpus marsupium*
Gum Assafotida	*Ferula assaa-foetida*
Gum Arabic	*Acacia arbica*
Gum Camphhor	*Cinnamomum camphora*
Gum Risino	Resin gum
Pix Burgundica ?	Exudation from *Abies excelsa*
Pix Liquida	Liquid from *Pinus sylvestris*
Saponis mollis	Soap made of Olive oil and Potash

Extracts

Extracts Gentiana	*Gentiana lutea*
Extracts Hummuli	Humulus sp. ?
Extracts Belladona	*Atropa belladonna*
Extracts Conii	*Conium maculatum*
Extracts Taraxaci	*Leontodon taraxacum*
Extracts Anthemidis	*Anthemis nobilis*
Extracts Lactoca	*Lactuca sativum ?*
Extracts Papaunis	*Papaver sommiferum*
Extracts Colocynthide	*Citrullus colocynthis*
Extracts Hyoscyami	Hyoscyamus nigra
Extracts Cinchona	*Cinchona calisaya*
Extracts Glycerrhiza	*Glycyrrhiza glabra*
Extracts Colchici semim	*Colchicum autumanale*
Extracts Colchici Acetic	*Colchicum autumanale*
Extracts Colchici Radix	*Colchicum autumanale*
Extracts Nux-Vomica	*Strychnos nux vomica*
Extracts Quassia	*Picraena excelsa*
Extracts Jalape	*Exogonium purga*
Extracts Sarsa	*Sarsaparila officinalis*
Extracts Aloe	*Aloe vera*
Extracts Colocynth. Put	*Citrullus colocynthis*

Pills

Pil. Hydropyri	Mercurial Pill.
Pil. Galbani	*Ferula galbaniflua*

Ointments

Ung. Hydrogyri fort.	Oin. of Mercury
Ung. Sabina	Oin. of *Juniperus sabina*
Ung. Verteria	Oin. of Cavadilla sp.
Ung. Procis. Alg.	-------
Ung. Elemi	*Canarium commune*
Ung. Flor. Sambuci	*Sambucus nigra*
Cetaceum	*Uncaria gambir*
Adeps Prepar.	Fat of *Sus scrofa* (hog)

Powders

Pulvis Jalap	Rosa sp.
Pulvis Ipecacoama	*Cephaelis ipecacuanha*
Pulvis Cubebs	*Piper cubebe*
Pulvis Mastich	*Pistacia lentiscus*
Pulvis Tragacanth	*Astragalus gummifer*
Pulvis Basilicus	*Ocimum basilicum*
Pulvis Cinchone flavre	Cinchona sp.
Pulvis Senna	*Cassia acutifolia*
Pulvis Calumba	*Jateorrhiza calumba*
Pulvis Aloes Sacotrine	*Aloe vera*
Pulvis Cassia fist	*Cassia fistula*
Pulvis Scamomonia	*Convolvulus scammonia*
Pulvis Sarsa	Sarsaparilla sp.
Pulvis Myrha	*Commiphora abyssinica*
Pulvis Rhei e. L.	Rheum sp.
Pulvis Hallibori albi	*Veratrum viride*
Pulvis Conf. Aromat.	
Pulvis Cinammomi	*Cinnamomum zeylonicum*
Pulvis Scilla	*Urginea maritime*
Pulvis Cascarilla	*Croton eluteria*
Pulvis Cardamomum	*Elettaria cardamomum*
Pulvis Kino	*Pterocarpus marsupium*
Pulvis pepris Longum	*Piper longum*
Pulvis Crete comf.	Com. Chalk + Opium
Pulvis Colichici Rad.	*Colchicum autumnale*
PulvisDigitalis	*Digitalis purpurea*
Pulvis Dolichos	*Mucuna pruriens*
Pulvis Colocyinthidis	*Citrullus colocynthis*
Pulvis Senega	*Polygala senega*
Pulvis Capsici	*Capsicum fastigiatum*
Pulvis Tormentilio	*Potentilla erecta*
Pulvis Galle	Com. P. of Gall
Pulvis Kino g. r.	*Pterocarpus marsupium*
Pulvis Aconite fol.	*Aconitum napellus*
Pulvis Zingiberis	*Zingiber officinale*
Pulvis Cassia	Cassia sp.
Pulvis Valeriana	*Valeriana officinalis*
Pulvis Aunylic	
Dextrine	Com. P. of Dextrine
Carbo Animalis	Com. P. of Animal Chorcal
Carbo Ligni praperat	Com. P. of Plant Chorcal
Calcis	Com. P. of Calcium
Calcis Chlorinate	Com. P. of Calsium Chloride

Roots, Barks, Leaves

Radix Valeriana	*Valeriana officinalis*
Radix Tormentilla	*Potentilla erecta*
Radix Ipecacuan	*Cphaelis ipecacuanha*
Radix Galanga	*Alpinia galanga*
Radix Althea	Althea sp.
Radix Sarsa	*Sarsaparilla officinalis*
Radix Mezreon	*Daphne mezereum*
Radix Hellebore	*Vertarum viride*
Radix Serpentaria	*Aristolochia serpentaria*
Radix Gentiana	*Gentiana lutea*
Radix Colchici	*Colchicum autumnale*
Radix Krameria	*Krameria triandra*
Ras. Guaiaci	*Guaiacum officinale*
Ras. Quassia	*Picraena exclesa*
Ras. Sassafras	*Sassafras officinale*
Folia Senna	Cassia sp.
Folia Spigelia	Indian Pink Leaves
Folia Buchu	Barosma sp.
Folia Uva ursi	*Arctostaphylos urva ursi*
Folia Stramonium	*Datora stramonium*
Folia Aconite	*Aconitum napellus*
Folia Tilia	Tilia sp.
Folia Arnicai	*Arnica montana*
Folia Lobelia	*Lobelia inflata*
Folia Digitalis	*Digitalis purpurea*
Ligni Pterociapic	*Pterocarpus santalinus*
Ligni Haematoxylon	*Haematoxylum campechianum*
Cortex Cusparia	*Galipea cusparia*
Cortex Cinchona lancif	Cinchona sp.
Cortex Simaruba	*Simaruba amara*
Cortex Cinmomomi	*Cinnamomum zeylanicum*

Ethers and Spirits

Spirits Atheris Chlorici	Sp. of Chloride Ether
Spirits Atheris Sulph.	Sp. of Sulfate Ether
Spirits Atheris Nitroni	Sp. of Nitrous Ether
Spirits Atheris Aromatici	Sp. of Aromatic Ether
Atheris Rictificate	Ether
Olei Athereal	Oil of Ether
Chloroform	Chloroform
Collodiano	Collodiano
Sp. Lavadula	*Lavandula vera*
Sp. Rosmarini	*Rosmarinus officinalis*
Sp. Myristica	*Myristica fragrans*
Sp. Ammoniaca fetid.	Ftide Sp. of Ammonia
Sp. Ammonia arm.	Arom. Sp. of Ammonia
Liquir Ammonia fort.	Solution of Ammonia strong

It may be said that this document of 1857 with the list of medicinal substances in the Mission Hospital in Jerusalem is historical proof of the turning point in the medical history of Palestine. It is one of the first written testimonies of modern medical and pharmacological activity in the Levant in general and Palestine in particular. For thousands of years the lists of medicinal substances used by humans contained a fixed proportion of substances according to their origin (plants, minerals, and animals). The composition of this list testifies above all to the increasing use of various chemicals as medicines or as a component in medications together with plants, minerals, and animal substances. The growing use of chemicals and minerals was at the expense of substances derived from animals and other substances of indefinite origin, which were more widespread in the past.

The medical activities of the Mission in Jerusalem are recorded in the rich archival collection of documents of the LJS, which are deposited in the Bodleian Library at Oxford. From them we drew many relating to medical activities in the hospitals in Palestine, including medical reports, plans for the construction of medical institutions, personnel matters, and publications concerning these institutions, as well as extensive correspondence. In this paper we will present one document from the LJS archival collection that throws light upon the medical methods practiced in the early period of the hospital.[80] It is an inventory of medications in the store of the dispensary at the Jerusalem hospital and is dated July 21, 1857. It lists 268 items on nine pages in partially legible handwriting and is entitled "List of Medicinal Preparations Found in Store and Dispensary on July 21, 1857".[81] Below is a chart presenting its composition (Table 4).

Table 10 - Composition of the 1857 list of medicinal preparations

Origin / Source	Number of substances	Percentage
Plants	147	54.8%
Chemicals and Minerals	117	43.7%
Animals	4	1.5%
TOTAL	268	100%

A comparative examination that we conducted showed that the list contains a quarter of the materia medica known and applied in that period in England,[82] and altogether about a third of the British pharmacopoeia of 1858, which contained 734 medicines.[83] Similarly, a comparison of the list with the standard inventory of clinics shows that the stores of the hospital and clinic in Jerusalem contained about 80% of the substances used at that time.[84] Most of the raw materials for preparing the medicines were imported from England, even those found in abundance in Palestine both in the open fields and in the markets. Among the substances derived from plants were several originating in Asia, mainly in India (Ipecaconha, Cajeputi), Africa (Kino), and America (Sassafras, Cinchona).

80 In the rich archives of the London Society stored at several sites in England and Jerusalem there are many protocols, which record the activities of the various institutions of the Society. In one of them there are the private medical diaries of the directors of the hospital in Jerusalem from May 1842 till December 1899. In the near future, a full account of this important historical source will be published.

81 The decipherment of the handwriting was done with the assistance of the following 19th century medical and pharmacological studies Woodville; Lewis, Duncan and British Pharmacopoeia. The writer wish to thank Dr. Tilli Tansey in the Academic Unit of the Wellcome Institute in London for her kind assistance.

82 Lewis.

83 British Pharmacopoeia.

84 Duncan.

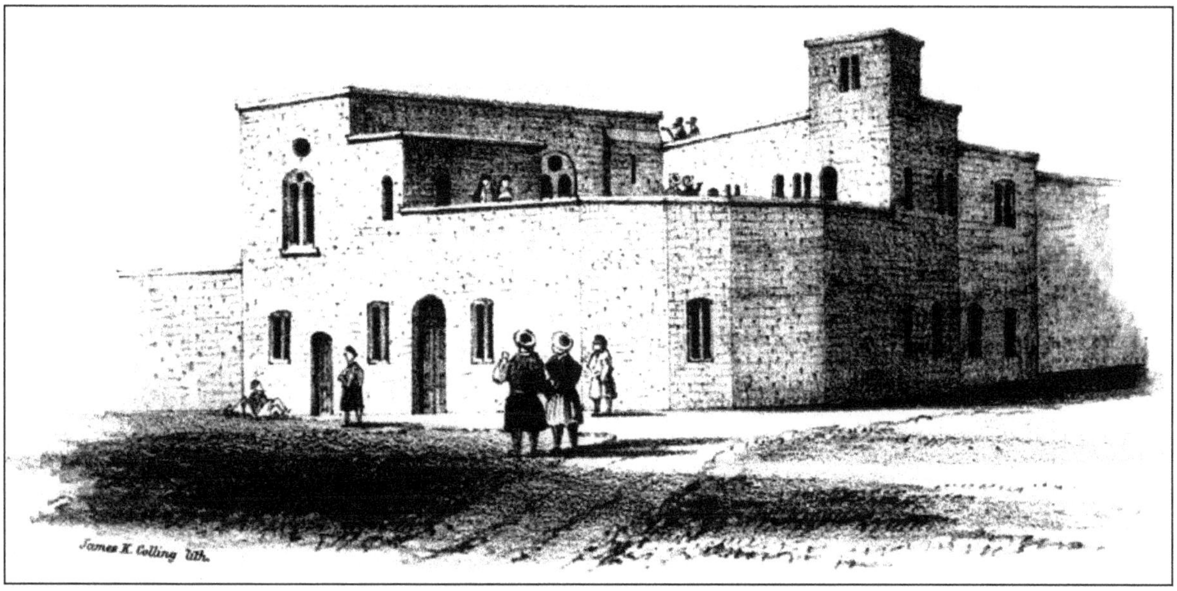

Figure 39 - The Hospital of the "The London Society for Promoting Christianity Amongst the Jews" in Jerusalem 1844

The use of substances from the New World was a characteristic of modern medicine, and the only evidence of such substances present in the Levant at the time was quinine, used by the Franciscan monks in Jerusalem in the 18th century.[85]

The only animal substances located in this list are ambergris (the intestinal secretion of the sperm-whale), Spanish fly (a medically active ingredient generally associated with reinforcing the sex drive), lard, and charcoal. These substances were widely used in the past as medications and are prevalent today in traditional medicine practiced throughout the Middle East. For comparison, note that in the region of Greater Syria during the Middle Ages the use of substances from 30 different kinds of animals has been recorded in the framework of scholarly medicine.[86]

Many of the substances found in the list could have been obtained in the Jerusalem marketplace, for example, cinnamon, nutmeg, pepper, camphor, aloe vera, sulphur, gall-nut, lead, iron, zinc, gum-arabic, galbanum, pine resin, soap, myrrh, rhubarb, cardamom, and galanga. Also listed were substances that could be found plentifully both in nature and in Palestinian agriculture, such as castor oil, almond, watermelon, bitter apple, bindweed, liquorice, pistachio, squill and laburnum.

Additional plants appearing in the list could easily have been grown in the garden of the British clinic in Jerusalem: rosemary, lavender, basil, anise, and saffron. The founder of the hospital, Dr. Edward Macgowan, made a proposal on this matter in February 1842. In his efforts to establish the hospital, he urged the LJS leaders to allow him to lease a plot of land and to employ a local worker to cultivate a garden adjoining the institution. Thus, "it would be possible for the Medical Department to save expenses by growing medicinal plants".[87] However, even if the hospital staff were to raise these plants in their garden, or collect them from the open fields, there would still be the need to extract the oils from them, to produce the powders, to collect the resinous juices, and so on. Such processes need professional skills, expensive training, and reliable workers over a prolonged period of time. The medical staff undoubtedly preferred to purchase the oils, essences, and powders in England, where these substances were produced in mass quantities by industrial processes and were of high quality.

An explanation for the facts given above might be the distance between the Jerusalem hospital and England, the methods of transport, and the risk they incurred for the medicinal substances and medications. A consignment took several weeks to arrive by ship from England, and after arrival it was transported from Jaffa to Jerusalem by mule-caravans. Another possible explanation could have been the financial situation of LJS, which permitted it to purchase only the main, basic substances. The traditional substances in the medical stores of the British Hospital in Jerusalem, constituting more than half of the listed items, were apparently a significant factor in the inventory of substances, so their medical importance was therefore relatively high. These substances seem gradually to have disappeared, and are hardly mentioned in the pharmacological framework of conventional medicine. However, they did not disappear entirely, and some of them were to occupy a major place in the stores of alternative medicine, which is very popular today among the sick and ailing.

Comparisons between the 1857 listing and the historical inventory of medicinal substances in the lengthy time span from the Muslim conquest in the 7th century to Napoleon's campaign on the end of the 18th century show a decline in the number of plants used as a basis for medications from 234 to 169 (plants were often used as ingredients in chemical

85 Horn, p. 181.

86 Lev, Animals.

87 Medical diaries, L.J.S Archive in Jerusalem, August 1845, p. 112.

compounds), and in the number of animal-based products from 30 to 4. In the 1857 listing, 117 chemicals and minerals were used - a new and significant factor in the inventory of medicines. These in fact replaced the minerals used in the medicines of earlier periods until the Middle Ages and generally constituted 5-10% of the general inventory.[88] This comparison of the historical inventory and conventional listings is introduced here for the sole purpose of assessment.

A comparison of the listing with the list of popular medicinal substances drawn up, as described above, by Tobler after his visit to Jerusalem in 1845 also proves that the substances in the Jerusalem markets and in the city dispensaries such as the Jewish, Greek, and Franciscan dispensaries, could have been of help to the British Hospital in time of need.

Conclusions

A level of medicine can be measured by a number of standards, mainly the public health system, medical training, and medicinal substances. Accordingly, a comparison of the medical services of the London Jews Society in 19th-century Palestine with the level of medicine conducted decades earlier, by the Ottoman medical system, and even by the Franciscan medical institution, the only foreign establishment operating in Palestine at that time is instructive. It shows that the British started a new era, that of modern medicine.

One of the best historical attestations to the turning point in the medical history of Palestine is a list compiled in July 1857 of medicinal substances stored in the hospital dispensary in Jerusalem. It was found in the rich archives of the London Jews Society in England. The document is one of the first written testimonies of modern medical and pharmacological activity in the Levant in general and Palestine in particular. For millennia the lists of medicinal substances, which were used by humans contained a fixed proportion of substances according to their origin (plants, minerals, and animals). The composition of the 1857 list testifies, above all, to the increasing use of various chemicals as medicines or as a component in medications together with plants, minerals, and animal substances. The growing use of chemicals and minerals was at the expense of substances derived from animals and others of indefinite origin, which had been more prevalent in the past. The presence of chloroform in the list is strong evidence for the first application in the Holy Land of modern techniques of anaesthesia.

88 Lev, Materials, p. 324.

Chapter IX
Traditional Drugs Sold in the Market of Jerusalem at the End of the 20th Century

A study of present-day uses of traditional medicinal materials in Jerusalem was conducted by the author and Dr. Zohar Amar.[1] The survey covered selected markets of medicinal materials belonging to various religious and ethnic communities, and also included questions put to the sellers and buyers about the healing characteristics of the various materials.

Aspects of the research program included days of touring the Jerusalem's markets, interviewing several drug salesmen, systematic recording (comprising listing and photography), choosing the main informants, and monitoring their business activity over a five-year period. This activity involved frequent visits, many conversations with and questioning of customers, purchasing of materials, learning the trading practices (use of imports from other countries or local purchase), identifying the materials scientifically, and learning how the medicine sellers work. This last involved checking their level of professionalism and knowledge, recording their family history, their methods of acquiring the profession, etc.

In the Roman period drug selling was known as an art, which included diverse fields of expertise; drug sellers were members of distinct professional and social organisations. In the Middle Ages, in the periods of Muslim and Christian rule in the Near East, herbalists and owners of stands for preparing and selling medicines were recognized as a body under professional supervision by the authorities.[2] By contrast, today most of the drug sellers do not usually have any formal education in the fields of medicine and pharmacy.

Some of them chose this profession by chance and gained the training and experience in the course of many years of working at selling the medicines. However, in the case of most sellers, especially the Muslims, whose stores are located in the old quarters of Jerusalem, this occupation is a family matter, passed on by inheritance (down three generations at least). Some of them still occupy the same *'atarin* shops where their ancestors used to sell. The most distinguished example is the members of the Tori family, whose tradition of selling folk medicines goes back through several generations. Their family store is in an old vaulted building; only recently was the store renovated and arranged in the modern style - losing, thereby, something of its unique character.

During the study, we discovered, to our sorrow, that this commercial field of selling folk medicines is indeed declining. The range of remedies in the stores has diminished with time; the quantities sold have dwindled; several stores have changed their character and started dealing in spices and ornaments. Businesses have even collapsed because of lack of customers and the stores have been sold or rented out. Without doubt, during the five years of this study the inventory of medicines diminished and a significant proportion of the medicinal substances that were available in the past are unobtainable today. Hence the importance of this research, which documents a traditional medical culture that is about to disappear from the world.

Final and definitive identification of the substances was usually based on scientific analyses developed in the natural sciences. For example, medicinal materials from plants required accurate botanical definition, minerals were analyzed by mineralogical tests, other materials were subjected to chemical analysis; some of these measures yielded chemical-pharmacological information about their composition and qualities.

During the research we grappled with many identification problems concerning popular names unknown in the classical Arabic dictionaries, and medications with names that did not match the accepted identification; we also found some fraudulent materials, some of which were deemed valuable.

The phenomenon of deception was common in the past. Pliny as well as Dioscorides presented evidence of its frequency, and described methods of faking various perfumes and medicinal resins. They offered means to discriminate among them. In the Middle Ages the *Hisba* was written, which

[1] Lev & Amar.

[2] Ibn Abi Usaybia, p. 601.

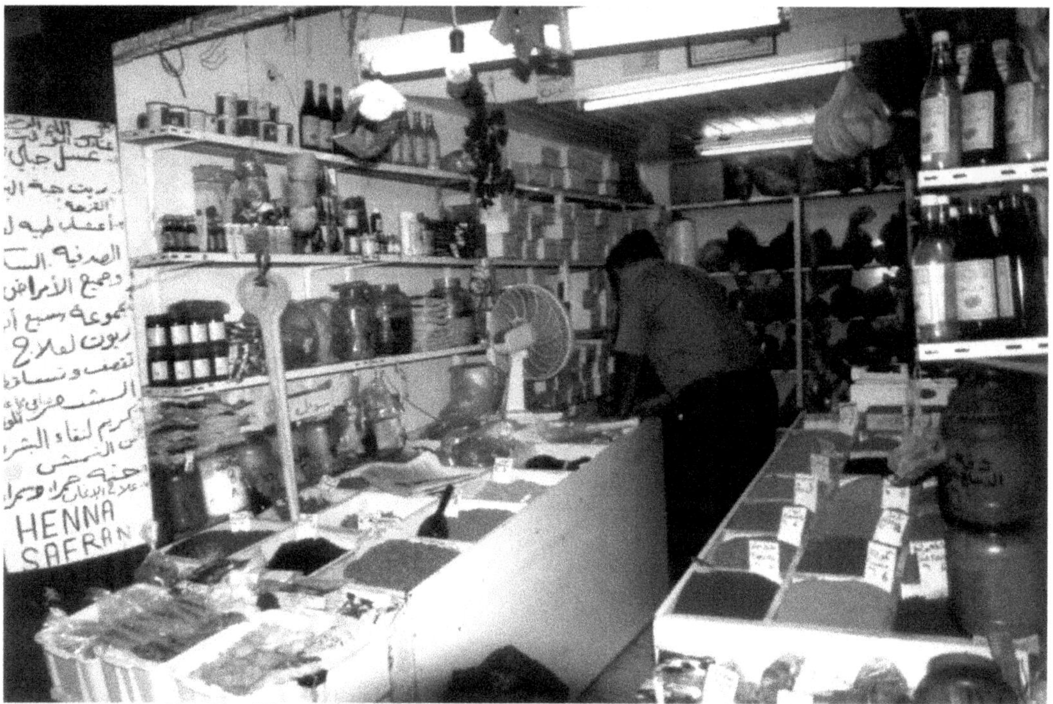

Figure 40 - Traditional Medicinal Substances Shop in *Suk al-Attarin*, Jerusalem

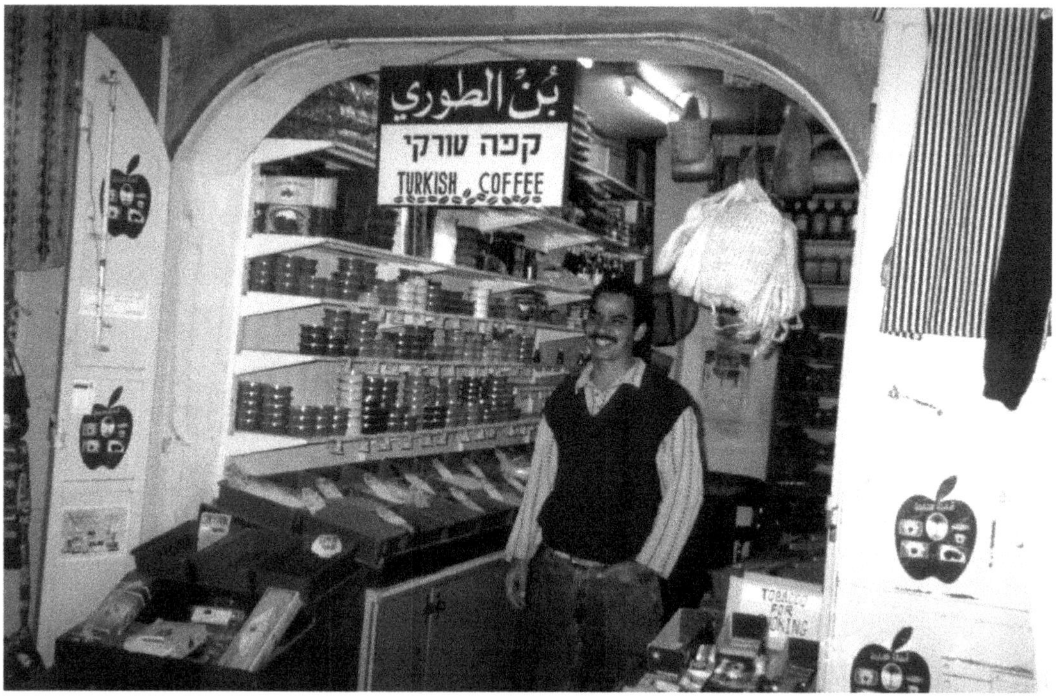

Figure 41 - Shop and Vendor *"Tori"* - Third Generation of Traditional Medicinal Substances in Jerusalem

included instructions for the inspectors of markets — the *muhtasab*. These concerned commercial cleanliness, supervision of weights, measures, and prices, and preventing the sale of counterfeit goods, including medicinal materials.[3] Examples of fakes that we saw during the research are the following:

1. Sometimes we found bottles of "Galena" (PbS), used for painting the eyes blue and for treating them, to contain ground charcoal.
2. Instead of the "skancor", identified as the medicinal lizard (*Scincus scincus*), some vendors sold the striped lizard (*Mabuya vittata*) or the spotted Negev lizard (*Eumeces s. schneideri*).

A comprehensive table (Table 1) contains the bulk of the information obtained from the intensive research. The materials are arranged in the alphabetical order of their scientific names rather than in a systematic scientific order, for the convenience of the reader.

3 Buckley.

Table 11 - Ethno-Medicinal Substances in Jerusalem (Late 20th century)

Plants

Scientific Name	**English Name**	**Part used or product**	**Medicinal Use**
Abrus precatorius	Indian liquorice	Seed	Personal problems
Acacia arabica	Gum-arabic tree	Resin	Voice refining, throat inflammations
Alkanna tinctoria	Alkanet	Root	Digestive problems, joint pains
Allium cepa	Onion	Seed	Colds, virility enhancement
Allium cepa	Onion	Oil	Sugar and cholesterol level reduction
Allium sativum	Garlic	Seed	Stomach soothing, anti-vomiting
Aloe vera	Aloe	Juice	Skin diseases, wound healing, purgative
Aloexyion agallochum	Aloewood	Wood	Strengthens nerves, brain, heart and senses, clears obstructions
Alpinia galanga	Galingale	Root	Cleansing digestive system, reproductive system problems
Amaranthus blitum	Blite	Seed	Fever, diarrhea, dysentery
Ammi majus	Bishopsweed	Seed	Urinary system stones and inflammations
Amomum granum paradisi	Black amomum	Seed	Back problems, arthritis
Anacylus pyrethrum	Pellitory of Spain	Root	Energizing drug, toothache
Anastatica hierochuntica	Rose of Jericho	Plant	Disinfectant and easing childbirth
Anchusa italica	Borage	Flower	Nerves, vision, arthritis
Anethum graveolens	Dill	Seed	Intestinal diseases, respiratory channels
Anona squamosa	Custard apple	Seed	General healing
Areca catechu	Areca nut	Seed	Preventing nausea
Artemisia arborescens	Artemisia tree	Branch	Stomach strengthening, reducing fever
Artemisia dracunculus	Tarragon	Branch	Diuretic, toothache, heart
Artemisia judaica	Wormwood	Branch	Stomach ache, stomach worms
Artemisia herba-alba	Wormwood	Branch	Asthma, sore throat
Astragalus gummifer	Tragacanth	Resin	Stomach ache, coughs
Astragalus sarcocolla	Sarcocolla	Resin	Incense, pains
Avena sativa	Oat	Seed	Laxative, chest and throat complaints
Beta vulgaris	Beet	Seed	General tonic, adds iron to body
Boswellia carteri	Frankincense	Resin	Flatulence, heart diseases, general tonic
Boswellia carteri	Frankincense	Oil	Flatulence, reducing fat in blood
Boswellia sp.	Olibanum	Resin	Flatulence, reducing fat in blood
Boswellia sp.	Black olibanum	Resin	Flatulence, reducing fat in blood
Brassica campestris	Bird rape	Seed	Potency, arthritis
Brassica oleracea	Cauliflower	Seed	General medicine
Caesalpina bonducella	Nikkar nut	Seed	Reducing fever, aphrodisiac
Calamintha incana	Basil	Leaf	Intestinal worms, stomach ache
Capparis spinosa	Caper	Fruit	Pain relief, rheumatism
Capsicum annum	Red pepper	Fruit	Arthritis
Capsicum annum	Sweet pepper	Fruit	Stomach reinforcing, aphrodisiac
Carthamus tinctorius	Safflower	Seed	Purgative, liver problems
Carthamus tinctorius	Safflower	Flower	Purgative, liver problems
Carum carvi	Caraway	Seed	Uterus constrictor, flatulence
Carum copticum	Ajava	Seed	Stomach ache, spleen illnesses
Cassia acutifolia	Senna	Leaf	Purgative
Cassia fistula	Indian laburnum	Fruit	Purgative, intestine cleansing
Ceratonia siliqua	Carob	Fruit	Stomach strengthening, phlegm clearing
Ceratonia siliqua	Carob	Jam	Tongue sores, stomach ache
Ceratonia siliqua	Carob	Seed	Purgative, toothache
Cicer arietinum	Chick-pea	Seed	Stomach problems, flatulence
Cinchona sp.	Quinine	Bark	Jaundice, stomach problems
Cinnamomum camphora	Camphor	Wax	Incense, skin diseases
Cinnamomum zeylanicum	Cinnamon tree	Bark	Cleansing the female genital system
Cinnamomum zeylanicum	Cinnamon tree	Oil	Digestive system strengthening, skin diseases
Citrullus colocynthis	Bitter apple	Fruit	Stomach and joint pains, diabetes
Citrus limon	Lemon	Fruit	Reducing blood sugar level
Citrus limon	Persian lemon	Fruit	Reducing blood sugar level
Citrus limon	Persian lemon	Small fruit	Reducing blood sugar level

Scientific Name	English Name	Part used or product	Medicinal Use
Cocos nucifera	Coconut palm	Oil	Hair strengthening, skin protection
Coffea arabica	Coffee	Seed peel	Sugar in blood, arteriosclerosis
Commiphora mukul	Bdellium tree	Seed	External sores, intestinal diseases
Commiphora myrrha	Myrrh	Resin	Sugar in blood, flatulence
Conium maculatum	Hemlock	Seed	Sedative, intoxicant, hallucinogen
Corchorus olitorius	Jews mallow	Leaf	Health food, general remedy
Corchorus olitorius	Jews mallow	Seed	Health food, general remedy
Coriandrum sativum	Coriander	Seed	Reducing sugar, stomach aches
Corylus avellana	Hazel	Fruit	Bleeding, eye diseases
Crocus sativus	Safran	Stigma	Sore throat, blood pressure
Croton tiglium	Purging croton	Seed	Purgative, emetic
Cucumis melo	Melon	Seed	General tonic
Cucumis melo var. chate	Chate-melon	Seed	General remedy
Cucumis sativum	Cucumber	Seed	Body tonic
Cuminum cyminum	Cumin	Seed	Flatulence
Curcuma longa	Turmeric	Root	Disinfecting sores
Daucus carota	Carrot	Seed	Aphrodisiac
Descurainia sophia	Arar Tree	Seed	Reducing fever, infections, headaches
Dorema ammoniacum	Ammoniacum	Resin	Incense, blood sugar reduction
Elaeagnus angustifolia	Oleaster	Fruit	Dysentery, diarrhea
Elettaria cardamomum	Cardamom	Fruit	Blood sugar, stomach acidity
Embelia ribes	Embelia	Seed	Headaches
Entada scandens	Entada	Seed	Backaches, aphrodisiac
Eruca sativa	Garden rocket	Seed	Aphrodisiac, intestinal cleaning
Eruca sativa	Garden rocket	Oil	Hair loss
Eucalyptus sp.	Eucalyptus	Seed	Reducing fever
Eucalyptus sp.	Eucalyptus	Oil	Opening respiratory canals
Eugenia caryophyllata	Clove	Flower	Local anaesthetic, general remedy
Eugenia caryophyllata	Clove	Oil	Toothache, warts, cosmetics
Ferula asa-foetida	Asafetida	Resin	Sugar reduction, abortifacient
Foeniculum vulgare	Fennel	Seed	Stomach aches, intestinal diseases
Glycyrrhiza glabra	Liquorice	Root	Heartburn, coughs, blood cleansing
Glycyrrhiza glabra	Liquorice	Juice	Expectorant, eases thirst
Hibiscus esculentus	Gambo okra	Seed	Purgative, tranquilizer
Hordeum vulgare	Barley	Seed	Purgative, chest and throat treatment
Hyssopus officinalis	Hyssop	Oil	Backaches, warms body
Illicium verum	Star anise	Fruit	Health spice
Inula viscosa	Elecampane	Leaf	Joint diseases, colds
Jasminum sp.	Jasmine	Oil	Medicinal oil, perfume
Juglans regia	Walnut	Seed	Tonic, hair strengthening, facial skin improvement
Lactuca sativa	Lettuce	Seed	Hair strengthening
Lactuca sativa	Lettuce	Oil	Hair treatment and strengthening
Lagenaria vulgaris	Bottle-gourd	Oil	Prostate treatment
Lallemantia royleana		Seed	Pneumonia, respiratory canals
Laurus nobilis	Laurel	Leaf	Arthritis, sugar in blood
Laurus nobilis	Laurel	Oil	Arthritis, sugar in blood
Lavandula officinalis	Lavender	Leaf	Migraines, preventing miscarriages
Lavandula officinalis	Lavender	Oil	Slimming, partial paralysis
Lawsonia inermis	Henna	Leaf	Wound healing, hemorrhages, fungi
Lawsonia inermis	Henna	Seed	General medicine
Lepidium sativum	Garden-cress	Seed	Stomach aches, hair strengthening, aphrodisiac
Lilium candidum	White-lily	Oil	Antiseptic, anticonvulsant
Linum usitatissimum	Flax	Seed	Hormonal regulation, calcium supplementation
Linum usitatissimum	Flax	Oil	Coughs
Liquidambar orientalis	Oriental sweet gum storax	Resin	Asthma, skin diseases, stimulant
Luffa cylindrica	Sponge gourd	Seed	Purgative, emetic

Scientific Name	**English Name**	**Part used or product**	**Medicinal Use**
Lupinus albus	Lupin	Seed	Blood sugar reduction
Majorana hortensis	Majoram	Leaf	Pain relief, easing childbirth
Majorana syriaca	Hyssop	Leaf	Respiratory channel illnesses, arthritis
Malva sp.	Mallow	Seed	Intestinal worms, urinary system stones
Matricaria aurea	Chamomile	Flower	Respiratory canals, stomach aches
Matricaria aurea	Chamomile	Seed	Digestive system
Melissa officinalis	Lemon balm	Branch	General medicinal tea
Mentha longifolia	Mint	Branch	Flatulence, acidity neutralization
Mentha piperita	Peppermint	Branch	Stomach aches
Mentha piperita	Peppermint	Oil	Backache, toothache
Mentha spicata	Mint	Branch	Flatulence, acidity neutralization
Mentha spicata	Mint	Seed	Arthritis, sugar in blood
Mentha spicata	Mint	Oil	Arthritis, sugar in blood
Moringa peregrina	Ben tree	Seed	Stomach aches, children's illnesses
Myristica fragrans	Nutmeg	Seed	Intoxicant, aphrodisiac
Myristica fragrans	Mace	Seed Peel	Pain killer
Nardostachys jatamansi	Spikenard	Root	Heart pain
Nardostachys jatamansi	Spikenard	Oil	Component of various medicines
Nicotiana tabacum	Tobacco	Leaf	Smoking
Nicotiana tabacum	Tobacco	Seed	Fragrant oil
Nigella sativa	Black cummin	Seed	Dizziness, sugar in blood
Nigella sativa	Black cummin	Oil	Lung diseases, arthritis
Ocimum basilicum	Sweet basil	Branch	Clearing halitosis, health food
Olea europaea	Olive tree	Oil	Skin diseases, many medications
Orchis sp.	Salep	Bulb	Sore throat, soothing coughs
Origanum vulgare	Wild majoram	Leaf	Stomach aches
Paeonia mascula	Garden peony	Root	Nerve diseases, nightmares
Pandanus odoratissimus	Screw pine	Seed	Cough treatment
Papaver sommiferum	Poppy	Seed	Refreshment, fertility enhancement, cough treatment
Paronychia argentea	Immortelle	Flower	Urinary tract infections and diseases
Peganum harmala	Syrian rue	Seed	Tonic, heart diseases, sugar in blood
Pelargonium graveolens	Rose pelargonium	Branch	Heartburn, nausea, eye diseases
Petroselinum sativum	Parsley	Seed	Kidney stones, impotence
Phagnalon rupestre	Phagnalon	Stem	Backache
Phaseolus vulgaris	French bean	Seed	Digestive aid
Picrenia excelsa	Bitter wood	Wood	Blood sugar reduction
Pimenta officinalis	Pimento	Fruit	Stomach aches, flatulence
Pimpinella anisum	Anise	Seed	Stomach aches, aphrodisiac
Pimpinella anisum	Anise	Oil	Flatulence, clearing lice
Pinus pinea	Stone-pine	Seed	Tonic
Piper cubeba	Cubebe pepper	Fruit	Flatulence, expectorant, diuretic
Piper longum	Long pepper	Fruit	Aphrodisiac, digestive system
Piper nigrum	Black pepper	Fruit	Colds, fever, pains
Piper nigrum	White pepper	Fruit	Cough, reinforcing stomach
Pistacia atlantica	Pistacia	Fruit	Stomach aches
Pistacia lentiscus	Mastic tree	Resin	Heartburn, stomach soothing
Pistacia sp.	Pistacia	Resin	General remedy
Pistacia vera	Pistacia	Fruit	Nourishing health food
Plantago ovata	Blond psyllium	Seed	Antiseptic, skin diseases and allergies
Portulaca oleracea	Common purslane	Seed	Blood cleansing, aphrodisiac
Prunus amygdalus	Almond tree	Seed	Hair strengthening, wart removal
Prunus amygdalus	Almond tree	Oil	Soothing eyes, face cleansing
Prunus mahaleb	Perfumed cherry	Seed	Digestive system, children's pains, flatulence
Pulicaria sp.	Flea-bane	Branch	Appetite stimulant
Punica granatum	Pomegranate	Peel	Diarrhea
Punica granatum	Pomegranate	Jam	Diarrhea
Pyrus malus	Apple	Vinegar	Fat removal, weight reduction
Quassia amara	Surinam quassia	Wood	Blood sugar level reduction

Scientific Name	**English Name**	**Part used or product**	**Medicinal Use**
Quercus sp.	Oak	Gall	Diarrhea, hair dye
Raphanus sativus	Radish	Seed	Warming medication, coughs, impotence
Raphanus sativus	Radish	Oil	Pain relief
Rheum officinale	Rhubarb	Root	Jaundice, liver pains
Rhus coriaria	Tanning sumach	Fruit	Perspiration stimulant, diarrhea, cholesterol reduction
Ricinus communis	Castor oil plant	Oil	Wound healing, purgative
Rosa sp.	Rose	Flower	General medicinal tea
Rosa sp.	Rose	Oil	Flatulence, stomach aches
Rosa sp.	Rose	Water	Perfume production, strengthening facial skin
Rosmarinus officinalis	Rosemary	Branch	Kidney stones, sugar in blood
Rosmarinus officinalis	Rosemary	Oil	Kidney stones, tonic
Rubia tinctorum	Madder	Root	Diuretic, abortifacient
Ruta sp.	Rue	Branch	Pacifying children
Saccharum officinarum	Sugar cane	Juice	Tranquilizer, tonic, respiratory canals
Salvia fruticosa	Sage	Leaf	Hemorrhages, intestinal diseases and pains
Sambucus nigra	Black elder	Flower	Asthma, breathing and chest diseases
Santalum album	Indian sandalwood	Wood	Incense
Santalum album	Indian sandalwood	Oil	Joint diseases
Saponaria officinalis	Soapwort	Root	Diabetes
Sesamum indicum	Oriental sesame	Seed	Coughs, sore throat
Sesamum indicum	Oriental sesame	Oil	Sore throat and coughs
Sinapis alba	Mustard	Seed	Pains and infections
Solanum melongena	Eggplant	Seed	Treating sterility, wart removal
Sorghum vulgare var.Technicum	Egyptian millet	Seed	General remedy
Spinacia oleracea	Spinach	Seed	Jaundice, tonic food, strengthens lungs and chest
Styrax benzoin	Gum benjamin	Resin	Incense, evil eye
Tamarindus indica	Indian date	Juice	Cleansing blood and stimulating circulation
Tamarindus indica	Indian date	Fruit	Cleansing blood and stimulating circulation
Terminalia horrida	Black myrobalan	Seed	Improving vision, heart, asthma, joint pains, sugar
Teucrium capitatum	Hulwort	Branch	Intestinal diseases, sugar reduction
Trigonella foenum-graecum	Fenugreek	Seed	Sugar reduction, diuretic
Trigonella foenum-graecum	Fenugreek	Oil	Slimming
Triticum sp.	Wheat	Seed	Arthritis, urinary tract
Urtica pilulifera	Nettle	Seed	General remedy
Vicia ervilia	Bitter-vetch	Seed	Tonic
Viola odorata	Sweet-violet	Oil	Relieving backaches
Vitex agnus-castus	Chaste tree	Seed	Headaches, stomach aches, joint pains
Vitis vinifera	Grapevine	Vinegar	Body strengthening, easing itches
Zingiber officinale	Ginger	Root	Flatulence, digestive system, impotence
Ziziphus jujuba	Common jujube	Fruit	Intestinal worms, blood cleansing
Ziziphus spina-christi	Christ thorn	Fruit	Colds, weight reduction
Ziziphus spina-christi	Christ thorn	Leaf	Blood pressure reduction

Animals

Scientific Name	**English Name**	**Part used or product**	**Medicinal Use**
Apis mellifera	Honey bee	Wax	Purgative, reducing eye inflammations, sore throat
Apis mellifera	Honey bee	Honey	Burns, coughs
Bos taurus	Cow	Cheese	Health food, potency
Cypraea sp.	Sea shell	Shell	Wart removal, treatment of skin irritations
Larinus sp.	Tegal fly	Cocoon	Medicinal drink, internal use
Moschus moschiferus	Musk deer	Musk oil	Medicinal drink, sugar in blood
Moschus moschiferus	Musk deer	Musk grain	Headaches, sugar in blood
Physeter catodon	Ambergris	Secretion	Reinforcing potency, kidneys, and general
Scincus scincus	Medical skink	Body	Fertility of men and women
Sepia officinalis	Cuttle fish	Skeleton	Skin diseases, mania
Strombus sp.	Snail	Operculum	Personal relations, evil eye
Tubipora musica	Coral	Skeleton	Stop bleeding, blue eye cosmetic
Unidentified	Deer	Horn	General tonic, drug addiction

Minerals

English Name	Medicinal Use
Alum	General tonic, reducing liver size, disinfectant
Antimony	Cosmetic, eye diseases
Citric acid	Digestive aid
Galena	Cosmetic, eye diseases
Hematite	Body cooling, treatment of dropsy and spleen complaints
Jew's stone	Kidney stones
Lead	Skin diseases, evil eye
Salt	Skin diseases
Soda	Unknown
Sulfur	Fertility, skin diseases
Vitriol	Unknown
Vitriol (Blue)	Poison, evil eye
Vitriol (Green)	Skin diseases, burns, hematomas

Other Materials

English Name	Part used or product	Medicinal Use
Flower water	Plant oil	Flatulence
Katarn	Cedar tar	Skin diseases
Lakka	Tree resin	Incense, coloring
Manna	Insect secretion	Mild laxative, swelling reduction
Mummy	*Mummy*	Bone healing, sugar and cholesterol reduction
Pine Tar	Pine tar	Treatment of burns, incense, evil eye
Soap	Plant soap	Disinfectant, softening, skin diseases

The survey has made it possible to prepare a summary list that includes all the materials in use today in traditional medicine. This list opens a window to a whole and usually hidden world of medicine, traditions and customs, which still persist as we enter the third millennium, in Jerusalem, Israel and neighboring countries. For analysis of the table the numerical data have been summarized in Table 2.

Table 12 - Composition of the Survey's Medicinal Materials List

Origin	No. of materials	Percentage
Plants	212	86.5%
Minerals	13	5.3%
Animals	13	5.3%
Others	7	2.9%
Total	245	100%

Anyone examining the list may criticise the absence of wild plants known to be used in folk medicine today, as they were in the past. These plants are still gathered by the popular healers or by the patients themselves in wild, and are not regularly sold in the markets or in the spice and drug vendors' stores, but we made a point of not ignoring their use. Also, a large proportion of the imported plants that appear in the list are spices originating in Asia, and are currently used for seasoning and cooking as well as in folk medicine.

A numerical analysis of the data in the list indicates that plants provide most (86.5%) of the medicinal materials. This is a stable trend, evident in the medical literature throughout the course of history.[4]

The use of animal organs did not flourish towards the end of the second millennium. This can be understood in light of changes in the patterns of medical practice – among consumers of folk medicine also – and perhaps also in relation to changes of moral standards and the attitude to animals and their use in medicine.

Use of minerals, too, is much less than that of plants. The explanation for this numerical discrepancy seems to lie in the users' perception that some of the minerals applied in the past are poisonous. Likewise, in all cultures in the past, minerals formed only a small part of the inventory of medicinal substances.

The data show that most of the popular medicinal materials sold in the markets of Jerusalem are of local origin, but it is a small majority. Almost half of the materials in the stores come from abroad as imported products.

The vast majority of the plants sold in the stores as popular remedies are cultivated, with only a minority of them wild. This fact is understandable particularly in relation to the claim that wild plants are collected privately and used widely on a non-commercial basis by the patients or folk healers; that is why they were not found in the shops, nor included in our lists.

4 Lev, Materials, p. 281.

In the context of the medicinal materials derived from animals, the data clearly show that most of them originate from wild species, and only a minority from domesticated species. A possible explanation for this finding is the huge range of animal products offered in the general stores. Also, patients and folk healers may prefer to buy products such as cheese, milk, meat, chicken and animal parts, and eggs, which are used in folk medicine, in non-specialist shops, where good quality is assured. Therefore, the folk remedy vendors in the markets of Jerusalem sell mainly traditional products derived from domesticated animals, such as honey, wax, and cheese, rather than products from wild species. Because most of the population in Israel is urban, and remote from wild animals, and because the nature preservation laws are strictly enforced, products of wild animals are found in only a few shops in Jerusalem. We may note that a large proportion of these materials are horns and bones of large mammals, of which very little use is made, and that the deleterious impact on their populations is slight.

In sum, the study of folk medicinal substances available in shops uncovered the remains of ancient medical practices which still exist in traditional societies in Jerusalem and Israel and in various other countries and cultures around the world.

In the modern age, it is very important to document and restore what survives of the ancient medical culture, which belongs to a vanishing world. Furthermore, the public is becoming increasingly aware of the findings of alternative, natural medicines.

In conclusion, it should be said that throughout ancient times in Israel, humans used various natural materials as sources of medicines. The knowledge of the properties of these materials and their medicinal use was acquired through many generations by trial and error. Historical and current studies indicate that the Land of Israel has been distinguished down the generations for its rich inventory of natural medical materials. Among the main reasons for this we may point out:

1. Israel's location (at a meeting point of three continents), and the country's special climate, thanks to the influence of the Mediterranean as a moderating factor on the one hand, and the deserts as a drying factor on the other. In addition, Israel's particular topographic structure has contributed to the country's richness in natural resources. Israel lies at the intersection of different phytogeographic and zoogeographic areas, where there are contacts among plants and animals that originate in differing and contrasting climates: temperate, tropical, desert, and scrubland.

2. Geological phenomena such as the Dead Sea Rift, and its climatic consequences, such as the Judaean desert, have also influenced the richness of the inventory of medicinal materials.

3. Israel's geographic location — between the Mediterranean Sea and the Arabian and Asian deserts, hence its position on a main trading junction between Mesopotamia and Egypt and between Arabia and Europe, have enriched the inventory of medicinal materials. Throughout history, a variety of medicinal substances have traversed Israel; they were discovered, put into medical use, and exported from cultures such as Egypt, Assyria, Babylon, India, and China; and in later times Europe and South America.

Appendix I
Table of the Historic Periods

Period Name	**Time Period**
Hellenistic Period	333 - 40 BCE
Roman Period	40 BCE – 324 CE
Byzantine Period	324 – 640
Early Islamic Period	640 - 1099
Umayyad	660 - 750
Abbas	750 - 969
Fatimid	969 - 1099
Crusader Period	1099 – 1291
Ayyubid Period	1187 – 1290
Mamluk Period	1260 – 1517
Ottoman Period	1517 – 1917

Note: The Ayyubid and Mamluk periods are also called the late Middle Ages or the Second or Later Islamic Period.

Appendix II
Physicians and Literary Sources for the Use of Medicinal Substances in Jerusalem of the 10th to 18th Centuries

This section contains a list of basic biographical information regarding physicians, scholars, geographers and pilgrims of different religious affiliations connected with natural medicinal substances related to Jerusalem, the Land of Israel and the surrounding regions. It also refers to historical and archaeological sources and commercial documents. The list is arranged alphabetically and gives the full name, period of activity and other important particulars regarding the main sources used or referred to in the text.

Abu al-'Abas al-Nabati
Abu al-'Abas Ahmad bin Mahmud bin Mafraj ibn Rumia al-Ashbili was a Muslim physician and herbalist who was active in Andalusia and died in 1239 CE. In 1215 he set out on a journey to the East, remained for some time in Greater Syria (al-Sham) and described many plants in the Land of Israel and Jerusalem. His treatise is not extant, but selections from it were quoted in the book written by his pupil Ibn al-Baytar.

Al-Ghassani
Abu al-Qassam ibn Mahmud Aluzir al-Ghassani was a 16th century Muslim physician who acted as the court physician of the Moroccan ruler. In 1586 he wrote a comprehensive treatise on medicinal plants and medications containing 379 articles on particular medicines.

Al-Ghazi
Muhammad b. Muhammad b. 'Abdallah Radi al-Din al-Ghazi al-Dimashqi al-'Amiri al-Qurashi al-Shaf'I was a Muslim scholar of the 15th/16th centuries originally from Gaza. He was active in many localities (Damascus, Egypt) and wrote a book on agriculture which also contains much information on medicinal plants in the al-Sham region.

Al-Biruni
Abu al-Reihan Muhammad ibn Ahmad al-Biruni al-Hawarzimi lived during the years 973-1051 CE and was considered one of the great Muslim scholars. He was well-versed in many fields such as mathematics, history, linguistics, philosophy and natural sciences. His many works were translated and published in several languages. The book *Pharmacy and Materia Medica* faithfully documents the medicinal drugs of his period and the work of scholarly pharmacists.

Al-Dimashqi
al-Dimashqi was an Arab geographer of the 14th century. He wrote a book called *A Selection of Periods and Wonders on Land and Ocean* which also includes information on the use of natural medicinal substances in Greater Syria.

Al-Ghafiqi
Abu Jafar Ahmad ibn Mahmud ibn al-Sid al-Ghafiqi was an important scholar and physician in Andalusia. He was considered an expert on the subject of medicinal substances, their names and uses. His well-known book *On Simple Drugs* was used by pharmacists and folk healers until modern times.

Al-Israeli
Kohen Attar al-Israeli was a Jewish physician who was active in Egypt in the 13th century. He wrote an important book on pharmacology which acquired a place of honour in the practice of traditional medicine until modern times.

Al-Kindi
Abu Yusuf Yaqub ibn Ishaq al-Kindi was a 9th century scholar who lived between the years 800-870 CE and was engaged in the study of philosophy, mathematics and astrology. He was born and lived in Iraq and acquired his scientific knowledge in Basra and Baghdad. As tutor to the son of the Caliph, he was exposed to the works of classical philosophers and physicians and later even translated them into Arabic. Most of his works are lost, except for the book *On the Chemistry of Perfume and Distillation* and his book *Medical Formulary* or *Aqrabadhin* which contains hundreds of medical prescriptions of his time.

Al-Magusi
Ali ibn al-'Abbas al-Magusi was a 10th century Persian Muslim physician who lived until 994 CE. He composed a comprehensive medical encyclopedia on the subject of Arab medicine. The book was translated into Latin in the 11th century and became a textbook in medical schools in Europe.

Al-Muqaddasi
Shams Aladin Abu Abdullah Mahmud ibn Abu Bakr al-Bana'a al-Bashari is known by the name of al-Muqaddasi (the Jerusalemite). He was born in Jerusalem and travelled widely throughout the Islamic Empire. His most famous work *The Best Divisions for Knowledge of the Region* which was completed in 985 CE was one of the best books on general geography. In it he describes the agricultural, industrial and medical resources of different regions, mainly that of the al-Sham region.

Al-Qazwini
Zakariya ibn Muhammad ibn Mahmud al-Qazwini was a 13th century Persian scholar who lived until 1283 CE. He was a member of a famous family of imams, a judge, and a scientist. He was interested in natural science and wrote a book called *Monuments of the Lands and Histories of Peoples* in which he described countries according to their geographical and historical aspects. Another important book that he wrote was called *Wonders of the Creation and Unique of the Existence*, which contains a description of minerals, plants and animals and their uses in daily life and in medicine.

Al-Razi

Abu Bakr Mahmud ibn Zakariya al-Razi was an Arab physician who lived during the years 865-925 CE. His medical education was acquired in Baghdad where he also served as the physician of the ruling authorities and director of the hospital. Al-Razi is considered to be among the most original and prolific writers during the Middle Ages. He wrote 184 books, 56 of which dealt with medical science. His works were translated into Latin and Hebrew and they served for centuries as medical textbooks.

Al-Tamimi

Abu Abdullah Mahmud ibn Sa'id al-Tamimi was a 10th century Muslim physician born in Jerusalem. His medical education was acquired in Jerusalem, Ramlah and Egypt. His numerous medicinal treatises were not preserved, but parts of his book *Almarshad* (the Guide) are extant in unpublished manuscripts, and other parts of it were quoted by later medical writers. al-Tamimi specialized in eye medicine and in theriac.

Al-'Uthmani

Shams Aladin al-'Uthmani was a kadi (judge) in Safed in the 14th century. He wrote a treatise describing the history of Safed and its surroundings. From this treatise the part mainly preserved describes various agricultural crops some of which served as remedies, as well as notable medicinal substances which were used in the region.

Al-Zaharawi

Abu al-Kassam Khalif ibn al-'Abas al-Zaharawi was an Andalusian Muslim physician who lived and worked in Cordoba during the second half of the 10th century. He wrote medical treatises and the best known among them was *al-Tasrif* parts of which was translated into Latin, Hebrew and French.

Assaph Harofe

Assaph Harofe was a Jewish physician whose exact period of life and place of activity are unknown. Researchers assume he was active in the north-east region of the Levant sometime between the 6th and 10th centuries. His teachings were apparently collected by his disciples in a book written in his name and which was based on the school of Hippocrates. His language was influenced by the Talmud and his books described medical principles, methods of treatment, medicinal substances and many, varied prescriptions.

Benevenutus Grassus

Benevenutus Grassus was a Frankish physician who was active during the period of the Crusader Kingdom of Jerusalem (12th –13th centuries). His religious affiliation is unknown (Jewish or Christian). In his important book dealing with eye medicine he calls himself the 'Jerusalemite' and made note of 'our Jerusalem medications.' His book influenced eye medicine in Europe.

Daud al-Antaki

Daud ibn Amar al-Antaki was a 16th century Muslim physician who lived until 1599 CE. He was born in Antioch and was blind and crippled from birth. He studied mathematics, natural science and medicine and was active in Damascus and Cairo. His medical treatise testifies to the wide knowledge he acquired from other doctors and to his personal experience and expertise in the study of animals, plants and minerals of Greater Syria in general and Jerusalem in particular.

David de Silva

Rabbi David de Silva (1684-1740) was a physician and one of the leaders of the Jewish community in 18th century Jerusalem. He studied medicine in Europe and practiced in Jerusalem. His book *Pri Megadim* provides us with information about the medicinal uses of the contemporary *materia medica* in Jerusalem.

Dioscorides

Pedanius Dioscorides of Anazarbus was a 1st century Greek physician, one of the fathers of medical botany, who served in the armies of Nero and Vespasian. During these military expeditions he collected plant, animal and mineral specimens and examined their medical qualities. He is famous for his treatise *Materia Medica* – a systematic medical codex which describes textually and graphically hundreds of medicinal plants and scores of animals and minerals which were used for curative purposes. This book became the basic text in the science of pharmacology and medicine for over 1600 years.

Ebers Papyrus

The Ebers Papyrus (named after the German Egyptologist Georg Ebers) is the term for the medical papyri which were discovered in the 19th century in the city of Thebes in Upper Egypt. These papyri were apparently written in the 16th century BCE and contain a considerable amount of theoretical and practical medical information. This includes 877 medical prescriptions which make use of a large variety of medicinal substances.

Eugene Roger

Eugene Roger was a 17th century French Franciscan monk from the region of Paris who specialized in pharmacology and medicine. During his stay in the Land of Israel in the years 1630-1635 he lived as a monk in Jerusalem, serving as physician to local governor and he had close connections with the ruling authorities. His travelogue contained a great deal of first-hand historical and geographical information, as well as a few references to the medicinal uses of wild and cultivated plants mainly in the region of Jerusalem and Hebron.

Felix Fabri

Felix Fabri was the son of an eminently respectable Zurich family who lived during the years 1438-1502. He was admitted into the Dominican Order in 1452 and became an emissary and preacher. After his first voyage to the Land of Israel he prepared himself for a second visit from 1480-1483 which he documented in great detail and in a serious and trustworthy manner. His book throws light on the landscape of the country, its inhabitants and their customs, and describes the flora and fauna and even the merchandise sold in the marketplaces.

Francesco Suriano

Francesco Suriano was born in 1450 to a wealthy trader family in Venice. At first he dealt with Levantine trade and so learnt Greek and Arabic. In 1475 he was accepted into the Franciscan

Order and was sent on a lengthy and varied mission to the monasteries in the Land of Israel and Lebanon, but mainly to Jerusalem. His wide knowledge was recorded in his book on the Holy Land and its landmarks and in it he describes in detail agricultural crops and their uses. He died later than 1528 after his return to Italy.

Frederick Hasselquist
Frederick Hasselquist was an 18th century Swedish scientist and nature researcher who lived during the years 1722-1752. He was an outstanding pupil of the naturalist Carolus Linnaeus and he set off on a journey of scientific research among Eastern countries. He visited Egypt, Syria, the Land of Israel, Cyprus, Rhodes and Turkey. He stayed in Israel for about five weeks during which time he documented 600 plants, animals, rocks and minerals. During his travels he died of tuberculosis at the age of thirty and his book was published posthumously by Linnaeus in 1757.

Hayim Vital
Rabbi Hayim ben Yosef Vital lived during the years 1543-1620. He was born in Safed and was the son of a Torah Scribe. He became the disciple and follower of Rabbi Isaac Luria (the Ari) and one of the great scholars and mystic kabbalists in Safed. He also engaged in the study of alchemy, astronomy and medicine. He worked alternatively in Jerusalem and in Damascus where he wrote a book on medicines and remedial cures. It contains significant information about curative methods, medicinal substances and remedial cures.

Hippocrates
Hippocrates was one of the greatest physicians in ancient Greece who is seen as the founder of modern medicine and is therefore called the 'Father of Medicine.' According to tradition he was born in 460 BCE to an Asclepian family in the island of Kos and his father was also a physician. Many medieval treatises are ascribed to Hippocrates and his disciples (we know of 70 today) and are called the Hippocratic Collection which contain medical principles, methods of treatment, medical ethics and medicinal substances. Hippocrates is also known as the author of the Hippocratic oath.

Hunian ibn Ishaq
Hunian ibn Ishaq was a 9th century Christian physician, the most famous among the pupils of Ibn Masawayh, who lived during the years 809-877 CE. He translated many medical works (about 150) from Greek to Syrian and Arabic. Among the well-known treatises that he translated was the *Material Medica* of Dioscorides and the book by Galen on simple drugs. Hunian also wrote many original works (about 100) which have mostly disappeared.

Ibn al-Baytar
Mahmud Abd Allah bin Ahmad ibn al-Baytar al-Malaki was born in 1197 CE in Malaga in Southern Spain and died in 1248 CE. He studied medicine and botany with Abu al-'Abas al-Nabati in Andalusia and set off on a study expedition around the Mediterranean after which he became court physician to the Ayyubid rulers in Egypt. His extensive knowledge in general and of the plants in the Land of Israel in particular, was recorded in his books, the most famous being the *Compendium on Simple Drugs* which also contains quotations from earlier physicians who have since been forgotten.

Ibn Masawayh
Ibn Masawayh was a 9th century Christian physician who lived until 857 CE. He worked in the Persian Academy of Jondshapur and in Baghdad, and was the head of a translation school. The most famous among his pupils was Hunian ibn Ishaq. He composed many medical works, some of which are still to be found in libraries and others which have disappeared over the years. He died in 857 CE.

Ibn Rushd
Abu al-Walid Mahmud ibn Rush lived and worked in Andalusia during the years 1126-1198 CE. He is considered one of the great Arab philosophers, but he was also a judge and a physician, and became a court physician in Marrakesh (Morroco). He wrote books on philosophy, law and medicine.

Ibn Sina
Abu Ali al-Hasin Abd Allah lived during the years 980-1037 CE. He is listed among the great Arab philosophers, and was an eminent physician who published books on philosophy, the sciences, and medicine. His most important medical work *Canon of Medicine* became a basic textbook for medieval physicians of all faiths. The book was translated into many languages and contains much information on the field of medicine and medicinal substances.

Ibn Wahshiya
Abu Bakr Ahmad ibn Wahshiya was a writer of the 10th century who wrote one of the most important books on Nabatean farming. His book brings together early and late traditions in which realistic and mystical descriptions are intermingled.

Ishaq ibn 'Amran
Ishaq ibn 'Amran was a Muslim physician who was active in Baghdad and was invited to Kairouan (in North Africa, now Tunisia) at the beginning of the 9th century to be a court physician. Ishaq was later executed by the prince when he fell out of favour. He wrote 12 books, one of which dealt with specific medicines and was extensively quoted by al-Ghafiqi.

Jacques de Vitry
Jacques de Vitry (1165-1240) was a Christian preacher and religious leader of French origin with a wide range of knowledge. He acted as Bishop of Acre during the years 1216-1225 CE. His great erudition which was based on his personal observations and the painstaking collection of earlier sources, mainly the writings of the Archbishop of Tyre (William of Tyre) was condensed into a treatise that also contained a little information about the medicinal uses of natural substances in the Land of Israel during his period.

Maimonides
Rabbi Moses ben Avraham ben Maimon (1135-1204) was a 12th century Jewish philosopher, halachic authority and physician of Spanish origin. He migrated to Egypt and lived in Cairo from 1166 in the service of the Ayyubid rulers. He

wrote halachic works as well as medical and pharmacological treatises including the books: *On Asthma*, *Poisons and their Antidotes*, *Aphorisms of Moses* and *Glossary on Medical Materials*. These books were translated into many languages and one may learn from them about the medical uses of various medicinal substances.

Moshe Bassola

Rabbi Moshe Bassola who lived during the years 1480-1560 was the rabbi of the Pisaro community in Italy and head of the Ancona Yeshiva. He was a kabbalist and author, and for messianic reasons he went on a two-year journey from 1521-1523 to the Land of Israel and to nearby Jewish communities. In his book he documented his travels in great detail, and it contains a large amount of important information about the state of the country, its inhabitants in general and the Jewish communities in particular.

Moshe Poriat

Rabbi Moshe Poriat was a 17th century Torah scribe. He was born in Prague and went to Jerusalem in the 1620's, but because of the dire conditions of the city he returned to Europe and earned his livelihood by book printing, including his own book *Darkei Zion* (The Ways of Zion). The book contains a description of the market places in the Holy City that tells us about the merchandise, their price and their uses.

Pliny the Elder

Plinius was a 1st century Roman soldier, scientific researcher, and writer who lived during the years 23-79 CE. Pliny published scores of books that have been lost, but his encyclopedic collection *Historia Naturalis* (Natural History) survived. It is composed of 37 books, and Books 20-37 deal with the medicinal use of plants, minerals and animals. Some of the medical information directly concerns well-known cultivations in the Land of Israel such as dates and balsam.

Refael Malki

Rabbi Refael Mordechai Malki was a 17th century Jewish scholar and physician. He was born in the Iberian Peninsula but spent most of his life in Italy where he also studied medicine. In 1677 he went to Jerusalem and became a halachist, a public figure and a physician. His halachic and medical works have been preserved and they contain much information regarding the state of medical care in the Jerusalem of his day, the illnesses and the frequently used medications as well as the medical standards of other physicians of this period. He died in Jerusalem in 1702.

Saladino d'Ascoli

Saladino Fiero of Ascoli was a Jewish physician and pharmacist who was active in Italy during the mid-15th century. He wrote a book in 1430 at the request of experienced pharmacists in order to prevent errors by young pharmacists. The book was based on the works of the great classical, Arabic and European physicians and pharmacists who preceded him. It was written in Latin and translated into Hebrew during the author's lifetime and contributed greatly to the knowledge of researchers studying European pharmacology of that period.

Shabtai Donolo

Shabtai Donolo was a 10th century Jewish physician and astronomer who lived in Southern Italy during the years 913-982 CE. Particulars about his life are not very clear, but his *Book of Pharmacology* provides much information. The book on pharmacology documents the practice of Jewish medical science in Europe before the inflow of Arabic medicine in the medical schools in Salerno during the 11th century.

Theophrastus

Theophrastus of Eresos was a Greek philosopher and a pupil of Aristotle, who lived during the years 370-287 BCE. According to legend, Theophrastus inherited Aristotle's garden of plants and devoted his life to the study of plants, publishing basic texts on their morphology, taxonomy, and physiology. He is considered the father of botanical science. But his most famous work is his *History of Plants* in which 500 medicines are mentioned.

Appendix III
List of Medicinal Substances in 10th -18th Century Jerusalem

(in alphabetical order of common names)

Animals

Common Name	Scientific Name
Adder, Ter	*Echis coloratus*
Beaver	*Castor fiber*
Bee, Honey	*Apis mellifica*
Coral	*Tubipora musica or Corallium rubrum*
Cow	*Bos Taurus*
Cuttle Fish	*Ossa sepia*
Desert partridge	Ammoperdix heyi
Earthworm	*Lumbricus sp.*
Fish	Unidentified
Fox	Vulpes sp.
Gazelle	Gazella sp.
Goat	*Capra hircus mambrica*
Goose	*Anser anser*
Hen	*Gallus gallus domesticus*
Human	*Homo sapiens*
Kermes	Unidentified
Lamb	Ovis
Musk Deer	*Moschus moschiferus*
Pearl	*Avicula margarittifera*
Scorpion	*Leiurus quinquestriatus hebraeus*
Spanish fly	*Lytta vesicatoria*
Sperm Whale (Amberigris)	*Physeter catodom*
Wolf	*Canis lupus*

Minerals

Name
Alum
Amonia
Arsenic Sulfide
Asphalt
Earth (Clay) sp.
Jews' Stone (Cidaris sp.)
Kohl (Galena, Antimony)
Mercury
Salt (Halite)
Sulphur
Tartrate
Thermal (mineral) water
Vitriol sp.
Zinc

Plants

Common Name	Scientific Name
Absinet	*Artemisia absinthium*
Agaric	Agaricus sp.
Almond	*Amygdalus communis = Prunus amygdalus*
Aloe	Aloe sp.
Anise	*Pimpinella anisum*
Apple	*Pyrus malus = Malus sylvestris*
Asafetida	*Ferula assa-foetida*
Asparagus	*Asparagus officinalis*
Autumn Mandrake	*Mandragora autumnalis*
Balsam	*Commiphora opobalsamum*
Barley	*Hordeum vulgare*
Basil	*Ocimum basilicum*
Ben Tree	*Moringa peregrina*
Bird Rape	*Brassica campestris*
Borage	Anchusa sp.
Bottle-gourd	*Lagenaria vulgaris*
Bugle	Ajuga sp.
Cabbage	*Brassica oleracea*
Camphor	*Cinnamomum camphora*
Carrot	*Daucus carota*
Cassia	Cassia (Senna) sp.
Celery	*Apium graveolens*
Celtic Spikenard	*Valeriana celtica*
Chamomile	*Matricaria recutita (chamamilla)*
Chate Melon	*Cucumis melo var.chate*
Cherry	Prunus (Cerasus) sp.
Chestnut	*Castanea sativa*
Chickpea	*Cicer arietinum*
Chicory	*Cichorium intybus*
Christ Thorn Jujube	*Ziziphus spina-christi*
Christmas Rose	*Helleborus niger*
Cinnamon	*Cinnamomum zeylanicum*
Clove	*Eugenia caryophyllata*
Cocoa	*Theobroma cacao*
Coconut Palm	*Cocos nucifera*
Coffee	*Coffea arabica*
Colocynth	*Citrullus colocynthis*
Common Ivy	*Hedra helix*
Common Liquorice	*Glycyrrhiza glabra*
Common Madder	*Rubia tinctorum*
Common Melon	*Cucumis melo*
Coral Peony	Paeonia sp.
Cretan Anise	*Pimpinella cretica*
Cucumber	*Cucumis sativus*
Cumin	*Cuminum cyminum*
Date	*Phoenix dactylifera*
Dead Sea Apple	*Solanum inacum*

Common Name	Scientific Name
Deer Balls	*Lycoperdon lividium*
Dill	*Anethum graveolens*
Dodder of Thyme	*Cuscuta epithymum*
Dog Rose (Wild)	*Rosa canina*
Dragon's Blood	*Daemomorops draco*
Dwarf Elder	*Sambucus ebulus*
Eastern Strawberry Tree	*Arbutus andrachne*
Eggplant	*Solanum melongena*
Elder	*Sambucus nigra*
European Nettle Tree	*Celtic australis*
Fig Tree	*Ficus carica*
Flax	*Linum usitatissimum*
Flea Wart	Plantago sp.
Flixweed	*Caltiris quadrivalvis*
Frankincense	*Boswellia carteri*
Garden Bean	*Vicia faba*
Garden Cress	*Lepidium sativum*
Garden Rocket	*Eruca sativa*
Garden Sorrel	*Rumex acetosa*
Garlic	*Allium sativum*
Garlic	*Allium sp.*
Ginger	*Zingiber officinale*
Grape Vine	*Vitis vinifera*
Guaiacum	*Guaiacum sanctum*
Gum Arabic	*Acacia arabica*
Hazel Nut	*Corylus avellana*
Headed Thyme	*Coridothymus capitatus*
Hedge-Mustard	Sisymbrium sp.
Henna	*Lawsonia inermis {alba}*
Hollyhock	Alcea sp.
Hyssop	*Hyssopus officinalis*
Indian Aloe-tree	*Aquilaria agallocha*
Jasmine	Jasminum sp.
Jericho Balsam	*Balanites aegyptiaca*
Job's Tears	*Coix lachryma-jobi*
Juniper	Juniperus sp.
Larch	Larix sp.
Laurel	*Laurus nobilis*
Leek	*Allium porrum*
Lemon	*Citrus limon*
Lentil	*Lens culinaris*
Lentisk	*Pistacia lentiscus*
Lettuce	*Lactuca sativa*
Lupins	*Lupinus termis*
Madonna Lily	*Lilium candidum*
Marjoram, Sweet	*Majorana hortensis*
Marjoram, Wild	*Origanum syriacum*
Mint	Mentha sp.
Mulberry	Morus sp.
Mustard	*Sinapis alba*
Myrobalan	Terminalia sp.
Myrrh	*Commiphora myrrha*
Myrtle	*Myrtus communis*
Nutmeg, Mace	*Myristica fragrans*

Common Name	Scientific Name
Oak	Quercus sp.
Oak Gall	Quercus sp.
Officinal Storax	*Styrax officinalis*
Olive Tree	*Olea europaea*
Onion	*Allium cepa*
Opium, Poppy Head	*Papaver somniferum*
Oriental Sesame	*Seasamum indicum*
Parsley	*Petroselinum sativum*
Peach	*Prunus persica*
Pear	*Pyrus communis*
Pepper	Piper sp.
Peruvian Bark	Cinchona sp.
Pine	Pinus sp.
Pistachio	Pistacia vera
Plum	*Prunus domestica*
Pomegranate	*Punica granatum*
Poplar	Populus sp.
Prickly Burnet	*Sarcopoterium spinosum*
Purging Cassia	*Cassia fistula*
Purslane	*Portulaca oleracea*
Quince	*Cydonia oblonga*
Radish	*Raphanus sativus*
Rhubarb	Rheum sp.
Rice	*Oryza sativa*
Rose of Jericho	*Anastatica hierochuntica*
Rosemary	*Rosmarinus officinalis*
Rue	Ruta sp.
Safflower	*Carthamus tinctorius*
Saffron	*Crocus sativus*
Sagafino	Ferula sp.
Sage	Salvia sp.
Sandalwood	*Santalum album*
Sarcocolla	*Astragalus sarcocolla*
Sassafras	*Sassafras officinale*
Savine	*Juniperus sabina*
Savory of Crete	*Satureja thymbra*
Scammony	*Convolvulus scammonia*
Sea Holly	Eryngium sp.
Sebesten	*Cordia myxa*
Seville Orange (Sour Orange)	*Citrus aurantium*
Spikenard	*Nardostachys grandiflora (jatamansi)*
Spinach	*Spinacia oleracea*
Spiny Broom	*Calicotome villosa*
Sugar Cane	*Saccharum officinarum*
Sweet Clover	*Melilotus albus*
Sweet Lime	*Citrus medica*
Sweet Sedge	*Acorus calamus*
Sweet Violet	*Viola odorata*
Tall Asphodel	*Asphodelus aestivus (ramosus)*
Tamarinds	*Tamarindus indica*
Tamarisk	Tamarix sp.
Tanning Sumach	*Rhus coriaria*
Tea	Thea sp.

Common Name	Scientific Name
Toadflax	Kickxia sp.
Tobacco	*Nicotiana tabacum*
Tormentil	*Potentilla tormientilla*
Tragacanth	*Astragalus gummifer*
Turmeric	*Curcuma longa*
Turpeth	*Ipomoea turpethum*
Varthemia	*Chiliadenus iphionoides*
Wall Pellitory	*Parietaria judaica*
Walnut	*Juglans regia*
Water Mint	*Mentha pulegium*
Watercress	*Coronopus squamatus*
Watermelon	*Citrullus vulgaris*
Wheat, Flour, Braed	Triticum sp.
White Mignonette	*Reseda alba*
White Water Lily	*Nymphaea alba*
Willow	Salix sp.
Wormwood	Artemisia sp.
Yarrow	Achillea sp.
Yellow Gentian	*Gentiana lutea*
Yellow Pond Lily	*Nuphar lutea*

Others

Name
Balsam of Jerusalem
Flower Water
Manna
Mummy
Oxymel
Theriac

Bibliography and List of Abbrevations

BSOAS – *Bulletin of the School of Oriental and African Studies*
EI – *Encyclopaedia of Islam*
HE – *Hebrew Encyclopaedia*
ITAC - *Israeli Trust of the Anglican Church*
LCL – The Loeb Classical Library, London–Cambridge
LJS – London Jewish Society
MIE – *Memoires Presentes a L'Institut d'Egypte*
PPTS – *Palestine Pilgrims Text Society,* London 1887–1897
RHC – *Recueil des Historiens des Croisades*
ZDPV – *Zeitschrift des Deutschen Palastina – Vereins*

Abu–Rabia: A. Abu–Rabia, *Folk Medicine among the Bedouin Tribes in the Negev*, Sde Boqer 1983. (Hebrew).

Adgington: S. Adgington, "Medical Knowledge in the Crusading Armies: The Evidence of Albert of Aachen and Others", in: M. Barber (ed.), *The Military Orders: Fighting for the Faith and Caring for the Sick*, London 1994, pp. 320–326.

al-'Asali, Ma'ahid: Kamil Jamil al-'Asali, *Ma'ahid al-'ilm fi Bayt al-Maqdis*, Amman 1981. (Arabic).

al-'Asali, Wata'iq: Kamil Jamil al-'Asali, *Waṯa'iq Maqdisiyya Tarikhiyya*, III, Amman 1989. (Arabic).

al-'Umari: Ibn Fadl Allah al-'Umari, *Masalik al-'absar fi Mamalik al-'Amsar*, A.F. Sayyid (ed.), Textes Arabes et Etudes Islamiques, Tome 23, Paris 1985. (Arabic).

al-'Uthmani: B. Lewis, "An Arabic Account of the Province of Safad–1", *BSOAS,* 15 (1953), pp. 477–488.

al-Antaki: Daud al-Antaki, *Tadhkirat Ula li-'Lbab wa 'l-Jami' al-'Ujab al-'Ujab*, Cairo 1935. (Arabic).

al-Ashbili: Ibn al-Khair al-Ashbili, *'Amdat al-Tibb fi Ma'rafat al-Nabat.* Rabat 1990. (Arabic).

al-Asfahani: 'Imad al-din al-Asfahani, *al-fatah al-qasi fi al-fatah al-qadsi*, Mohmad Sabah (ed.), Cairo 1965.

al-Badri: Taqi al-Din al-Badri, *Nuzhat al-Anam fi Mahasin al-Sham.* Beirut 1980. (Arabic).

al-Baghdadi: *'Abd al-Latif* al-Baghdadi, *Kitab al-Ifadah wa-'l-I'tibar*, London 1965. (Arabic).

al-Biruni: H.M. Said & R.E. Elahie (eds.), *Al–Biruni's Book on Pharmacy and Materia Medica*, Karachi 1973.

al-Dimashqi: Shams al-Din Muhammad al-Dimashqi, *Kitab Nukhbat al-Dahr fi 'Aja'ib al-Bar wal-Bahr,* A.F. Mehren (ed.), Leipzig 1923. (Arabic).

al-Ghafiqi: M. Meyerhof & G.P. Sobhy (ed. & trans.), *The Abridged Version of "The Book of Simple Drugs", of Ahmad Ibn Muhammad Al–Ghafiqi by Gregorius Abul–Farag (Barhebraeus)*, I–IV, Cairo 1932–1940.

al-Ghassani: al-Ghassani, *Hadaqat al-Azhar fi Mahiyyat al-'Ushab wa-l-'Aqqar*, Beirut 1990. (Arabic).

Ali & Mahdihassan, Mineral: S.A.M. Ali & S. Mahdihassan, "Bazaar Medicine of Karachi Inorganic Drugs", In: S. Mahdihassan (ed.) *Bazaar Drugs and Folk Medicine in Pakistan*, Karachi 1984, pp. 82–89.

Ali & Mahdihassan, Animal: S.A.M. Ali & S. Mahdihassan, "Bazaar Medicines of Karachi: The Drugs of Animal Origin", In: S. Mahdihassan (ed.), *Bazaar Drugs and Folk Medicine in Pakistan*, Karachi 1984, pp. 69–73.

Ali et al: S.A.M. Ali, H.S.J. Bakht & S. Mahdihassan, "Simples of Unani Pharmacy", In: S. Mahdihassan (ed.), *Bazaar Drugs and Folk Medicine in Pakistan*, Karachi 1984, pp. 52–63.

al-Idrisi: al-Idrisi, *Opus Geographicum*, (Cerulli E. et al, eds.) IV. Naples-Rome 1974.

al-Israili: Abul-Muna Dawud b. Abi Nasr Kohen al-Attar al-Israili, *Minhag ad-Dukkan.* Cairo 1940. (Arabic).

al-Kindi: M. Levey, *The Medical Formulary of the Aqrabadhin of al–Kindi*, Madison 1966.

Allan: N. Allan, "Hospice to Hospital in the Near East: an Instance of Continuity and Change in Late Antiquity", *Bulletin of the History of Medicine*, 64 (1990), pp. 446–462.

al-Mas'udi: Ali b. al-Husayn al-Mas'udi, *Muruj al-Dhahb* C. Barbier de Meynard (ed.), Paris 1861-1877. (Arabic).

al-Muqaddasi: al-Muqaddasi, *Ahsan al-Taqasim fi Marifat al-Aqalim,* (ed.) De Goeje, Leiden 1906. (Arabic).

al-Nuwayri: Shihab al-Din Ahmad al-Nuwayri, *Nihayat al-Arab fi Funun al-Adab.* Cairo 1924.

al-Qalqashandi: al-Qalqashandi, *Subh al-'Asha fi Sina'at al-Insha*, Cairo 1913-1919. (Arabic).

al-Qazwini: al-Qazwini, *'Ajab-al-Makhluqat*, Beirut 1981. (Arabic).

al-Rawi & Chaakravarty: A. al-Rawi & H.L. Chaakravarty, *Medicinal Plant of Iraq*, Ministry of Agriculture Technology, Bulletin no. 146, Baghdad 1964.

al-Razi: Abu Bakr Muhammad ibn Zakariya al-Razi, (Rhazes), *Kitab al-Hawi fi Tibb,* Hyderabad 1967-1968.

al-Tamimi: al-Tamimi, *al-Mursid ila Jawahir al-Aghdhiya wa-Quwa al-Mufradat min al-Adwiya*, MS Paris, Bibliotheque Nationale, no. 2870. (Arabic).

al-Wasti: Abu Bachr Muhammad Ibn Ahmed al-Wasti, *Fadhal al-Bayt al-Maqdis*, Y. Hason (ed.) Jerusalem 1979.

al-Ya'qubi: Ahmad ibn Abu Ya'qub al-Ya'qubi, *Kitab al-Buldan* (M.J. De Goeje, ed.). Leiden 1892. (Arabic).

al-Zahari: Abu Abd-Alla Mahmad Ben Abi Bahar al-Zahari, *Kitab al-J'arafiya,* (Mahmad haj Zadak edition), in: *Bulletin d' Etudes Orientales*, 21(1968), pp. 1–312. (Arabic).

Amar & Lev, Jerusalem: Z. Amar & E. Lev, *Physicians, Drugs and Remedies in Jerusalem from the 10th to the 18th Centuries,* Tel-Aviv, 2000 (Hebrew).

Amar & Lev, Survey: Z. Amar & E. Lev, *A Historical Survey of Medicinal Substances of the al-Sham Region during the Middle Ages (640-1517 CE)* , Tel-Aviv 1999.

Amar & Lev, Tobler: Z. Amar & E. Lev, "The Traditional Materia Medica in Jerusalem According to Titus Tobler", *Harefuah*, 138 (2000), pp. 604-607. (Hebrew).

Amar & Seri: Z. Amar & Y. Seri, *The Land of Israel and Syria According to al-Tamimi's Description*. Ramat Gan (Hebrew, forthcoming).

Amar, al-Baytar: Z. Amar, "Ibn al-Baytar and the Study of the Plants of al-Sham", *Cathedra*, 76 (1995), pp. 49-76. (Hebrew).

Amar, Colocynthis: Z. Amar, "*Citrullus colocynthis* in the Economy of Gaza at 19-20 Century", (forthcoming).

Amar, de Silva: Z. Amar *Pri Megadim* of Rabbi David de Silva. (Hebrew, forthcoming).

Amar, Dibs: Z. Amar, "Dibs in the Land of Israel during the Middle Ages", in: *Judea and Samaria Research Studies,* V, Kedumim-Ariel 1996, pp. 241-248. (Hebrew).

Amar, Herbalist: Z. Amar, "Abu al-'abas al-Nabati – Andalusian herbalist in the Land of Israel in the Ayyubid Period", *Ariel,* 100-101 (1994), pp. 235-239. (Hebrew).

Amar, Industrial: Z. Amar, "Agricultural Products and Industrial Plants in the Land of Israel during the Middle Ages, *Ariel,* 112-113 (1996), pp. 46-70. . (Hebrew).

Amar, Grapes: Z. Amar, "Grape Cultivation and Wine Production in Judea and Samaria during the Middle Ages", in: *Judea and Samaria Research Studies – Proceedings of the Fourth Conference,* Kedumim-Ariel 1995, pp. 247-261. (Hebrew).

Amar, Landscape: Z. Amar, "Testimonies about the Natural Landscape of Judea and Samaria during the Middle Ages", *Shomron v' Binyamin 3,* (Z.H.Erlich, ed.) Ariel 1993. pp. 110-124. (Hebrew).

Amar, Preservation: Z. Amar, "The Preservation of Sacred Healing Sites in Jerusalem", in: *Judea and Samaria Research Studies – Proceedings of the Seventh Conference,* Kedumim-Ariel 1997, pp. 207-222. (Hebrew).

Amar, Production: Z. Amar, *Agricultural Production in the Land of Israel During the Middle Ages: An Agro-historical Study of their Transformations,* Ph.D. Thesis, Bar-Ilan University, Ramat-Gan, Israel 1996. (Hebrew).

Amar, Substances: "Medicinal Substances in Eretz-Israel in the Times of the Bible, the Mishnah and the Talmud in Light of Written Sources", in: *Illness and Healing in Ancient Times*, Haifa 1996. pp. 52-62. (Hebrew).

Amar, Theriac: Z. Amar, "The Export of Theriac from the Land of Israel and its Uses in the Middle Ages", *Korot,* 12 (1996-1997), pp. 16-29. (Hebrew).

Amar, Traditions: Z. Amar, "Traditions and Realia in the Writing of a Tenth Century Physician in Jerusalem" *Cathedra,* 81 (1996), pp. 23-34. . (Hebrew).

Amarna: W.L. Moran (trans. & ed.), *The Amarna Letters*, Baltimore and London 1987.

Antonini: Antonini Placentini, Itinerarium, P. Geyer (ed.), "Itineraria et alia Geographica", *Corpus*, *Christianorum Series Latina*, CLXXV, Turnholti 1965.

al-Ansari: 'Ali Ahan 'Abd al-Athim al-Ansari, *Dhaker Theriaq al-Faruq,* National Library of Medicine, Maryland, No. 16. See in: S.J. Greenberg, *A Shelf list of Islamic Medical Manuscripts at the National Library of Medicine*, Maryland 1996.

Arce: A. Arce, *Miscellanea de Tierra Santa*, I, Jerusalem 1950.

Ashkenazi, Church : Y. Ashkenazi, "Church Involvement in Medical Services in Byzantine Eretz-Israel", in: *Illness and Healing in Ancient Times*, Haifa 1996. pp. 46-51. (Hebrew).

Ashkenazi, Curing: Y. Ashkenazi, "Curing and Nursing in the Church of Jerusalem during the Byzantine Period" in: Z. Amar, E. Lev and J. Schwartz (eds.) *Medicine in Jerusalem throught the Ages*. Tel-Aviv 1999. pp. 33-50. (Hebrew).

Ashtor, Levant: E. Ashtor, "The Crusaders Kingdom and Trade in the Levant", in: B.Z. Kedar (ed.), *The Crusaders in their Kingdom*, Jerusalem 1978. pp. 30-54. (Hebrew).

Ashtor, Spices: E. Ashtor, "Spice Prices in the Near East in the 15th Century", *Journal of the Royal Asiatic Society*, 1967, pp. 26–41.

Ashtor, Sugar: E. Ashtor, "Levantine Sugar Industry in the Late Middle Ages", In: A.L. Udovitch (ed.), *The Islamic Middle East, 700–1900: Studies in Economic and Social History*, New Jersey 1981, pp. 91–132.

Ashtor, Trade: E. Ashtor, "European Trade in the Late Medieval Land of Israel", in: B.Z. Kedar, T. Dothan, S. Safrai, (eds.) *Commerce in Palestine throughout the Ages*, Jerusalem 1990. pp. 280-299. (Hebrew).

Assaph: S. Muntner, "Assaph (ha-Rofe) the Physician, 'Sefer Refuoth'" *Korot* (1965) 3:396-422, 533-560; (1967-1969) 4:11-40, 170-207, 389-443, 531-572; (1970) 5(1):27-68, 160-187, 295-330, (1971-1972) 5(2):435-473, 603-649, 773-807. (Hebrew).

Assises: A. Beugnot (ed.), "Les Assises de Jerusalem", *RHC,* Lois I–II, Paris 1841–1843.

Bagatti: B. Bagatti, "Father Anthony Manzani of Cuna (1650–1729), of Inventor 'The Balm of Jerusalem', *Franciscan Studies*, 6 (1946), pp. 250–361.

Bassola: I. Ben-Zvi, *A Pilgrimage to Palestine by Rabbi Moshe Bassola of Ancona*, Jerusalem 1938

Beach: D.C. Beach, "History, Production and Uses of Tragacanth", *Advances in Chemical Series*, 11 (1954), pp. 38–44.

Bedford & Holbeche: W.K.R. Bedford and R. Holbeche, *The Order of the Hospital of St. John of Jerusalem*, London 1902.

Benajahu: M. Benajahu, "Extracts from the Medicine and Properties Manuscript of Rabbi Hayim Vital", *Korot* 9(5-6): (1987) pp. 91-112. (Hebrew).

Benevenutus: C.A. Wood, *Benevenutus Grassus of Jerusalem, De Oculis*, California. 1929.

Ben-Yakov: A. Ben-Ya'akov, *The Traditional Medicine of the Babylonian Jews*, Jerusalem 1992. (Hebrew).

Berman: A. Berman, "The Persistence of Theriac in France", *Pharmacy in History*, 12 (1970), pp. 5–12.

Bresc: G. Bresc–Bautier, *Le Cartulaire du Chapitre du Saint–Sepulcre de Jerusalem*, Paris 1984.

Bodenheimer: S. Bodenheimer, *ha-Hai be-Artsot ha-Mikra,* Jerusalem 1967. (Hebrew).

Borchard: J.C.M. Laurent (ed.), *Peregrinatores Medii Aevi Quatuor*, Leipzig 1864, pp. 1–95.

Bown: D. Bown, *Encyclopedia of Herbs & Their Uses*, London 1995.

British Pharmacopoeia: *British Pharmacopoeia* 1858, 4th ed. London 1880.

Bryan: C.P. Bryan, *Ancient Egyptian Medicine – The Papyrus Ebers*, London 1930.

Buckley: R.P. Buckley,."The Muhtasib". *Arabica*, 39 (1992) pp 59-117.

Budge: E.A.W. Budge, *Syrian Anatomy Pathology and Therapeutics or the School of Medicine*, London 1913.

Calahorra: Calahorra, *Chronica della Provincia de Syria, y Tierra Santa de Gerusalem*, Madrid 1684.

Canaan, Plant-lore: T. Canaan, "Plant-Lore in Palestinian Superstition", *Journal of Palestine Oriental Society*, 8 (1928), pp. 129–168.

Canaan, Saints: T. Canaan, "Mohammedan Saints and Sanctuaries in Palestine", *Journal of the Palestine Oriental Society*, 5 (1925), p. 188.

Cawston: F.G. Cawston, "Antimony and Sulphur in the Treatment of the Lepers", *The Journal of Tropical Medicine & Hygiene*, 25 (1922), pp. 345–346.

Challenger: F. Challenger, *Aspects of the Organic Chemistry of the Sulphur*, London 1959.

Chandler et al: R.F. Chandler, S.N. Hooper & M.J. Harvey, "Ethnobotany and Phytochemistry of Yarrow, *Achillea millefolium*, Compositae", *Economic Botany*, 36 (2) (1981), pp. 203–223.

Chaplin: T. Chaplin, 'The Fever of Jerusalem', *The Lancet*, 2 (1864), pp. 236-238.

Chizik: B. Chizik, *Otsar ha-Tsmahim*, Herzlia 1952. (Hebrew).

Chopra et al: B. Chopra, K. Abrol & K.L. Handa, *Medicinal Plants of the Arid Zones,* Unesco 1960.

Cirelli: A. Cirelli, *Gli Annali di Terra Sante*, Karachi 1918.

Cohen, 18 Century: A. Cohen, E. Simon-Pikali & O. Salama, *Jews in the Moslem Religious Court* (in the XVIIIth Century), Jerusalem 1996. (Hebrew).

Cohen, Economy: A. Cohen, *Economic Life in Ottoman Jerusalem*, Cambridge 1989.

Connan et al: J. Connan, A. Nissenbaum & D. Dessort, "Molecular Archaeology Export of Dead Sea Asphalt to Canaan and Egypt in the Chalcolithic–Early Bronze Age", *Geochimica et Cosmochimica Acta*, 56 (1992), pp. 2743–2759.

Crowfoot & Baldensperger : G.M. Crowfoot & L. Baldensperger, *From Cedar to Hyssop*, London 1932.

D' Arvieux: D'Arvieux: *Voyage dans la Palestine*, Paris 1717.

Dafni, Dudaim: A. Dafni, ha-Dudaim Natnu Re'ah, Haifa 1984. (Hebrew).

Dafni, Edible: A. Dafni, *Edible Plants of the Land of Israel.* Tel-Aviv 1985. (Hebrew).

Danin: A. Danin, "'al ha-Ribas Shelanu ve-Shel Aherim " *Teva' va-Arets* (1969) pp.89-90. (Hebrew).

Darwish-Said et al: M. Darwish–Sayed, S.I. Balbaa & M.S. Afifi, "The Glycosidal Content of the Different Organs of *Citrullus colocynthis*", *Planta Medica*, 26 (1974), pp. 293–298.

Delaville: J. Delaville le Roulx, *Les Hospitalaris en Terre Sainte et a Chypre*, Paris 1904.

Demirhan: A. Demirhan, "The Evolution of Opium in the Islamic World and Anatolian Turks", *Studies in History of Medicine*, 4 (1980), pp. 73–97.

Dietrich: A. Dietrich, *Zum Drogenhandel Im Islamischen Agypten*, Heidelberg 1954.

Dinsmore & Dalman: J.E. Dinsmore & G. Dalman, "Die Pflanzen Palastinas", *ZDPV*, 34 (1911), pp. 1–38, 147–172, 185–241.

Dioscorides: R.T. Gunther (trans.), *The Greek Herbal of Dioscorides*, New–York 1959.

Donolo: S. Muntner, *Rabi Shabtay Donolo*, Jerusalem 1949. (Hebrew).

Ducros: M.A.H. Ducros, "Essai sur le Droguier Populaire Arabe de L'Inspectorat des Pharmacies du Caire", *MIE*, 15 (1930).

Duke: J.A. Duke, *Medicinal Plants of the Bible*, London 1983.

Duncan: A. Duncan, *The Edinburgh New Dispensatory,* Edinburgh 1804.

Durdola: J. Durdola, "Tumor Inhibitory Effects of Crude Extracts from *Poterium spinosum*", *Planta Medica*, 27 (1975), pp. 231–234.

Earles & Pharm: M.P. Earles & B. Pharm, *Early Theories of the Mode of Action of Drugs and Poisons*, 1974, pp. 97–110.

EL-Gammal: S.Y. El-Gammal, "Garlic in History", *Hamdard,* 28 (1985), pp. 85–89.

Epstein: J.N.Epstein (ed.), *The Gaonic Commentary on the Order Toharoth.* Berlin 1921-1924. (Hebrew).

Ernoul: Ernoul, "L'estat se la Citez de Iherusalem", In: H. Michelant & G. Raynaud (eds.), *Itineraires a Jerusalem*, Geneva 1882.

Estes: J.W. Estes, *The Medical Skills of Ancient Egypt*, New York 1989.

Feinbrun-Dothan: N. Feinbrun-Dothan, A. Danin, *Analytical Flora of Eretz-Israel*, Jerusalem 1991. (Hebrew).

Feldman: A. Feldman, *Plants of the Bible*, Tel-Aviv 1957. (Hebrew).

Feliks, Afarsemon: Y. Feliks, "Concerning the Expression 'Hei Ganeiv Zevutei De-Hevrei' in the En-Gedi mosaic pavments", *Tarbits* 40 (1971), pp. 256-257. (Hebrew).

Feliks, Balsam: Y. Feliks, "The History of Balsamom Cultivation in the Land of Israel", in: S. Dar and Z. Safrai (eds.), The Village in Ancient Israel, Tel-Aviv 1997. pp. 275-295. (Hebrew).

Feliks, Fruit Trees: Y. Feliks, Fruit trees in the Bible and Talmudic Literature, Jerusalem 1994. (Hebrew).

Feliks, Kilayim: Y. Feliks, *Mixed Sowing Breeding and Grafting 'Kilayim',* Tel-Aviv 1967. (Hebrew)

Feliks, Shevi'it: Y. Feliks, *Mishna Tractate Shevi'it,* Jerusalem 1987. (Hebrew)

Feliks, World: Y. Feliks, *Plant World of the Bible*, Ramat-Gan 1976. (Hebrew).

Feliks, Yerushalmi: Y. Feliks, *The Jerusalem Talmud (Talmud Yerushalmi) tractate Shev'iit (critically edited)*, Jerusalem 1980-1987. (Hebrew).

Fernie: W.T. Fernie, *Animal Simples Approved for Modern Uses of Cure*, London 1899.

Fleisher et al: A. Fleisher & Z. Fleisher, "Identification of Biblical Hyssop and Origin of the Traditional Use of Oregano–group Herbs in the Mediterranean Region", *Economic Botany*, 42 (1988), pp. 232–241.

Fleisher: A. Fleisher, N. Senir, G. Fleisher and A. Yafee, "Hidat ha-Ezov ha-Mikra'i", *Mada'* 24(6) (1980), pp. 272-275. (Hebrew).

Foust: C.M. Foust, "Mysteries of Rhubarb: Chinese Medicinal Rhubarb through the Ages", *Pharmacy in History*, 36 (1994), pp. 155–159.

Freidin: I. Freidin, 'Bikur Holim Perushim in Jerusalem – From Society to Hospital', *Cathedra* 23 (1983), pp. 117-140. (Hebrew).

Frencken et al: J.E. Frencken, P. Rugarabamu & J. Mulder, "The Effect of Sugar Chewing on the Development of Dental Caries", *Journal of Dental Research*, 68 (6) (1989), pp. 1102–1104.

Frenkel: J. Frenkel, "Early Arabic period (632-1099)", in: B.Z. Kedra (ed.), *The Crusaders in their Kingdom*, Jerusalem 1978. pp. 223-238. (Hebrew).

Frescobaldi: T. Bellorini, E. Hoade & B. Bagatti (eds.), *Visit to the Holy Places of Egypt, Sinai, Palestine and Syria in 1384 by Frescobaldi*, Gucci and Sigoli, Jerusalem 1948.

Gal: M. Gal, "Zaqum Mitsri" *Teva' va-Erets* 15 (1973) pp. 147-149. (Hebrew).

Ghaleb: E. Ghaleb, *Dictionnaire des Sciences de la Nature*, Beirut 1966.

Gidney: W.T. Gidney, *The History of the London Society for Promoting Christianity Amongst the Jews, from 1809 to 1908*, London 1908.

Gil: M. Gil, *Palestine during the first Muslim Period (643-1099)*, Tel-Aviv 1983. (Hebrew).

Goitein, Jewry: S.D. Goitein, *Palestinian Jewry in Early Islamic and Crusader Times*, Jerusalem 1980. (Hebrew).

Goitein, Society: S.D. Goitein, *A Mediterranean Society*, Berkeley 1967–1988.

Goor, Rose: A. Goor, *The History of the Rose In the Holy Land Throughout the Ages*, Jerusalem 1981. (Hebrew).

Goor, Fruits: A. Goor, *Fruits of the Land of Israel*, Tel-Aviv 1974. (Hebrew).

Goor, Wines: A. Goor, "Yeinot Erets-Israel bi-Mey Kedem", *Teva' va-Erets* 3 (1961), pp. 33-39. (Hebrew).

Gordon, Medicine: B.L. Gordon, *Medicine Throughout Antiquity*, Philadelphia 1949.

Gordon, Medieval: B.L. Gordon, *Medieval and Renaissance Medicine*, New York 1959.

Goren: H. Goren, *'Go View the Land' German Study of Palestine in the 19th Century*, Jerusalem 1999. (Hebrew).

Grabois: A. Grabois, "From 'Holy Geography' to 'Palestinography': Changes in the Descriptions of Thirteenth Century Pilgrims", *Cathedra* (1984) 31:43-66.

Greenberg: Z. Greenberg, "The Turkish Municipal Hospital in Jerusalem," *Cathedra* 78 (1995), pp. 49-64. (Hebrew).

Grieve: M. Grieve, *A Modern Herbal*, London 1994.

Groom: N. Groom, *Frankincense and Myrrh: A Study of the Arabian Incense Trade*, London 1981.

Gucci: T. Bellorini, E. Hoade & B. Bagatti (eds.), *Visit to the Holy Places of Egypt, Sinai, Palestine and Syria in 1384 by Frescobaldi, Gucci and Sigoli*, Jerusalem 1948.

Hakim: M. Hakim, *Hamdard Pharmacopoeia of Eastern Medicine*, Karachi 1970.

Haller: J.S. Haller, "A Drug for All Seasons: Medical and Pharmacological History of Aloe", *Bulletin of the New York Academy of Medicine*, 6 (1990), pp. 647–659.

Hamarneh, Chemical: S. Hamarneh, "Climax of Chemical Therapy in 10th Century Arabic Medicine", *Der Islam*, 38 (1980), pp. 283–288.

Hamarneh, Ibn al-Quff: S. Hamarneh, "Ibn Al–Quff's Contributions to Arab–Islamic Medical Sciences", *Hamdard*, 34 (1991), pp. 27–36.

Hamarneh, Origins: S. Hamarneh, *Origins of Pharmacy and Therapy in the Near East,* Natio Foundation, Tokyo 1973.

Hamarneh, Plants: S. Hamarneh, "Medical Plants, Therapy and Ecology in Al–Ghazzi's Book on Agriculture", *Studies in History of Medicine*, 2 (1978), pp. 223–263.

Harrison: R.K. Harrison, *Healing Herbs of the Bible*, Leiden 1966.

Hartwell: J.L. Hartwell, "Plants Used Against Cancer – A Survey", *Lloydia* (1967–1971), 30:395, 407; 31:142; 32:28, 94, 168, 278, 292; 33:144; 34:113, 234, 328, 386.

Hasselquist: F. Hasselquist, *Voyages and Travels in the Levant*, London 1866. The original text was published as - F. Hasselquists, *Iter Palaestinum*, Stockholm 1757

Heim: H. J. Heim, *Dr. Titus Tobler: der palastinafahere. Ein oppenzellisches Lebensbild.* Zurich, Trogen 1879.

Heyd: W. Heyd, *Histoire du Commerce du Levant au Moyen–Age*, Leipzig 1936.

Hill: A.E. Hill, *Economic Botany*, New York 1952.

Hooper: D. Hooper, *Useful Plants and Drugs of Iran and Iraq*, Field Museum of Natural History, Publ. 387, Chicago 1937.

Horn: E. Horn, *Ichnographiae Monumentorum Terrae Sanctae*, E. Hoade & B. Bagatti (eds.), Jerusalem 1962.

Hospitalier: J. Delaville le Roulx (ed.), *Cartulaire General de L'ordre des Hospitaliers de S. Jean de Jerusalem, 1100–1310*, Paris 1894–1906.

Houh et al: L. Houh, J.K.N. Jones & W.H. Wadman, "Constitution of Gum *Myrrh*", I, *Journal of the Chemical Society* (1952), pp. 796–800.

Howe: F.N. Howe, "Age–Old Resins of the Mediterranean Region and Their Use", *Economic Botany*, 4 (1950), pp. 307–316.

Howes: F.N. Howes, *Vegetable Gums and Resins*, New York. 1949.

Hunian: Hunian ibn Ishaq, *The Ten Treatises on the Eye*, M. Meyerhof (ed. & trns.) Cairo 1928.

Ibn Abi Usaybia: Ibn Abi Usaybia, *Uyun al-Anba fi Tabaqat al Atibba.* Beirut 1965. (Arabic).

Ibn al-Baytar, al-Jami: Ibn al-Baytar, *Kitab al-Jami' li-Mufradat al-Adwiya wa-'l-Aghdhiya*, Bulaq, Cairo 1874. (Arabic).

Ibn al-Baytar, Tafsir: Ibn al-Baytar, *Tafsir Kitab Diasquridus* (ed.) Ibrahim ibn Murad, Beirut 1989. (Arabic).

Ibn Qayyim : Ibn Qayyim al–Jawziyya, *Medicine of the Prophet*, M. al–Akili (ed.), Philadelphia 1993.

Ibn al-Qifti: 'Ali ibn Yusuf, Ibn al-Qifti, *Tarikh al-hukama'*, (ed.) J. Lippert, Leipzig 1903. (Arabic).

Ibn Battuta: Ibn Battuta, *Voyages d'Ibn Batoutah* (C. Defremery and B.R. Sanguinetti, ed. and tran.) Paris 1854.

Ibn Jubayr: Abu al-Husayn Ibn Jubayr, *Rihlah,* (ed.) De Goeje, Leiden 1907.

Ibn Katir: Ibn Kaṯir, 'Isma'il ibn 'Amr, *al-Bidaya wa-al-nihaya*, Beirut 1977. (Arabic).

Ibn Khaldun: Ibn Khaldun, *The Muqaddimah* (F. Rosenthal trans.), III, London 1958

Ibn Masawayh: Ibn Masawayh, *Kitab al-Azmina,* (P. Sbath ed. & trans.) *Bulletin de l' Institute di Egypte* (1932-1933) 15:235-257.

Ibn Rushd: Ibn Rushd, *Kitab al-Kulliyat.* Madrid 1939. (Arabic).

Ibn Sina: Ibn Sina, *Kitab al-Qanun fi 'l-Tibb*, Beirut 1877. (Arabic).

Ibn Wahshiya: M. Levey (tran.), *Medieval Arabic Toxicology, The Book of Poisons of Ibn Wahshiya and its Relation to Early Indian and Greek Texts*, Philadelphia 1966.

Isaacs: H. Isaacs, "The Impact of Western Medicine on Muslim Physicians and their Writing in the 17th Century", *Bulletin of the British Association of Orientalists*, 11 (1979–1980), pp. 52–57.

Ishaq: Ishaq b. Sulayman al-Israili, *Kitab al-Aghdiya wal-adwiya,* Beirut 1992. (Arabic).

Issa: A. Issa Bey, *Dictionnaire des Noms des Plantes*, Cairo 1930.

Jacob: W. Jacob, "Medicinal Plants of the Bible – Another View", In: I. & W. Jacob (eds.), *The Healing Past*, Leiden 1993.

Jones & Nunn: J.K.N. Jones & J.R. Nunn, "The Structure of Frankincense Gum", *Journal of the American Chemistry Society*, 77 (1975), pp. 5745–5746.

Josephus, JA: Josephus, *Jewish Antiquities* (R.Marcus tran.), London 1966

Josephus, JW: Josephus, *The Jewish War* (H.J.Thackeray tran.), London 1967

Kamal, Encyc.: H. Kamal, *Encyclopedia of Islamic Medicine*, Cairo 1975.

Kamel, Zakom: M.S. Kamel, "Studies on Balanites Aegyptiaca Fruits: An Antidiabetic Egyptian Folk Medicine", *Chemical and Pharmaceutical Bulletin*, 39 (1991), pp. 1229–1233.

Kaplan, Asphalt: D. Kaplan, "Asphalt in the Dead Sea: Its Use in Ancient Times", *Korot* 3(5-6) (1964) pp.230-237.

Kaplan, Bitumen: D. Kaplan, "Bitumen in Ancient Epochs of Israel", *Korot* 3(1-2) 1962 pp.80-83. (Hebrew).

Kass, Montefiore: M. A. Kass, "Sir Moses Montefiore and Medical Philanthropy in the Holy Land", in: *Health and Disease in the Holy Land*, eds. M. Waserman and S. Kottek, New York 1996.

Kass, Western: E. Kass, "Western Medicine in Nineteenth-Century Jerusalem", *Journal of the History of Medicine and Allied Sciences* 44 (1989), pp. 447-461.

Kedar: B.Z. Kedar, "Benevenutus Grassus of Jerusalem, an Oculist in the Era of the Crusades", *Korot*, 11 (1995), pp. 14–41. (Hebrew).

Kermers & Urdang: E. Kremers & G. Urdang, *History of Pharmacy*, Philadelphia 1976.

Kramer: S.N. Kramer, "First Pharmacopeia in Man's Recorded History", *American Journal of Pharmacology*, 126 (1954), pp.76–84.

Khusraw: Nasir-I Khusraw, *Sefer nameh* (C. Schefer, ed. and tran.) Amsterdam 1970 (Paris 1881).

Kislev: M. Kislev, "The Identification of the Harhevina and 'Akrabanim", *Leshonenu* 58 (1994-1995), pp. 105-117. (Hebrew).

Klein-Franke: F. Klein-Franke, "Health and Healing in Medieval Muslem Palestine", in: M. Waserman & S. Kottek (eds.), *Health and Disease in the Holy Land*, New York 1996, pp. 103–134.

Kohen & Shemid'a: 'A. Kohen and A. Shemid'a, "Sigal Tsanu'a", *Tev'a va-Erets* 32(2) (1990), pp. 18. (Hebrew).

Kottek & Schwake: S. Kottek and N. Schwake, "The First Jewish Hospital in Jerusalem", *Medicine's Geographic Heritage*, 4 (1988), pp. 3-10.

Krispil: N. Krispil, *Bag of Plants*. Jerusalem 1983-1989. (Hebrew).

Kroner: H. Kroner, "Die Haemorrhoiden in der Medizin des XII und XIII Jahrhunderts", *Janus*, (1911), pp. 645– 718.

Kupper: A. Kupper, "Kontras Erets Israel" *Kvets 'Al Yad*, 7(17) (1968), pp. 101-123. (Hebrew).

Le Strange: 1890. G. Le Strange, *Palestine under the Moslems*, London

Leclerc: L. Leclerc (trans.), *Ibn al–Baytar, Traite Des Simples* (3 vol.), Paris 1983.

Lev & Amar: E. Lev and Z. Amar, "Ethnopharmacological Survey of Traditional Drugs Sold in Israel at the End of the 20th Century". *Journal of Ethnopharmacology* (2000) 72: 191-205.

Lev & Amar, Traditional: E. Lev, and Z. Amar, *Traditional Medicinal Substances of Israel*. Jerusalem 2002. (Hebrew).

Lev, Animals: E. Lev, "The Medicinal uses of Animals and their Products in the Medieval Levant", *Harefua* 139 (2000), pp. 483-487. (Hebrew).

Lev, Jerusalem: E. Lev, "Medical Materials in Jerusalem during the Tenth to the Eighteenth Centuries" in: Z. Amar, E. Lev and J. Schwartz (eds.) *Medicine in Jerusalem throughout the Ages*. Tel-Aviv 1999. pp. 51-78. (Hebrew).

Lev, Kebara: E. Lev, *The Vegetal Food of the "Neanderthal" Man in Kebara Cave, Mt. Carmel in the Middle Palaeolithic Period*, M.Sc. Thesis, Department of Life Sciences, Bar-Ilan Univesity 1992. (Hebrew).

Lev, Materials: E. Lev, *Medicinal Substances of the Medieval Levant*, Tel-Aviv 2002. (Hebrew).

Levi Ben Yefet: Levi Ben Yefet, *Sefer ha-Mitsvot*, Ms. Leiden (Or. 4766), Institute of Microfilmed Hebrew Manuscripts, National Library Jerusalem, # 2805. (Hebrew).

Levey, Beduins: S. Levey, *Medicine, Hygiene and Health among the Sinai Beduins*, Tel-Aviv 1978. (Hebrew).

Levey, Chemistry: M. Levey, *Chemistry and Chemical Technology in Ancient Mesopotamia*, Amsterdam 1959.

Levey, Ibn Masawiah: M. Levey, "Ibn Masawiah and his Treatise on Simple Aromatic Substances", *Journal of the History of Medicine and Allied Science*, 6 (1961), pp. 394–410.

Levkowitz: M.Y. Levkowitz, "ha-Nahash shel Asklepiyus ke-Semel ha-Refua",*ha-Rofe ha-'Ivryi* 36(2) (1963), pp. 156-159. (Hebrew).

Levy, Frenkel: N. Levy, "Dr. Simon Frenkel (1809-1880) the First Jewish Physician in the Land of Israel", *Harefua* 118 (1990), pp. 489-494 (Hebrew).

Levy, Medicine: N. Levy, *Chapters in the History of Medicine in Palestine, 1799-1948*, Haifa, 1998. (Hebrew).

Lewis: W.A. Lewis, *A Complete Dictionary of the Whole Materia Medica*, London 1810.

Little: D.P. Little, *A Catalogue of the Islamic Documents from al–Haram al–Sharif in Jerusalem*, Beirut 1984.

Loewenfeld & Back: C. Loewenfeld & F. Back, *The Complete Book of Herb and Spices*, London 1978.

Low: I. Low, *Die Flora der Juden*, I-IV, Vienna-Leipzig 1924-1934.

Lutfi: H. Lutfi, *al–Quds al–Mamlukiyya*, Berlin 1985.

Maimonides, Answers: Moshe Ben Maimon (Maimonides), *Medical Answers (Responsa)*, S. Muntner (ed.), Philadelphia 1969.

Maimonides, Aphorisms: Moshe Ben Maimon (Maimonides), *The Medical Aphorisms of Moses Maimonides*, F. Rosner & S. Muntner (eds.), New York 1970.

Maimonides, Asthma: Moshe Ben Maimon (Maimonides), *Treatise On Asthma*, S. Muntner (ed.), Philadelphia 1963.

Maimonides, Glossaire: Moshe Ben Maimon (Maimonides), *Un Glossaire de Matiere Medicale Compose par Maimonide*, M. Meyerhof (ed.) *Memoires Presentes a l'Institut d'Egypte*, 41 (1940).

Maimonides, Hemorrhoids: Moshe Ben Maimon (Maimonides), *Treatise On Hemorrhoids*, S. Muntner (ed.), Philadelphia 1969.

Maimonides, Mishna: Moshe Ben Maimon (Maimonides), *Mishna 'im Perush Rabeno Moshe Ben Maimon*, Y. Kapah (ed.), Jerusalem 1963-1967. (Hebrew).

Maimonides, Poisons: Moshe Ben Maimon (Maimonides), *Poisons and their Antidotes* (S. Muntner, ed.), Jerusalem 1942. (Hebrew).

Maimonides, Regimen: Moshe Ben Maimon (Maimonides), *Regimen Sanitatis*, S. Muntner (ed.), Jerusalem 1957. (Hebrew).

Maimonides, Sexual: Ben Maimon, Moshe (Maimonides), Sexual Life, (S. Muntner ed.), Jerusalem 1965. (Hebrew).

Malki: M. Benajahu (ed.). *Medical Works of Rabbi Refael Mordecai Malki*, Jerusalem 1985. (Hebrew).

Margalit: D. Margalit, "The Snake as a Symbol of Medicine", *Korot* 6(9-10) (1974) pp. 615-618. (Hebrew).

Masterman: E. W. G. Masterman, *Hygiene and Diseases in Palestine – in Modern and Biblical Times,* London 1925.

Matossian: M.K. Matossian, *Poisons of the Past*, New Haven 1989.

Mazor: 'I. Mazor, *Geulogya be-Patish Israely,* Tel-Aviv 1980. (Hebrew).

Medical Report: Medical Report, "Syrian Medical Aid Association", *British and Foreign Medical Review,* 13 (1842), pp. 579-590.

Michelant & Raynaud: H. Michelant & G. Raynaud, *Itineraires a Jerusalem*, Geneva 1882.

Michie & Cooper: C.A. Michie & E. Cooper, "Frankincense and Myrrh as Remedies in Children", *Journal of the Royal Society of Medicine*, 84 (1991), pp. 602–605.

Miller: T.S. Miller, *The Birth of the Hospital in the Byzantine Empire*, Baltimore and London 1985.

Mitchell: P. Mitchell, "Pathology in the Crusader Period: Human Skeletal Remains from Tel Jezreel", *Levant*, 26 (1994), pp. 67–71.

Mishra et al: R.K. Mishra, R.B. Arora & S.D.S. Seth, "Anti-inflammatory Activity of Musk", *Journal of Pharmacy and Pharmacology,* 14 (1962), pp. 830–831.

Moldenke: H.N.&. A.L. Moldenke, *Plants of the Bible*, Waltham 1952.

Morton: J.F. Morton, *Major Medicinal Plants*, Illinois 1978.

Moussaieff: A. Moussaieff, Jerusalem Balsam – from the Franciscan Pharmacy to Maritndail 32: Pharmacognosy Research. M.Sc. thesis, The Hebrew University, Jerusalem 2001.

Mujir al-Din: 'Abd al-Rahman ibn Muhammad Mujir al-Din, *al-'Uns al-jalil bi-tarikh al-Quds wa-al-Khalil*, Amman 1973.

Muntner: S. Muntner, "Pharmaceutical Composition in Ancient Hebrew Literature", *Korot* 5(7-8) (1971) pp. 550-552. (Hebrew).

Nahmias: B.Nahmias, *Hamsa*: *Amulets, Beliefs and Traditional Medicine in the Old City of Jerusalem.* Tel-Aviv 1996. (Hebrew).

Nissenbaum, Monster: A. Nissenbaum, "The Dead Sea Monster", *International Journal of Salt Lake Res*., 1 (2) (1992), pp. 1–8.

Nissenbaum, Asphalt: A. Nissenbaum, "ha-Asphalt shel Yam ha-Melah", *Lada'at* 20(6) (1990), pp. 17-20. (Hebrew).

Nissenbaum, Mummies: A. Nissenbaum, "Molecular Archaeology: Organic Geochemistry of Egyptian Mummies", *Journal of Archeological Science*, 19 (1992), pp. 1–6.

Nissenbaum, Dead Sea: A. Nissenbaum, "The Dead Sea – An Economic Resource for 10,000 Years", *Hydrobiologia*, 267 (1993), pp. 127–141.

Nissenbaum, Utilization: A. Nissenbaum, "Utilization of Dead Sea Asphalt Throughout History", *Review Chemistry England*, 9 (3–4) (1993), pp. 365–383.

Norris: H.H. Norris, *The Origin, Progress and Existing Circumstances of the London Society for Promoting Christianity Amongst the Jews, An Historical Inquiry*, London 1925.

Nunn: J.F. Nunn, *Ancient Egyptian Medicine*, London 1996.

O'Hara: J. O'Hara–May, "Food or Medicine", *Transactions of the British Society for the History of Pharmacy*, 1 (1971), pp. 61–70.

Osborn: D.J. Osborn, "Notes on Medical and Other Uses of Plants in Egypt", *Economic Botany*, 22 (1968), pp. 168–177.

Palevitz et al : D. Palevitz, Z. Yaniv. A. Dafni and Y. Fridman, *Ethnobotanical survey of the Flora of Israel as a Source for Drugs*, Jerusalem 1985. (Hebrew).

Palevitz: D. Palevitz, "Tsimhye-Marpe ve-'Erkam ba-Refua ha-Modernit", *Mad'a*, 26(6) (1978), pp. 264-269. (Hebrew).

Palmer: B. Palmer (ed.), *Medicine and the Bible*, Devon 1986.

Pegolotti: F.B. Pegolotti, *La Pratica Della Mercatura*, A. Evans (ed.), Cambridge Mass. 1936.

Perelman: M. Perelman, *Midrash Refuah*, Tel-Aviv 1926. (Hebrew).

Perry: Y. Perry, *British Mission to the Jews in 19th Century Palestine* (Forthcoming).

Perry & Lev: Y. Perry and E. Lev, "Medical Activities of the British Mission to the Jews in 19th Century Palestine" *MDliSal ḥ istᶜ ry* 2003.

Piloti: P.H. Dopp (ed.), *Traite d'Emmanuel Piloti sur le Passage em Terre Sainte (1420)*, Paris 1958.

Plants & Animals: A. Alon (ed.), *Plants and Animals of the Land of Israel*, I-XII, Tel-Aviv 1982-1990. (Hebrew).

Plessner: M.Plessner, "On Daud al-Antaki's Medical and Magical Encyclopaedia and Some of its Sources", *Eretz-Israel*, 7 (1964), pp. 138-141

Plinius: G. Plinius, *Naturalis Historia,* W.H.S. Jones (trns.) (*LCL*) London 1992.

Post & Dinsmore: G.E. Post & J.E. Dinsmore, *Flora of Syria, Palestine and Sinai,* Beirut 1932–1933.

Prawer, Colonial: J. Prawer, *The Crusaders - a Colonial Society*, Jerusalem 1985. (Hebrew).

Prawer, History: J. Prawer, *The History of Eretz Israel Under Moslem and Crusader Rule (634-1291),* Volume 6: The Middle Ages. Jerusalem 1981. (Hebrew)

Prawer, Jerusalem: J. Prawer, *The Latin Kingdom of Jerusalem,* London 1972.

Preuss: J. Preuss, *Biblical and Talmudic Medicine*, F. Rosner (trans.), NewYork 1983.

Pringle: D. Pringle, *The Red Tower*, London 1986.

Putsiynakova: P. Putsiynakova, *Apitherapy, Ripuy be-Motsarei Kaveret*, M. Almalyiah (trns.), Haifa 1993. (Hebrew).

Raba: J. Raba, *Russian Travel accounts on Palestine*, Jerusalem 1986. (Hebrew).

Rauwolf: L. Rauwolf, *Aigentliche Beschreibung der Raiss inn die Morglenlaender,* Graz 1971. (facsimile of 1583 edition).

Raz: E. Raz, *The Book of the Dead Sea*, Jerusalem 1993. (Hebrew).

Reiani: Y. Reiani, *Medicinal Substances of the Yemenite Jews*. M.Sc. Thesis submitted to the School of Pharmacology, Hebrew University, Jerusalem 1963. (Hebrew).

Riaz: M. Riaz & F.M. Chaudhary, "Chemistry of Medicinal Plants of the Genus Cinnamomum", *Hamdard*, 32 (1989), pp. 57–71.

Riddle, Dioscorides: J.M. Riddle, *Dioscorides on Pharmacy and Medicine*, Austin 1985.

Riddle, Research: J.M. Riddle, "Methodology of Historical Drug Research", In: J.M. Riddle, *Quid pro quo: Studies in the History of Drugs*, 1992, pp. 1–19.

Riddle, Tradition: J.M. Riddle, "Folk Tradition and Folk Medicine Recognition of Drugs in Classical Antiquity", In: J. Scarborough (ed.), *Folklore and Folk Medicine*, Wisconsin 1987, pp. 33–61.

Roger: F.E. Roger, *La Terre Sainte, ou Description topographique tres particuliere des Saints Lieux & de la Terre Promission*, Paris 1664.

Rosner: F. Rosner, *Medicine in the Bible and the Talmud*, New Jersy 1994.

Saladino: S. Muntner, (ed.) *Saladino d' Ascoli, Book of the Pharmacists (1430),* Tel-Aviv 1963, (Hebrew).

Sandoli: S. de Sandoli, *Itinera Hierosolymitana Crucesignatorum* (saec. XII–XIII), I–II, Jerusalem 1978–1980.

Schick: C. Schick, "For the Sake of Jerusalem", *Ariel*, 130-131 (1998), p. 225. (Hebrew).

Schittny: H.R. Schittny, "Die Historische Apotheke der Franziskaner in Jerusalem", *Geschichte der Pharmazie*, 45 (1993), pp. 41–45.

Schreiber: W. Schreiber, "Plant Poisons in Medieval Warfare", *Medical Bulletin*, 38 (1981), pp. 23–29.

Schur: N. Schur, "Franciscan Physician and Pharmacists in Jerusalem" " in: Z. Amar, E. Lev and J. Schwartz (eds.) *Medicine in Jerusalem throughout the Ages*. Tel-Aviv 1999. pp. 99-106. (Hebrew).

Schwake: N. Schwake, "Hospitals and European Colonial Policies in the 19th and early 20th Centuries", in M. Waserman and S. Kottek (eds.) *Health and Disease in the Holy Land,* New York 1996, pp. 231-262.

Schwartz: E. Schwartz, *Kyrillos Von Skythopolis*, Leipzig 1939.

Seetzen: U.J. Seetzen, *Reisen durch Syrien, Palestina etc*, ed. Fr. Kruse, Berlin 1854.

Serapion: P. Guigues, "Le noms Arabes dans Serapion, 'Liber de Simplici Medicina", *Journal Asiatique*, 6 (1905), pp. 49–112, 479–546.

Shahnaz et al: A. Shahnaz, M.A. Kalhoro, Z. Kapadla & Y. Badar," 'Aloe' A Biologically Active and Potential Medicinal Plant", *Hamdard*, 36 (1993), pp. 108–115.

Shalmovitz: N. Shalmovitz, *The Pharmacological Qualities of Plant Extracts of Anchusa sp. and Echium sp. (Boraginacea),* M.Sc. Thesis, Tel Aviv University 1973.

Shani et al: Y. Shani, B. Yosef and G. Zolman, "Sira Kotsanit ve-Hashimush Ba be-Tipul be-Sakeret", *Tev'a va-Erets* 4 (1975), p. 185. (Hebrew).

Shapira, Sugar: N. Shapira, "The Part Played by Jews in the Production of Sugar" *Korot* 2(3-4) (1959) pp. 133-144. (Hebrew).

Shapira, Wine: N. Shapira, "The Wine Industry as to the Ancient Hebrew sources", *Korot* 3(1-2) (1962) pp.40-71. (Hebrew).

Shapira, Musk: N. Shapira, "'Al Homrie ha-Bosem me-ha-Hai ba-Mekorut ha-'Ivri'im ha-Kedumim", *ha-Rofe ha-'Ivri* 32(2) 1959 pp. 95-103.

Shoshan: S. Shoshan, *Mekoroth Refuah,* Rehovot 1979. (Hebrew).

Shvarts: S. Shvarts, "Messianism and Politics in the Establishment of Jewish Medical Services in Jerusalem during the 19th Century", in *Medicine in Jerusalem throughout the Ages,* A. Zohar, E. Lev and J. Schwartz (eds.), Tel Aviv 1999. (Hebrew).

Sickenberger: E. Sickenberger, *Les plantes Egyptiennes d'Ibn El Beithar*, Cairo 1890.

Singer: Y. Singer, "'The Garlic", *Korot* 3(5), (1960) p. 77. (Hebrew).

Singh: R.S. Singh & A.N. Singh, "Impact of Historical Studies on the Nomenclature of Medicinal and Economic Plants with Particular Reference to Clove (LAVANGA)" *Ancient*, 2 (1) (1982), pp. 227–232.

Steinmetz: E.F. Steinmetz, *Materia Medica Vegetabilis*, Holland 1954.

Stapleton: H.E. Stapleton, "Chemistry in Iraq and Persia in the Tenth Century", *Memoris Asiatic Society of Bengal*, 7 (1927), pp. 317–418.

Stern & Goren: S. Stern and H. Goren, "A Bibliography of Titus Tobler", *Cathedra,* 48 (1998), pp. 46-48. (Hebrew).

Stern, Description: S. Stern, "A Description of Medicinal Conditions in mid-19th Century Jerusalem", in Z. Amar, E. Lev and J. Schwartz (eds.), *Medicine in Jerusalem throughout the Ages*, Tel Aviv 1999. pp.107-127. (Hebrew).

Stern, Tobler: S. Stern, "Titus Tobler, 19th Century Researcher of Eretz Israel", *Cathedra* 48 (1998), pp. 30-45. (Hebrew).

Stetter: C. Stetter, *The Secret Medicine of the Pharaohs*, Chicago 1990.

Suriano: T. Bellorini, E. Hoade & B. Bagatti (eds.), *Fra Francesco Suriano Treatise on the Holy Land*, Jerusalem 1949.

Tal: P. Tal, *Medicinal Plants,* Tel-Aviv 1981. (Hebrew).

Theodosios: H. Usener (ed.), *Der Heilige Theodosios*, Leipzig 1890.

Theophrastus: Theophrastus, *Enquiry into Plants,* A. Hort (trns.) (*LCL*) London 1990.

Thompson, Art: C.J.S. Thompson, *The Mystery and Art of the Apothecary*, London 1929.

Thompson, Texts: R.C Thompson, *Assyrian Medical Texts*, London 1923.

Tobler , Beitrage: T. Tobler, *Beitrage zur Medizinischen Topographie von Jerusalem*, Berlin 1855.

Tobler, Denkblatter: T. Tobler, *Denkblatter aus Jerusalem*, Konstanz 1853.

Tobler, Descriptions: T. Tobler, *Descriptiones Terrae Sanctae*, Leipzig 1874.

Tobler, Journey: T. Tobler & A. Molinier, *Itinera Hierosolymitana*, I, Geneva 1879.

Tolkowsky: S. Tolkowsky, *Citrus Fruits: Their Origin and History throughout the World,* Jerusalem 1966.

Troilo: Troilo, *Troilo's Orientalische Reisebechreibng*, Leipzig 1717.

Tuhfat: H.P.J. Renaud & S. Colin, *Tuhfat Al-Ahbab, Glossaire de La Matiere Medical Marocaine*, Paris 1934.

Ulman: S. B. Ulman, "Tsimhei Refua ba-Mikra", *Sinay* 26 (1960), pp. 194-205; 27 (1960), pp. 372-382. (Hebrew).

Uphof: J.C. Uphof, *Dictionary of Economic Plants*, New York 1968

Venice Laws: *Nuovo Archivio Veneto*, N.S., IV.

Vilnai: Z. Vilnai, "Shemot Mekomot Lekuhim Me'olam ha-Tsmahim"' *ha-Teva' va-ha-Erets* 5 (1939), pp. 453-460. (Hebrew).

Vohora & Khan: S.B. Vohora & S. Y. Khan, *Animal Origin Drugs Used in Unani Medicine*, New Delhi 1979.

Volney: M.C.F. Volney, *Travels through Syria and Egypt in the Year 1783, 1784 and 1785*, London 1972

Wadding: L. Wadding, *Annales Minorum,* VII, Karachi 1932.

Watson, Innovation: A.M. Watson, *Agricultural Innovation in the Early Islamic World*, London–New York 1983.

Watson, Theriac: G. Watson, *Theriac and Mithridatium*, London 1966.

Wilkinson: J. Wilkinson, *Jerusalem Pilgrims before the Crusades*, Jerusalem 1977.

Witztum & Gruber: A. Witztum and M.I Gruber, "Kuranit Kuranit'a ve-Kuranya, Hebrew, Aramaic and Arabic Names for Plants in the Mint Family", *Leshonenu* 56 (1992), pp. 147-151. (Hebrew).

Woodville: W. Woodville, *Medical Botany,* London 1819.

Ya'ari, Travels: A. Ya'ari, *Travels in the Land of Israel*, Ramat-Gan 1976. (Hebrew).

Ya'ari, Igrot: A. Ya'ari, Igrot Eretz Israel [Letters of the Land of Israel], Tel-Aviv 1943. (Hebrew).

Yadin & Naveh: Y. Yadin & J. Naveh, *Masada I, The Yigael Yadin Excavations 1963–1965: Final Reports*, Jerusalem 1989. (Hebrew).

Yaniv: Z. Yaniv, "Tsimhei Refua be-Re'i ha-Dorot" *Mada'* 26(1) (1982), pp. 10-22. (Hebrew)

Yaqut: Ibn Abd Allah al-Hamawi Yaqut, *Jacut's Geographisches Worterbuch,* (ed.) F. Wustenfeld, Leipzig 1870.

Yates & Kerns, Gazette: W. H. Yates and T. Kerns, "Medical News from the East", *London Medical Gazette* 31 (1842-3), pp. 905-908.

Yates & Kerns, Lancet: W. H. Yates and T. Kerns, "Medical News from the East", *Lancet* 1 (1842-3), pp. 867-870.

Zayyda: Y. Zayyda, "ha-Botanika ha-Refu'it be-Ysrael mi-Yemei ha-Mikra ve'ad Sof Yemei ha-Benayim", *ha-Rofe ha-'Ivri,* 1 (1956), pp. 82-90. (Hebrew).

Zilberstein: TS. Zilberstein, "'Al Shlosha Tsimhei Refua 'Atikim", *Teva' va-Erets (*1959), pp. 76-80. (Hebrew).

Zohary & Hopf: D. Zohary & M. Hopf, *Domestication of Plants in the Old World*, Oxford 1994.

Zohary: M. Zohary, *The Plant World: Morphology, Taxonomy, Evolution, Biology,* Jerusalem 1978.

Index of Main Arabic Names

Index of English Names

Index of Hebrew Names

Index of Scientific Names

www.ingramcontent.com/pod-product-compliance
Lightning Source LLC
LaVergne TN
LVHW071215210926
848482LV00015B/818